FORENSIC
EMERGENCY
MEDICINE

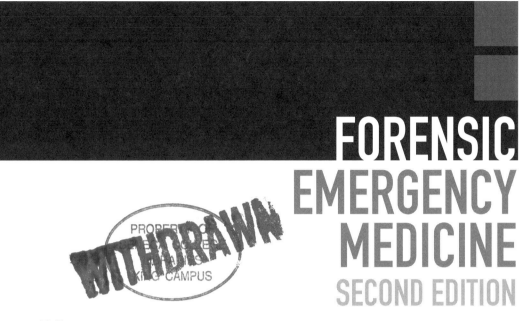

FORENSIC EMERGENCY MEDICINE

SECOND EDITION

Editors

■ **JONATHAN S. OLSHAKER**, MD, FAAEM, FACEP

Professor and Chairman, Department of Emergency Medicine
Boston University School of Medicine
Chief, Department of Emergency Medicine
Boston Medical Center
Boston, Massachusetts

■ **M. CHRISTINE JACKSON**, MD, FACEP

Assistant Professor, Department of Emergency Medicine
University of Maryland School of Medicine
Medical Director, Sexual Assault Forensic Examiner Program
Department of Emergency Medicine
Mercy Medical Center
Baltimore, Maryland

■ **WILLIAM S. SMOCK**, MD, MS, FAAEM, FACEP

Professor and Co-Section Chair, Division of Protective Medicine
Medical Director, Clinical Forensic Medicine Training Program
Department of Emergency Medicine
University of Louisville School of Medicine
Louisville, Kentucky

Editorial Coordinator

■ **LINDA J. KESSELRING**, MS, ELS

Technical Editor/Writer, Department of Emergency Medicine
University of Maryland School of Medicine
Baltimore, Maryland

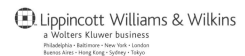
Lippincott Williams & Wilkins
a Wolters Kluwer business
Philadelphia · Baltimore · New York · London
Buenos Aires · Hong Kong · Sydney · Tokyo

Acquisitions Editor: Frances R. DeStefano
Managing Editor: Nicole T. Dernoski
Marketing Manager: Angela Panetta
Project Manager: Nicole Walz
Senior Manufacturing Manager: Ben Rivera
Design Coordinator: Holly Reid McLaughlin
Cover Designer: Larry Didona
Interior Designer: Karen Quigley
Production Services: Laserwords Private Limited, Chennai, India
Printer: Edwards Brothers

Library of Congress Cataloging-in-Publication Data
Forensic emergency medicine / editors, Jonathan S. Olshaker, M. Christine Jackson, William S. Smock ; Linda J. Kesselring, editorial coordinator.—2nd ed.
    p. ; cm.
  Includes bibliographical references and index.
  ISBN-13: 9-780-78179-274-5
  ISBN-10: 0-7817-9274-6
 1. Assault and battery. 2. Emergency medicine. 3. Medical jurisprudence. I. Olshaker, Jonathan S. II. Jackson, M. Christine. III. Smock, William S.
  [DNLM: 1. Emergency Medicine—methods. 2. Forensic Medicine—methods. 3. Expert Testimony. 4. Sex Offenses. 5. Violence. W 700 F7147 2007]
RA1122.F67 2007
614′.1—dc22

                                                                                          2006018684

To my wonderful wife and best friend Kelly;
To my two best dreams come true, my sons Scott and Eric;
To my mother, Thelma, for her unconditional love and teaching me to always try harder and reach higher;
To my brothers Mark and Robert for their goodness and guidance;
And to the memory of my father Bennett Olshaker, MD, as fine a man and physician as ever could be.

JSO

I dedicate this book to the many survivors of sexual assault, abuse, and incest and to the many people in the health profession, law enforcement, and the judicial system who try to eradicate the problem of sexual violence. I thank the SAFE examiners at Mercy Medical Center, who are constantly teaching me about sexual assault patients. I also dedicate this book to my family, Peggy, Ellie, and Donnon, and to my parents and my extended family, whom I love dearly.

MCJ

I dedicate these efforts to my loving wife, Cathy, and our wonderful children, Mariah, Skye, and Forrest Their support, patience, encouragement, and understanding have made my academic dreams a reality. To my mother, Carita Ackerly Warner, for her support, guidance, and love and to my grandfather, S. Spafford Ackerly, MD, the kindest and wisest physician, teacher, and guide I have ever known.

WSS

CONTENTS

Mary-Theresa L. Baker, MD
Medical Director, Baltimore Child Abuse Center
Associate Professor, Department of Pediatrics
University of Maryland, Baltimore, Maryland
Child Sexual Assault: The Acute Assessment

Patrick E. Besant-Matthews, MD
Self Employed, Dallas, Texas
Forensic Photography in the Emergency Department

Rosalind Bowman, BS
Forensic Scientist
Laboratory Section
Baltimore City Police Department
Baltimore, Maryland
Serology and DNA Evidence

John E. Douglas, EdD (Retired)
FBI Unit Chief
National Center for the Analysis of Violent Crime
FBI Academy
Quantico, Virginia
Perpetrators

K. Sophia Dyer, MD
Assistant Professor
Department of Emergency Medicine
Boston University School of Medicine
Medical Toxicologist/Attending Physician
Department of Emergency Medicine
Boston Medical Center
Boston, Massachusettts
New Drugs of Abuse

Carroll Ann Ellis, MA
Director, Victim Services Section
Fairfax County Police Department
Fairfax, Virginia
The Victims of Violence

Adam J. Geroff, MD
Assistant Professor, Department of Emergency Medicine
University of Maryland School of Medicine
Clinical Director, Emergency Care Services
Baltimore Veterans Affairs Medical Center
Baltimore, Maryland
Elder Abuse

M. Christine Jackson, MD, FACEP
Assistant Professor
Department of Emergency Medicine
University of Maryland School of Medicine
Medical Director
Sexual Assault Forensic Examiner Program
Department of Emergency Medicine
Mercy Medical Center
Baltimore, Maryland
Forensic Examination of Adult Victims and Perpetrators of Sexual Assault

Peggy L. Johnson, MD
Assistant Professor
Division of Psychiatry
Boston University School of Medicine
Vice Chair of Clinical Psychiatry
Department of Psychiatry
Boston Medical Center
Boston, Massachusetts
Interviewing Techniques

V. Jill Kempthorne, MD
Assistant Professor
Department of Pediatrics
University of Maryland
Baltimore, Maryland
*Sexual Abuse and
Sexual Assault of Adolescents*

Teri J. Labbe, BS
Forensic Scientist
Laboratory Section
Baltimore City Police Department
Baltimore, Maryland
Serology and DNA Evidence

Richard Lichenstein, MD
Associate Professor
Department of Pediatrics and Family Medicine
University of Maryland School of Medicine
Director, Division of Pediatric Emergency Medicine
University of Maryland Hospital for Children
Baltimore, Maryland
Child Abuse/Assault

Judith A. Linden, MD, SANE

Assistant Professor, Associate Residency Director
Department of Emergency Medicine
Boston University School of Medicine
and Boston Medical Center
Boston, Massachusetts
*Forensic Examination of Adult Victims and Perpetrators
of Sexual Assault*

Sharon A. H. May, JD

Assistant Public Defender
Office of the Public Defender for Baltimore City
Baltimore, Maryland
Testifying

Kimberly A. Mullings, BS

Forensic Scientist, Laboratory Section
Baltimore City Police Department
Baltimore, Maryland
Serology and DNA Evidence

John S. O'Brien, II, MD, JD

Clinical Assistant Professor, Department of Psychiatry
University of Pennsylvania, Pennsylvania Hospital
Philadelphia, Pennsylvania
Interviewing Techniques

Annie Lewis-O'Connor, PhD, MPH, ARNP

Assistant Professor
Department of Emergency Medicine
Boston University
Nurse Practitioner, Emergency Services
Boston Medical Center
Boston, Massachusetts
*Forensic Examination of Adult Victims and Perpetrators
of Sexual Assault*

Jonathan S. Olshaker, MD

Professor and Chairman
Department of Emergency Medicine
Boston University School of Medicine
Chief, Department of Emergency Medicine
Boston Medical Center
Boston, Massachusetts
Elder Abuse

Mark Olshaker

Author, Novelist, and Filmmaker
Washington, District of Columbia
Perpetrators

Daniel J. Sheridan, PhD, RN, FAAN

Assistant Professor, School of Nursing
Johns Hopkins University
Baltimore, Maryland
*Treating Survivors of Intimate Partner Abuse: Forensic
Identification and Documentation*

William S. Smock, MD

Professor and Co-Section Chair
Division of Protective Medicine
Medical Director
Clinical Forensic Medicine Training Program
Department of Emergency Medicine
University of Louisville School of Medicine
Louisville, Kentucky
Forensic Photography in the Emergency Department

Donald E. Steinhice

Investigator, Sex Offense Division
Baltimore City State's Attorney's Office
Detective (Retired), Baltimore City Police Department
Baltimore, Maryland
Law Enforcement

Adrienne H. Suggs, MD

Director, Pediatric Emergency and Inpatient Services
Department of Pediatrics
Franklin Square Hospital Center
Baltimore, Maryland
Child Abuse/Assault

Since the publication of the first edition of *Forensic Emergency Medicine* in 2001, acts of sexual assault, child and elder abuse, and domestic violence have remained at epidemic levels. The National Violence Against Women Survey documented a lifetime prevalence of rape of 17.6% among women and 3% among men. Adolescent sexual victimization is a significant problem. In the 2003 CDC Youth Risk Behavior Survey of high school students, 12% of the female respondents and 6% of the male respondents gave a history of having been forced to have sex. The National Clearing House on Child Abuse and Neglect Information statistics for 2003 document an estimated 2.9 million referrals to child protection services, with approximately 30% substantiated. An estimated 1,500 children died of abuse and neglect that year. Elder abuse remains a troubling reality in American society, and its incidence could increase in proportion to the projected growth in older age groups. At least 4 million women experience domestic violence (physical, psychological, sexual, and/or financial abuse) from a male intimate partner each year in the United States. The number of men abused by female intimates is estimated in the tens of thousands.

The emergency department remains the most likely place where the healthcare system will encounter these victims and, in many cases, offers the only chance to identify a serious problem and prevent tragic outcomes. Certainly there has been progress in recognizing individuals at risk as well as ensuring the availability of resources, including child protection services, domestic violence councilors, sexual assault nurse examiners, and elder services. But other trends make the job in this arena more difficult. The steady increase in emergency department overcrowding allows less time with individual patients, leads to long waits for evaluation, and causes great difficulty in finding inpatient beds. In many jurisdictions, funding for essential services such as SANE nurses, mental health interventions, and drug and alcohol abuse treatment programs has been cut drastically. In addition, the aging of the American population is putting more stress on emergency services from both increased utilization and complexity of comorbid diseases in the elderly population.

Still, the tasks of recognizing, evaluating, treating, and understanding acts of violence or neglect remain essential in the practice of emergency medicine. Proper documentation, meticulous collection of evidence, and careful adherence to protocols regarding the chain of custody of that evidence can clearly help law enforcement officials convict the guilty and exonerate the innocent.

The goal of the second edition of *Forensic Emergency Medicine* is to provide an up-to-date reference containing the information necessary to complete these important missions. In addition to updating chapters from the first edition, we have added new chapters on the topics of motor vehicle trauma, drugs of abuse, and DNA use and analysis.

Despite the present-day challenges of emergency department overcrowding and strained medical resources, the emergency physician can still successfully recognize that a problem exists, deliver competent and compassionate care, and use available resources for appropriate referrals and disposition. We hope and believe the second edition of *Forensic Emergency Medicine* will significantly aid emergency medicine practitioners as they perform these crucial tasks.

Jonathan S. Olshaker, MD

Although total violent crime is currently on a decline in this country, acts of child and elder abuse and neglect, sexual assault, and domestic violence remain at epidemic levels. In 1998, three million referrals for child maltreatment were made. More than one-third of these cases were substantiated. At least four million women experience ongoing physical, psychological, sexual, or violent abuse from male intimate partners each year in the United States. The 1998 National Institute of Justice Center for Disease Control survey on violence against women documented that an estimated 302,100 women and 92,000 men are forcibly raped each year in the United States. The National Elder Abuse Incidence Study showed that at least 450,000 elders each year are victims of abuse or neglect.

Emergency physicians have frequent opportunities to play a major role in the identification, evaluation, and treatment of these patients whose care involves significant forensic issues. The emergency department is clearly the most likely place where the healthcare system will encounter the unfortunate victims just described. For many victims, this will be the only chance to identify a serious problem before more tragic results ensue.

In some cases of abuse or sexual assault, the diagnosis will be obvious. In addition to evaluation and treatment, our role includes insuring proper documentation and evidence chain of custody to maximize law enforcement's chances of successful prosecution. Most importantly, we must realize that we are among the victim's first encounters with "the system." Therefore, we must carry out our evaluation and treatment in a compassionate, supportive, nonthreatening manner that gives the victims the best chance of getting through their nightmarish experience as psychologically whole as possible.

Many cases of abuse and neglect, however, are subtle and go unrecognized. While healthcare professionals have become increasingly aware of the incidence of child abuse and its manifestations, until recently, domestic violence and elder abuse have been largely ignored. Physicians fail to make the diagnosis for a variety of reasons: for example, they may lack proper training as medical students or residents, or they may not consider the diagnosis in cases with nontrauma chief complaints. Hence, these serious issues go unnoticed because physicians have not been taught the significance of less obvious clues or do not think to ask some basic questions.

This book was developed with the goal of providing all emergency physicians with a reference that will give them the necessary information to perform the essential tasks of recognition, evaluation, treatment, documentation, and understanding of victims of acts of violence, abuse, or neglect.

Importantly, it is unnecessary for emergency physicians to become judge and jury or to spend inordinate amounts of time with individual patients in an already busy environment. First and foremost, we must simply recognize that a problem exists. This will lead to appropriate referrals and disposition. The various chapters in this text describe at length the myriad of victim services immediately available in most jurisdictions, including child and adult protective services, social workers, sexual assault nurse examiners, and police forensic technicians. In addition, we included chapters on the relevant aspects of the legal system and guidance to medical personnel on testifying in court. This discussion should prove beneficial not only to emergency care providers involved in criminal evidentiary matters, but also to anyone called upon to give expert witness testimony.

We are greatly indebted to the authors of *Forensic Emergency Medicine* for their informative and passionate contributions. We sincerely hope this text will significantly aid emergency physicians in providing compassionate treatment, thorough forensic support, and, most importantly, early recognition of victims of sexual assault and other acts of violence, abuse, and neglect.

Jonathan S. Olshaker, MD

We thank the contributors to *Forensic Emergency Medicine* for the tremendous effort and passion put forth in their chapters, whether new in this edition or an update of their work in the first edition. We are grateful to Brian J. Browne, MD, Acting Chair of the Department of Emergency Medicine at the University of Maryland School of Medicine and Chief of Emergency Medical Services at the University of Maryland Medical Center, whose leadership and guidance played a major role in the initial plans for this book. Linda J. Kesselring, MS, ELS, technical editor/writer in the Department of Emergency Medicine at the University of Maryland School of Medicine, and our editorial coordinator, provided significant help to every author in the editing of their chapters and truly made this edition a better book. We are also thankful for the continued faith and support of the editorial staff at Lippincott Williams & Wilkins.

1

JOHN E. DOUGLAS ■
MARK OLSHAKER ■

WHERE DO WE BEGIN?

Early in the 1980s, when one of the authors (JED) was conducting in-depth interviews with incarcerated serial offenders that would help form the basis for the behavioral profiling and criminal investigative analysis program of the Federal Bureau of Investigation (FBI) (1 [pp ix–xiii, 15]), he interviewed an inmate of the Joliet Penitentiary in Illinois who had been convicted of murdering a woman by inflicting multiple stab wounds. Throughout the extensive interview, the 5-feet, 9-inch tall white man in his mid-20s maintained a soft, inappropriate affect, smiling frequently. He displayed what FBI special agents referred to as "the look"—darting eyes, nervous twitches, continual hand rubbing. His primary concern was how he had looked in a CBS television interview the day before. When told he had come across well, he laughed, relaxed considerably, and was much more forthcoming.

After the interview, the special agent sought out the prison psychiatrist to find out how the inmate was doing. The psychiatrist gave a positive reaction, stating that the inmate was responding very well to medication and therapy, adding that he had joined a Bible study group in prison and that if the progress continued he would be ready for parole.

The special agent asked the psychiatrist if he knew the specifics of the crime the inmate had committed. "No, I don't want to know," he replied. "I don't have the time, with all the inmates I have to deal with here." And, he added, he did not want to unfairly influence his relationship with his patient.

Before the psychiatrist could protest, the agent related how this asocial person had joined a church group and how after a meeting, when everyone else had gone, he propositioned the young woman who had hosted the meeting. She rejected his advances, at which point he knocked her to the floor, went to the kitchen and retrieved a knife, and stabbed her numerous times. Then, as she lay bleeding to death on the floor, he inserted his penis into an open wound in her abdomen and ejaculated.

"You're disgusting, Douglas!" the psychiatrist declared. "Get out of my office!"

"I'm disgusting?" the agent countered. "You're in a position to make a recommendation that this individual is responding to therapy and could be freed, and you don't know who in the hell you're talking to when you're dealing with these inmates. How are you supposed to understand them if you haven't taken the time to look at the crime scene photographs or reports, to go over the autopsy protocols? Have you looked at the way the crime was committed? Do you know if it was planned? Do you understand the behavior leading up to it? Do you know how he left the crime scene? Do you know if he tried to get away with it? Did he try to establish an alibi? *How in the hell do you know if he's dangerous or not?*" (2 [pp 335–337]).

At the heart of the dilemma is the fact that much of psychiatric therapy is based on self-reporting, and although a patient coming to a therapist under normal circumstances has a vested interest in revealing his true thoughts and feelings, a jailed convict desirous of early release has a vested interest

1

in telling the therapist what he wants to hear. To the extent that the therapist takes the report at face value without correlating it with other information about the subject, there is grave danger of a fundamental and perilous misevaluation. Edmund Kemper in California and Montie Rissell in Virginia, two of the serial murderers the author (JED) has interviewed and studied, were in court-mandated therapy as a condition of parole while they continued committing new crimes. Both managed to remain undetected and both showed "progress" to their therapists. On at least one occasion, Kemper attended a meeting with state psychiatrists while the severed head of his most recent victim lay in the trunk of his car (3).

The point of this experience and research is clear. Neither the law enforcement nor the medical/health community can effectively deal with violent, predatory, and often repeat or serial criminals or even evaluate the critical question of their current or future level of dangerousness, until the effort is made to *understand* the nature and type of each offender.

There can be many reasons certain individuals—almost exclusively males—become violent sexually oriented predators, having do with both "nature" and "nurture," "hard wiring," and environment. But studies have shown common elements that are too prominent to ignore. Among these are factors such as family history of alcoholism and psychiatric disorders, instability of residence, mother as the dominant parent, and negative relationship with father or male caretaker. All of these factors came into play in significantly more than half of the instances in the author's study. In addition, other important indicators such as family members with criminal histories, father leaving before the subject's twelfth birthday, negative relationship with the mother, the subject's ongoing perception of unfair treatment, and no older sibling role model all showed up in roughly 50% of the cases. Approximately 40% of the subjects were physically abused as children or adolescents, and nearly 75% experienced some form of psychological abuse; various forms of sexual abuse were also common, but in lower percentages (1 [pp 17–26]).

Not surprisingly, what this type of upbringing led to in the subjects studied was a tendency to fail in interpersonal relationships; aggressiveness and other antisocial behavior patterns; inappropriate emotional responses, including absence of guilt or conscience, chronic lying, and rebelliousness; underperformance in school and underemployment; active fantasy life and preoccupation with fantasies of violence, domination, and control (1 [pp 28–43]). It is therefore not difficult to see the type of background, combined with whatever is inherent in the child's physical/neurologic/emotional makeup, as part of a template for the adult violent offender.

Is early environment the only determining factor? Certainly not. Many have posed the question, in one form or another, of whether certain people are simply "evil." Although each of us may have personal views on the subject, we are not qualified, nor is it relevant to this discussion, to pass judgment on that issue. The one thing we can state empirically is that there are many complexities to individual personality that we do not understand or know how to evaluate, some of which do seem to be "inborn" and, together with other influences, unquestionably play a significant role in the formation of the adult criminal. Combining the environmental template with these inherent traits and characteristics, what we often see is an individual whose personality incorporates deep-seated feelings of inadequacy with equally deep-seated feelings of grandiosity and entitlement—that he is better than anyone else and is being held back by society and the people around him.

Once the antisocial behavior begins (often with acts such as starting a fire or causing cruelty to animals and other children), a series of "feedback filters" come into play: the subject justifies the act in his own mind; he sorts out errors in his performance of the act so that he can do it "better" and more efficiently next time; he finds that in performing the act he experiences an increased state of arousal; he discovers increased areas of dominance, power, and control in his life; he learns how to continue these acts without detection or punishment; he progresses to a larger, more elaborate, and harmful acting out of his fantasies (1 [p 70]).

But let us add a word of caution here, because it would be easy to misinterpret the data. As with other aspects of medicine, it is critical to keep in mind that although nearly all the affected subjects conform in greater or lesser degree to these and many other related traits, *most* of the individuals who have suffered similar backgrounds and upbringing are in no way criminally motivated and, in fact, grow up to lead "normal," productive lives. This is true not only for this population at large but more specifically for the siblings of criminal offenders, many of whom experienced the same negative influences.

Stated simply, various studies and our own experience have led us to several conclusions: although the background described in the preceding text could certainly result in an adult with serious psychological problems and emotional unhappiness, it does not follow that this adult would then be compelled to perpetrate violent, predatory acts on others. Why, then, do serial predatory offenders do what they do? It is because this act of manipulation, domination, and control—be it rape, murder, arson, or any other criminal enterprise—gives them a feeling of power, satisfaction, and fulfillment that they cannot obtain anywhere else in life. In this one moment, a "loser" or "nobody" who feels that he has no power or influence in normal life can exert the ultimate power over another human being, can make that other human being suffer and bend to his will, and can decide whether that other human being will live or die. For this type of individual, there is no greater sense of empowerment.

So vital is the sense of self-importance derived by some offenders and the need for recognition that it can lead directly or indirectly to their apprehension. The self-styled "BTK Strangler" terrorized Wichita, Kansas, beginning in January 1974. The name originated with the communications he sent to law enforcement and media, proudly explaining that his technique was to bind, torture, and kill. After some years, the case went cold and the killings ceased. His last communication was in 1979. Then in 2004, the communications began again, containing information that appeared to authenticate the sender as BTK, including crime scene photographs of an unsolved murder. There had been no official police photographs of this scene, owing to the quick removal of the body, but the new communication confirmed the statement in the author's original profile of BTK that sketches included in the early communications signified he was photographing his victims as "trophies."

Dennis Rader, a former municipal ordinance official from nearby Park City, was arrested and charged several months after the communications resumed. Among the pieces of evidence that led to his arrest was the tracing of an electronic imprint on a computer disk he had sent to a local television station (4). In a similar manner, Theodore J. Kaczynski was identified as the notorious Unabomber in 1996 after his brother David recognized familiar phrasing in an extensive rambling manifesto the subject insisted be published in national newspapers (5).

This discussion applies primarily—almost exclusively—to male individuals. A girl who appears to have a background identical to that of a boy who goes on to a troubled life of crime will almost never develop into the same type of sexual predator. The types of violent crimes committed by women are different in character from those committed by men, as are preference for weapons and means of murder. For reasons often speculated on but not yet clearly understood, girls and women from dysfunctional and abusive backgrounds tend to direct their rage, anger, and despair inward. Rather than being outwardly aggressive toward others, they often engage in self-destructive or self-punishing behaviors, such as alcohol or drug abuse, suicide attempts, prostitution, and attraction to abusive men (6). What this means, of course, is that violent predatory crimes are almost always committed by men; therefore, men are the focus of our examination.

Are individuals who derive satisfaction from forcibly controlling, assaulting, and killing *sick*? Depending on one's definition of the term, this can be a pretty safe bet. Are such individuals mentally ill? We would be more than willing to concede that anyone who derives his life's satisfaction from inflicting pain and suffering has severe mental problems. But is this individual *insane*? In other words, is he incapable of understanding the wrongness of his actions and resisting the impulse to follow through on his fantasies? In almost all cases, we believe the answer to that question is no. To our knowledge, there are no recorded cases of the hypothetical "policeman at the elbow," for example, in which an individual is so compelled to perform a predatory criminal act that he does so knowing that a uniformed police officer is watching him.

Although this may be a rather glib restatement of an important and admittedly controversial issue, our conclusion is that the critical operative word is *choice*. Regardless of family background and all other formative influences and regardless of intelligence or level of emotional stability, the overwhelming number of predatory criminals *choose* to do what they do because of the way it makes them feel. They are fully aware of what they are doing, often plan it, and understand that it is wrong and contrary to society's rules. They simply do not care. Or if they do care, that care is outweighed by the desire to do it anyway.

It is also important to keep in mind that, by definition, a serial criminal is a successful criminal. The more times he is able to get away with a particular offense, the better will be his ability to refine his *modus operandi* (MO) to continue to get away with the same crime. In any given case, this may be because the offender is above average in intelligence, despite his record of underachievement. Many serial offenders, particularly of the organized variety (a distinction explained later in this chapter), are reasonably bright. But success at avoiding detection and capture can also be related to the obsessive amount of time and energy the offender puts into fantasizing, planning, and evaluating the crime. When one of the authors was a teenaged agricultural intern, he noted with amazement the uncanny ability of cows to wander out of seemingly secure enclosures. He finally concluded that if the cow had nothing else on its mind, it could devote all of its mental resources to the task of finding a way out, however long it took. The situation of the sexual predator who spends an inordinate amount of his time, intellect, and emotional resources on his crimes turns out to be an analogous situation.

Therefore, besides being armed with an understanding of the commonalities among criminal sexual predators, it is equally important to understand the differences. Only then will we be equipped to evaluate the offender as an individual, lend aid and support to his victims, assist in his prosecution, and make an attempt to predict the likelihood of future violence. The method and manner in which a crime is committed relate directly to the criminal's personality type.

SEXUAL VIOLENCE

Rape is one of the most common predatory crimes to which emergency medical personnel respond; therefore, it is important that they have a fuller understanding of the rapist than of any other type of perpetrator. We will therefore devote the largest share of our discussion to this subject.

There is an ongoing debate within and between the law enforcement community, the health care community, and the women's movement about whether rape should be classified as a crime of sex or violence, and this discussion will not abate any time in the foreseeable future. In either category, rape almost always has the key component of anger.

We have heard of no better definition than the one provided by the distinguished prosecutor Linda Fairstein, Esq., former head of the New York County District Attorney's Office Sex Crimes Unit and now a successful novelist (7,8): rape is a crime of violence in which sex is the weapon. In an interview, Fairstein explained, "There is a sexual element to this that isn't part of any other crime, and that can't be denied. It's very much the piece of the crime that the victim doesn't want to happen or is afraid of. And so to me, it was about the one weapon that this type of offender had that other offenders don't use and victims don't want used against them" (9).

Rape of any kind is a horrible event. Any sexual assault leaves its victim and her partner, friends, and loved ones devastated. But we do a grave disservice to all victims and potential victims if we do not invest the time and effort to distinguish between types of rape and rapists. It may seem more sympathetic and caring to proclaim, for instance, that date rape is the same as stranger rape, but it is not true. So much depends on the circumstances of the assault. To assert that a date rape that does not involve a weapon and does not cause the victim to fear for her life is the same as a stranger abduction–rape at knifepoint or gunpoint in which the victim is brutally beaten dangerously oversimplifies the situation and hinders our ability to defend against both crimes and their different types of perpetrators. All sexual assaults share certain elements, but what they do not share is, in some ways, even more important if we are to learn prevention strategies from them and help victims recover from their individual traumas. Many things are required of the diligent, sensitive emergency medicine practitioners who respond to sexual assault (10). Besides delivering excellent medical care, by far the most important of these are providing emotional support and empathy to the victim.

CRIME CLASSIFICATION: CATEGORIES OF RAPISTS

In 1992, after more than 10 years of investigation and study by the Behavioral Science and Investigative Support Units of the FBI Academy in Quantico, Virginia, together with the pioneering research of Dr. Ann Burgess, Professor of Psychiatric Nursing at the University of Pennsylvania, Douglas et al. organized categories of sexual assault, with breakdowns similar to those of homicide and arson, into the *Crime Classification Manual* (11). Critical research was also conducted by Special Agents Roy Hazelwood and Ken Lanning of the Behavioral Science Unit (12). This research involved the review of numerous case files, victim statements, police reports, court testimony, school reports and psychiatric evaluations, parole and probation records, and records of family and developmental history. Following the analysis, rapists were broken down into four basic types, with the crime of rape further broken down into more than 50 subgroups (13 [pp 93–99]). Over the years, different researchers have assigned their own labels to the typologies, but the behavior is so consistent within each that the types should be recognizable regardless of how they are named.

The Power-Reassurance Rapist

The *power-reassurance rapist* (numerically, the most common type of rapist) feels inadequate, not being the type with whom women would voluntarily become involved. He compensates for these feelings of male inadequacy by forcing women to have sex with him. All the while, as the designation suggests, he is looking for reassurance of his own power and potency. This type has sometimes been referred to as the "gentleman rapist," or even classified as an "unselfish" rapist, in large part because his offenses, although traumatic, are usually physically less damaging to his victim than those of other types of sex offenders. Such a rapist may even apologize during the assault or ask the victim if he is hurting her—a question that serves his own need for reassurance more than it expresses a genuine concern for the victim. Therefore, the terms "gentleman" and "unselfish" are applicable only within the context of the full spectrum of the types of rapists (14).

This type tends to be a loner who fantasizes that his victim actually enjoys the experience and might even fall in love with him. He may go so far as to contact the victim after the assault and ask her to go out with him. Of course, the reality of rape cannot live up to his fantasies: instead of winning over a reluctant lover, he has terrorized, hurt, and angered an innocent person. Most rapists of the power-reassurance variety will admit later that they did not enjoy the sex with their victims. The experience did not satisfy the underlying obsession; therefore, he will have to try again with another woman.

Victims of choice are generally about the same age as or younger than the perpetrator and usually of the same race. If the rapist dates at all, the women he dates will be younger and less sophisticated than he; this is the only way he can feel equal. Because of his feelings of inadequacy, he gains control by surprise; he does not have the self-confidence or skills to con his way into a victim's apartment smoothly, so he is more likely to break into the victim's home in the middle of the night. When we delve into the past of this type of perpetrator, we generally see a history of unusual or bizarre masturbatory fantasies, often voyeurism, exhibitionism, cross-dressing, or making obscene phone calls. He frequents adult bookstores or movies and collects pornography. If he has a specific sexual dysfunction, it is likely to be premature ejaculation, which would be exhibited in consensual relationships and which he would report as a problem (from his point of view only) in his rapes.

He will tend to prefer the night and operate in his own residential or work area—in other words, within a very prescribed comfort zone—and will usually travel to the crime scene on foot. If he is a serial offender, this is particularly true of his first offense. He uses a weapon of opportunity, often something he finds at the crime scene. His patterns of crime are generally consistent, and the entire act, from the time he overpowers his victim until the time he leaves, is relatively brief, sometimes as short as 5 or 10 minutes. He will not use profanity or try to demean or humiliate his victim to the extent that the other rapist types will, but he may require her to recite a "script" in which she praises his lovemaking or expresses desire for him. He might cover the victim's eyes or mask his own features, both for the self-preservation motive of preventing identification and the possibility that he knows he should be ashamed of his actions. He is timid and will do whatever the victim allows him to. Rather than tear off her clothes or force her to strip, he may expose only the parts of the victim's body he intends to assault.

He is apt to keep a journal, news clippings, or some other record of his assaults to reassure himself of his potency. For the same reason, he may take souvenirs, such as pieces of the victim's underwear. Afterward, he may feel guilty or remorseful. But unless he is a first-timer who tries it, does not

like it, and decides never to do it again, he *will* do it again. He will continue with his acts of rape until he is caught or stopped by being arrested and incarcerated or killed or seriously injured in another crime or an unrelated incident. He tends to live alone or with his parents or in some type of dependent relationship. His mother probably was—or is—very domineering. He is employed below his ability level in a job that does not require a lot of contact with the public. Although he is physically the least dangerous type of rapist, if he is successful over a series of attacks, his confidence may be boosted and he may become more physically aggressive.

The Exploitative Rapist

The *exploitative rapist* (the second most common type of rapist) is a more impulsive predator. His crimes result from seizing an opportunity that presents itself rather than by fantasizing about the act ahead of time. He might approach a potential victim with a ruse or con, or might employ a direct, overpowering, blitz-style attack. Unlike the power-reassurance rapist, this type will not appear in any way concerned with the victim's welfare. He is selfish—verbally, physically, and sexually. He may suffer from some form of sexual dysfunction, and if he does, it will be just as apparent with his wife, girlfriend, or any other consenting partner as it will be with a victim of force. Often such sexual dysfunction is because of retarded ejaculation or difficulty in reaching climax.

Victims of preference tend to be around his age. He is on the prowl for a victim of opportunity, and this activity could take place in a bar or neighborhood he has targeted. Once he has a woman under his control, his only concern is getting her to submit sexually to him. That is the real thrill for him—the sex act is satisfying as an act of domination and control rather than providing what we think of as sexual gratification. Once he has forced submission, as far as he is concerned, the experience is over. But during that encounter, he can be expected to inflict multiple assaults on the victim. Anal assaults are common. Masks or attempts at disguise or hiding his face are uncommon. With this type of offender, often there will be an interval between rapes—a day, a month, 6 months—until he goes on the hunt once again; however, unlike the power-reassurance rapist, he will not try to maintain any contact with or come back to a victim once he has left her, although he often threatens to return if she reports the assault to police.

This type is very body conscious. He wants a macho reputation, to be known as a man's man, and therefore is likely to have some physically oriented employment. He is interested in sports. His vehicle reflects that image, too. In some regions of the country, it would be a Corvette or other muscle car; in others, it might be a pickup truck, well equipped for hunting. He does not take well to criticism or authority. He probably did not do well in high school or go to college. If married, he has a history of cheating on his wife and paying scant attention to his children. When we look into the background of such offenders, very often we find that his father has treated his mother in the same way the offender treats women.

The Anger Rapist

For the *anger rapist*, also referred to as the anger-retaliatory rapist, sexual assault is a displaced expression of rage and anger. For this type of rapist, the victim represents a person—or group of people—the offender hates. This could be a mother, wife, or girlfriend, even women in general. But his anger and resentment need not be rooted in an actual or legitimate wrong ever perpetrated against him.

It would not be unusual for this type to be involved in an ongoing relationship with a woman. Because he is driven by rage, the consequences of the anger rapist's attack can be anything from verbal abuse, to severe beating, to murder, although the fact that his conscious or subconscious intention is to get the anger out of his system means that this type usually will not kill. His attacks will be episodic, not at predictable intervals, triggered by precipitating stressors involving the woman or women at whom his rage is actually directed. In almost all cases, the displacement means he will not attack that person. He may attack someone else he knows, using weapons of opportunity such as kitchen knives or even his own fists if he is strong enough. Because he wants not just to overpower but to humiliate his target, there could be anal sex followed by oral sex and a great deal of profanity, and the context of his behavior will be an intention to degrade, such as by ejaculating on the victim's face or clothing.

Therefore, it is important for the examiner to realize that DNA and other crucial evidence can be found on many parts of the victim's body and her clothes. Whenever this is a possibility, a delicate but thorough line of questioning on this topic is indicated, with the twin goals of preserving the chain of evidence while ensuring the victim's emotional well being.

This type is far less common than the two described previously, possibly accounting for as few as 5% of rapists.

The Sadistic Rapist

The *sadistic rapist* is the least common type of rapist but in many ways he is the most dangerous sexual predator of all. The purpose of his attack is to live out his sadistic sexual fantasies on the unwilling victim. With this type, sexual fantasy and aggression merge, which is why he is also referred to as an *anger−excitation rapist*. Aggression and sadistic fantasy feed on each other, so, as the level of aggression rises, his level of arousal rises accordingly. His aggression is not anger based, as it is with the previous category. In fact, he can be quite charming and seductive as he lures the intended prey into his web. He is completely self-centered. The only thing he cares about is his own pleasure and satisfaction. He derives satisfaction from hurting people and having them in his power (15). Therefore, with this type, we expect to see various forms of mental and physical torture, and the physical torture may be directed particularly at sexually significant parts of the body such as mouth, breasts, genitals, buttocks, and rectum. His weapon of choice is frequently a knife, because it is so intimidating and causes mental anguish on the part of the victim. He often cuts or tears off his victim's clothing because he figures she will not need it after he has finished with her. Depending on his preferences, there may be much sexual activity, probably highly perverse in nature, or even none. He could, for example, prefer to penetrate with a sharp object rather than with his penis. His language will be commanding and degrading, but impersonal. The victim is merely there as an actress in his self-scripted drama, and her role is to show fear and respond to pain. Therefore, there is often a victim of preference, symbolic to him in some way, be she old or young, white, black, or Asian, slim-figured or full-figured, black-haired or blonde, redhead or brunette.

The sadistic rapist anticipates his crime and has perfected his MO over the course of his criminal career. As his fantasy evolves and he gains more experience with different victims, he will take more time planning ahead for successive crimes. He brings his weapon(s) with him and may have a torture kit made up in advance, including pliers or other sharp instruments, whips, manacles, needles, or whatever object he needs to fulfill his fantasy. Because his assault unfolds over a long period of time, he will have a place to which he can take his victim, where he knows they will not be disturbed. This might be an obscure cabin in the woods or a specially outfitted and soundproofed van. He may tell the victim that if she does what he tells her he will not hurt her further or will let her go, but this is only a ruse to control her and get her to cooperate. Because his satisfaction lies in the act of tormenting and dominating his victim, he may take photographs or record the scene as it unfolds on either audiotape or videotape. For the same reason, he may also take souvenirs to help him relive the experience and demonstrate to himself that he "owns" the victim. These souvenirs might include jewelry, items of clothing or underwear, or even body parts.

The attack itself will tend to be highly symbolic. There will be no remorse because the rapist has totally depersonalized his victim; he does not even think of her as a human being. This is the type of rape that most often ends in murder. In fact, killing the victim may be an integral part of the sadistic fantasy scenario. He may even continue to engage in activity with the body after death. It is generally impossible for the victim to play on his sympathy, because he has none. He wants her to suffer. The only instance in which he might relent is if the victim can somehow break through the depersonalization and get him to regard her as an individual. This occurred, for example, in one instance in which a victim stated that her husband had cancer. It happened that the rapist's brother was battling cancer, and he let her go. Another time, a sadistic rapist revealed in a prison interview that one of his victims reminded him of his mother and so he had released her. Unfortunately, this is a very uncommon scenario with the sexual sadist.

The sadistic type is usually white, with above-normal intelligence, and may be college-educated with a good middle-class job. He has a dominant personality and likes to collect bondage and sado-masochistic pornography. He may also collect related items, such as knives, guns, or Nazi memorabilia, and read military, law enforcement, or survivalist literature. He may have a large attack-type dog, such as a German shepherd, Doberman, or Rottweiler. Because of his intelligence and planning, he will be difficult to apprehend.

ADVICE TO VICTIMS

As we all know, human nature is not exact, and not every rapist fits neatly into one of the four categories described in the preceding text. There is often a mixed presentation, with elements of one classification grafting onto the general description of another, which is why it is so difficult to give specific advice to potential victims as to how to react to a sexual criminal, particularly under the acute stress of the attack itself. But in most cases, one category will dominate, and our reaction should be molded around the understanding of what motivates that specific type of rapist and what he is after (12 [pp 358–363]).

In any discussion of criminal personality, the cautions and cautionary tales are as important as the conclusions. Montie Rissell, mentioned earlier, was in some ways an unusual rapist. He attacked and murdered five women near his home in Alexandria, Virginia, while still in his teens, later blaming his

criminal behavior on having to live with his mother rather than his father after his parents' troubled marriage broke up when he was 7 years old. By the time he was in high school, he had a rap sheet detailing driving without a license, burglary, car theft, and rape.

Rissell's first killing was savagely instructive of the dangers of misinterpreting offender behavior. While still in high school, on being put on probation and during the course of receiving psychiatric counseling as a provision in that probation, he heard from his girlfriend—a year ahead of him and then away at college—that their relationship was over. A trigger emotional event of this nature is generally the precursor to a serial sex crime. Rissell promptly drove to the college, where he spotted the young woman with her new boyfriend. Rather than express his rage on the person he felt he was hurt by, he drove back home, fortified himself with beer and marijuana, and spent hours sitting in his car in the parking lot of his apartment complex. Several hours later, another vehicle appeared, driven by a single woman. On the spur of the moment, Rissell decided to get back what he had just lost. He approached the other car, pulled a handgun on the woman, and forced her to go with him to a secluded area nearby.

As it happened, Rissell's victim was a prostitute, which is significant for two reasons: she would not have the same fear of having sex with a stranger as would someone outside the profession and, although frightened, she would probably draw on a strong and well-developed survival instinct. Her behavior, according to the prison interview with Rissell, reflected this. When she was alone and defenseless and it was clear that her attacker intended to rape her at gunpoint, she attempted to diffuse the situation by hiking up her skirt, asking him how he liked it and in what position he wanted her.

Rather than making him gentler or more sensitive to her, this behavior enraged him. As an anger (or anger-retaliatory) rapist, Rissell was set off by what he perceived as his victim's attempt to *control* the situation. In fact, when she subsequently feigned orgasm in an attempt to gratify him, he became greatly upset that she was "enjoying" the experience. This reinforced in him the notion that all women are whores. Because he was able to depersonalize her, it was easy for him to think about killing her, an idea that solidified in his mind when she attempted to run away, thereby further "controlling" the situation (2 [pp 137–142], 16).

Had the attacker been a power-reassurance rapist, resistance or struggle might have prevented the attack, and acquiescence might have mitigated its severity. However, in the case of this anger-retaliatory rapist, the opposite was true. And once this type has killed, found the act satisfying, and realized he can get away with it, he escalates the crimes to those of a serial rapist–murderer. He will not stop until something stops him.

In light of these and other considerations, the only nearly absolute advice we feel comfortable in imparting to victims relates to a few key behavioral indicators on the part of the rapist or potential rapist. If an offender wears a mask or otherwise attempts to disguise his identity, that is a "good" sign. In most cases, it signifies that he intends to get away with the crime, leaving his victim alive but unable to identify him. If he does not attempt to prevent identification, this could signify at least two scenarios, neither of them good. The first is that he is disorganized, "making it up as he goes along," which means that his actions may be unpredictable, even to himself. The second, even more dire, is that he plans to get away with his crime and, to ensure this, he does not intend to leave a victim alive to identify him. This being the case, resistance of whatever kind the victim can muster would be indicated. Unfortunately, this does not mean she might not be hurt, but just that the consequences of not resisting are even riskier. Likewise, another indication where resistance by any means possible is required would be if an offender orders his victim into a car, intending to take her away from the abduction point, because once in the vehicle she loses all control, all possibilities of alerting others, and therefore all possibilities of intervention (13 [pp 358–361]).

THE PROSPECT OF REHABILITATION

In terms of evaluating a perpetrator of sexual assault for amenability to "rehabilitation" or future dangerousness, it is critical to look at the behavior exhibited during the crime and whether that behavior is representative of a pattern.

Rehabilitation and dangerousness are inextricably intertwined. On the general subject, we can do no better than to quote the distinguished clinical psychologist Dr. Stanton E. Samenow. Samenow, in collaboration with the late psychiatrist Samuel Yochelson, undertook a pioneering study of violent criminals at St. Elizabeth's Hospital in Washington, DC, and published the landmark work *The Criminal Personality* (17). In his own penetrating book, *Inside the Criminal Mind* (18), Samenow wrote, "Rehabilitation as it has been practiced cannot possibly be effective because it is based on a total misconception. To rehabilitate is to restore to a former constructive capacity or condition. *There is nothing to which to rehabilitate a criminal.* There is no earlier condition of being responsible to which to restore him."

In an interview (19), Samenow further stated, "If you've worked with sex offenders—people who

have committed these offenses again and again and again—you know that we do not in psychiatry and psychology have a way to change sexual orientation. People who molest kids, for example, they've done it and they've done it and they've done it, and they haven't been caught for a fraction of what they've done. To turn these people back in to the community knowing that we have nothing to offer them that is going to ensure the safety of kids is unconscionable."

Are there, then, any good candidates for rehabilitation? As a matter of fact, there are—a notion with which Samenow agrees (20). As far as rapists are concerned, such candidates would fall overwhelmingly into the power-reassurance category. An exploitative rapist also might possibly see the error of his ways and atone if he has committed only one offense that was highly opportunistic in nature. In this case, factors such as age and the sophistication of the crime would weigh in the evaluation.

The far better candidate is the power-reassurance rapist, but again, we must look closely at the individual indicators: is this a first offense, or has he already raped several times? With each crime, the likelihood of turning him around decreases substantially. Were there extraordinary stressors in his life at the time? Was his behavior overtly violent? What was his behavior after the offense? Did he readily admit his crime or did he immediately establish an elaborate alibi? Did he show remorse? All these considerations are critical in determining whether rehabilitation is even possible, or if the possibility of future dangerousness is simply too great (13 [pp 114–115]).

VICTIMIZERS OF CHILDREN

If there is any crime more odious than sexual violence against women, it would be sexual violence against children. Our own view, based on examination of data and strong personal conviction, is that the number of brutalizations and murders of children will not diminish significantly until sentencing becomes more "realistic" in terms of recidivism and understanding of the continuing dangerousness of habitual offenders.

Children are "ideal" victims: curious by nature, trusting, easy for adults to manipulate and influence, hungry for affection and attention, eager to assert independence from their parents, and taught to obey adults (21). Again, offenders display varying personality types and a continuum of behaviors, all of which go into the evaluation of the individual case.

As with other such criminals, predators against children often represent a cycle of abuse. They themselves may have been victims of abuse as children, and their young victims may, in turn, either become future victimizers or be chronically victimized by others (22 [p 330]).

Some pedophiles, like other sexual predators, spend enormous amounts of time and energy planning and executing an abduction. Others are relatively harmless until placed in a situation of opportunity. For example, a shy, timid individual without social skills or deep, peer-oriented personal relationships may seem "creepy" if we notice him gazing at young children on the pony ride at the local fair, possibly even photographing them. But he would not steal a child from such a public environment and attempt to take him or her away with him.

Suppose that we alter that scenario. Now let us say that a young girl of interest to him rings his doorbell, selling Girl Scout cookies. If, upon answering the door, the man sees that a parent or some other competent adult is right there or watching from a car, nothing will happen. If, on the other hand, the child appears to be by herself, it is quite possible that on the spur of the moment, the man might pull her inside, close the door, and commit a horrible crime. Before that moment, it might not have occurred to him that he might someday act on his fantasies. But when the situation presents itself, he does so. The added risk is that, as in the feedback loop of the rapist, if the subject gets away with the crime, he may be encouraged to continue and escalate his behavior.

Predators of children use their advantages (23). They are bigger and stronger than their victims. They may impersonate police officers, teachers, or priests to legitimize themselves. They may manipulate a child's emotions by showering him or her with attention and then threaten to isolate the child from parents and others. Like the hunting lion surveying an entire herd of antelope at a watering hole, the sophisticated, experienced predator will identify and target the one vulnerable potential victim, the emotionally needy child. Therefore, the best single defensive strategy is for parents to instill a sense of self-esteem and confidence in their children. Strong, confident children are not the ones predators choose to victimize, given a choice.

In addition, it is critical for parents to teach children age-appropriate safety skills and to take careful note of any changes in their child's attitudes, behavior, or self-confidence. These changes include withdrawal or fearfulness; sleep disturbances, such as nightmares or bed-wetting; sexual "acting out" or unusual interest in sex; aggressiveness or rebelliousness; regression or infantile behavior; fear of specific people, places, or activities; and/or pain or injury in private regions (24).

Basic survival and safety skills involve teaching the child how to be something of a profiler. If a child becomes lost or separated from her parents or other guardian, she must know how to profile the types of adults most likely to be safe for her to approach for aid. These include an adult wearing a uniform or name tag, someone working behind a store counter, a bus driver, a pregnant woman or mother with her own children, or an elderly woman. Certainly, each of these personas has been used as a disguise by a child molester in an attempt to fool a potential victim. But the odds can be shifted considerably in the distressed child's favor because she is the one doing the selecting; she is choosing the authority figure to go to, rather than the other way around.

Children should be taught never to get into anyone's car unless a parent or guardian has specifically approved. They should be taught to be instantly wary if an adult stranger asks them for help or offers to take them somewhere or show them something (like a puppy). They should know it is good, not disobedient, to run away from anyone who tries to take them somewhere, and they should scream for attention (25).

Types of Child Molesters

As with predators of adults, child molesters fall into several categories and subcategories, and it is important to understand the distinctions. It is also important to note that not all pedophiles molest children; we suspect that most of them manage to keep their feelings in check. Pedophiles may have sexual relationships with adults and satisfy their urges in other ways, such as through fantasy, masturbation with dolls, or choosing lovers who are childlike, such as a small and/or flat-chested woman or one who engages in baby talk or similar behavior (21 [p 3]). But like other fetishes, pedophilia has the potential for becoming a danger if and when the fantasy element is no longer sufficient.

First, we must distinguish between the true pedophile—someone who prefers sex with children and has them as the subjects of his fantasies—and the situational pedophile, whose primary sexual drives and fantasies are directed at adults, but who will have sex with a child to fulfill some other need (22 [p 324], 26). For example, this second type may feel too inadequate to approach the true object of his desires, so he uses a child as a substitute.

We believe there are considerably more situational child molesters than preferential child molesters. A pedophile who molests will likely molest far more children over the course of his life, because that is where his primary sexual urges lie. This is what he thinks about all the time. It is possible for a situational offender to molest only one child, one time, or it could become a long-term behavior for him.

In *Child Molesters: A Behavioral Analysis for Law Enforcement Officers Investigating Cases of*

Child Sexual Exploitation (21 [pp 6–7]), Special Agent Kenneth Lanning of the FBI's Behavioral Science Unit outlines four types of *situational child molesters*: repressed, morally indiscriminate, sexually indiscriminate, and inadequate.

The *repressed molester* may abuse his own children because they are most readily available. Not surprisingly, he tends to have low self-esteem and has sex with children as substitutes for adults he does not feel he can approach. This subject is likely to use a lure or con rather than force to get a child to go with him, and the incidents are usually linked to some precipitating stressor in his life.

The *morally indiscriminate molester* would also molest his own children, although he will manipulate, lure, or even use force to obtain other victims. This subject tends to be abusive in virtually all areas of his life: he abuses his wife and friends, is a liar and a cheat at home and at work, and has no qualms about stealing something he wants. Because this type has no conscience, it is not difficult for him to act on impulse. If asked why he molested a child, he might respond, "Why not?"

The *sexually indiscriminate molester* would answer the question in the same manner but takes the thought a step further. He abuses children because he is bored and the experience seems new, exciting, and different to him. Lanning has described this type as a "try-sexual," implying that he will try anything (21 [p 7]). These offenders might pursue group sex with adults, spouse swapping, or bondage—acts that are not criminal among consenting adults—but then may involve a child (even his own) in that sexual experimentation. Compared with the other types of situational child molesters, these subjects are generally from a higher socioeconomic level and are more prone to molest multiple victims. Whereas the other types indulge in child pornography, this type might have a much more diverse collection of "erotica."

The *inadequate molester* is much like other inadequate subjects. He is a social outsider, has had few friends his own age as a teenager, and may continue to live with his parents or an older relative as he grows older. For this subject, children are nonthreatening, like his other potential targets—the elderly and prostitutes. His victim could be a child he knows well or a stranger whom he can use as a substitute for an unapproachable peer. The subject is not so much naturally sexually attracted to children, as he is sexually curious but insecure around adults. If he collects pornography, it likely involves adults, not children. Because he is so withdrawn from society, the danger is that hostility and anger could build up until he finds an outlet for them. This subject can be very dangerous; if his rage explodes, he is often compelled to torture and kill his victim.

Lanning classifies *preferential child molesters* into three categories: seduction, introverted, and sadistic (21 [pp 8–9]).

The *seduction molester* courts his victim with attention and gifts, attempting to slowly win trust and lower inhibitions. He is adept at communicating with children and at choosing the most vulnerable targets. This type is insidious and may be involved with children as a popular teacher, coach, or scout or youth group leader. Alert parents may be able to spot the potential for trouble.

The *introverted molester*, the closest to the stereotype of the creepy stranger in a raincoat, does not possess the interpersonal or social skills to lure or con potential victims. His sexual activity is limited to brief encounters, and he usually targets strangers or young children.

The *sadistic molester* is physically the most dangerous type because, like the sadistic rapist of adults, his satisfaction derives from having total control and seeing the victim's response to the suffering inflicted. He must cause physical and/or psychological pain to become sexually aroused. This molester uses trickery or force to obtain victims and then tortures them when they are under his control. He is the type of molester most likely to abduct and murder his victims.

Like other sexual predators, child molesters are often difficult to recognize. In most cases, they look like the rest of us. However, a number of indicators should arouse suspicion—particularly if, taken together, they form a long-term pattern of behavior. A teenager with unusual interest in children and little social contact with his peers would be a prime example. An adult who tends to move frequently and unexpectedly or has a less than honorable military discharge with no reason given would be another example. Additional pedophile behavioral traits include extreme relationships with women—being either domineering or weak, dependent, and child-like; having sexual problems with any woman in his life; collecting child pornography; hanging out in malls, playgrounds, and other places frequented by children; and indulging in idealization and objectification of children (21 [pp 16–17]).

Child Abductors

Child abductors tend to be social misfits who would have shown signs of trouble even as children. Usually unmarried—too incompetent socially to maintain a relationship with a woman, even as a cover—they have no regular contact with children. Their poor social skills make it difficult for them to manipulate, lure, or seduce a child, so they might carry weapons to intimidate or control a victim. They are also likely to harm the victim.

Female child abductors have motivations and behaviors distinct from those of their male counterparts. A woman who abducts a child on her own—as opposed to being the compliant victim of a male offender—almost always does so not because of sexual urges but because of her emotional need to have a child. Therefore, the remainder of our discussion of molesters and abductors applies to men.

Lanning describes four phases of child abduction: buildup, abduction, postabduction, and recovery/release (27). In the buildup and abduction phases, the fantasy creates the need, and the precipitating stressor or stressors fuel the action. The level of planning and the chances of success depend on the type of abductor. The *thought-driven* abductor plans ahead, weighs risks, and exercises discipline in selection of the victim, whereas the *fantasy-driven* abductor answers his specific emotional needs and follows his own ritual, although this might increase his risk of being caught.

In the postabduction and recovery/release phases, the treatment of the child depends on the motivation for the abduction and on the competence of the offender. As pressure grows, the abductor must somehow rid himself of the victim. The longer a child is missing, the smaller the chances of a positive outcome.

As with other types of violent criminals, we categorize abductors as organized, disorganized, and "mixed." Behavior and physical evidence help us in making this categorization. A fuller discussion appears later in this chapter, but it is important here to understand these distinctions:

The *organized* abductor likely possesses average or above-average intelligence and social skills, targets strangers as victims, and plans ahead. He may transport his victim—alive or dead—over a significant distance. Body dumpsites are difficult to find, and evidence may be destroyed. He may try to make a statement, going for shock value in disposing of the body. He is likely to be aggressive in sexual activity and may kill either for thrill or to avoid detection.

The *disorganized* offender is of lower intelligence, chooses victims he knows personally or has observed closely, and does not plan well. He may kill inadvertently or if he loses control of the situation. Sexual assault may occur after the child is unconscious or dead. Bodies are not moved far from the crime scene—the subject may not have the means to transport a body—and are not well covered or hidden and therefore tend to be found quickly (25 [pp 157–158], 27).

Incestuous molesters can cross the spectrum of types. An introverted pedophile may marry with the intent of producing children whom he can molest. A seduction molester may marry a woman with

children so as to become a "father figure" and have access to them (21 [p 12]). One tip-off is that he engages in sex with his spouse only as often as necessary to preserve the illusion of normalcy. Incestuous molesters, of course, are not only fathers. They can be grandfathers, uncles, or any other relative.

Child molestation can be a particularly difficult problem for health care providers, social workers, and law enforcement officers, because children are often hesitant or reluctant to report incest and molestation. The sad fact is that society may inadvertently punish the victim. Consider the best case: when a child reports the abuse and corrective action is taken. In addition to shame and embarrassment—including taunts from some people and disbelief from others—there is the potential for separation from everything important and familiar to the victim. As Peter Banks, Director of Outreach at the National Center for Missing and Exploited Children, observed (28): "Think of what happens when you report that you've been abused by a family member. Your whole entire life is disrupted. You're taken out of your home. You lose your friends, your school, your dog, everything." Banks noted, too, that sometimes in the face of all this disruption and pressure, victims even recant. Then, in addition to the problems in the current situation, the child essentially becomes a victim for the rest of his life, suffering long-term damage from the trauma of the abuse, as well as from the stigma of being branded a liar. And if a child reports abuse to someone who cannot or will not help, the abuser's threats are reinforced. There is also the issue of emotional blackmail: the child's original feeling of being flattered by attention turns to fear, confusion, and humiliation.

Children need to be reminded that their feelings are important—that they have the right to say "no" to things that feel bad or wrong. They must know that if someone touches them in a way they do not like—or makes them touch someone else in a way they do not like—it is not their fault; and if they tell an adult but do not receive help, they should tell another adult.

When a molester is accused, particularly for the first time, there are certain behaviors that we see frequently. He will deny, acting shocked, surprised, and indignant. He may blame the accusation on the child's misunderstanding, saying something like, "Is it a crime to hug a child?" Depending on his social support structure, he may bring in character witnesses to back him up. He will try to minimize events and may be aided in this strategy inadvertently by the victim's reluctance to admit the extent of the molestation because of embarrassment or discomfort. The molester often attempts to justify or reinterpret what happened or patently falsify the truth. He may pursue a strategy to lessen the impact or punishment, such as agreeing to plead to a lesser crime or claiming temporary insanity. Accused molesters in this phase tend to be high suicide risks (21 [pp 37–40]).

PARENTS AS MURDERERS AND ABUSERS

Unfortunately, some parents kill their children. Investigators find that the younger a child victim, if forensic evidence does not indicate otherwise, the more likely a relative rather than a stranger was involved. Regardless of cause, the behavioral indicators of parental involvement in a homicide are often clear to a trained investigator. Parents are not usually as detached about body disposal as strangers are, taking care with the body, wrapping it up, and showing it tenderness. Parents are also far more likely than strangers to feel remorse, leading investigators to recover the body for proper burial (27 [p 32]).

More common than murder by parents, of course, is the less extreme but more chronic type of harmful behavior. The nature of the offense tells us much about the perpetrator and the probability of future violence.

For certain types of situational abusers of children, we believe that rehabilitation through education and coping strategies is possible. This potential for success is almost strictly limited to abuse by parents, guardians, or other regular caretakers and applies more to physical and psychological abuse than to sexual abuse. Sometimes, mistreatment is caused by the adult's feelings of stress and responsibility. For example, a single working mother who beats her misbehaving child out of frustration and physical and mental exhaustion may be amenable to intervention that alleviates some of her burden without removing the child. In such instances, the chances for cessation of the cycle are more positive.

This may also be true for those who mistreat the elderly—our next topic of focus.

VICTIMIZERS OF THE ELDERLY

People are often surprised when we group children, prostitutes, and the elderly together as victims. But it is a fact that these three groups are uniquely linked because of their vulnerability. A given predator may view children (boys, girls, or either), or prostitutes, or elderly women as his preferential victim. But he may also use any of these three groups as a "warm-up," a practice before moving on to more challenging victims. A young (probably teenaged) beginning rapist, for example, may target an elderly woman because, at this point, such a victim is all he can handle. Once he learns what to do, he will go after his true victim of preference.

An elderly woman is particularly vulnerable, not only because of physical weakness or infirmities, but also because of her dependence on others for helping with home maintenance and repair, running errands, doing chores, and providing transportation. The individuals providing such services are often not well known to her. A stranger let into the house or apartment to deliver something or make a repair can gather valuable intelligence information for a future assault, burglary, or scam. Because it is often difficult for senior citizens to get to a bank regularly, they may keep large amounts of cash at home—an attractive target for a young, unsophisticated offender.

An early case in which one of the authors (JED) was called to consult involved the 1977 murder of an elderly woman, Anna Berliner, in her home in Oregon. Local police had also sought help from a clinical psychologist about the type of offender they were dealing with in this crime. Among the victim's injuries were four deep pencil wounds in the chest. The psychologist had interviewed approximately 50 men charged with or convicted of homicide. Most of these examinations had been done in prison. On the basis of his experience, he predicted that the offender would be someone who had spent a fair amount of time in prison, probably a drug dealer, because only in prison is a sharpened pencil widely considered a deadly weapon.

The author disagreed, believing that the age and vulnerability of the victim, the overkill, and the facts that it was a daytime crime and nothing of great value was missing suggested that an inexperienced juvenile offender was involved. The pencil was there—a weapon of opportunity requiring no great analysis or skills to employ. The killer turned out to be an inexperienced 16-year old who had gone to the victim's house scheming to get a contribution to a walkathon in which he was not actually participating.

The key feature of this crime scene was that all behavioral evidence suggested the involvement of an offender who was unsure of himself. An experienced felon attacking an elderly woman in her home would be very sure of himself. Merely picking up on a single piece of evidence does not give the entire picture. This is something we must keep in mind throughout our evaluations of offenders in crimes against the elderly (2 [pp 349–350]).

DOMESTIC VIOLENCE: STALKING

Domestic violence cuts across all socioeconomic, cultural, and racial groupings. The rates of recidivism are sickeningly high. This problem is discussed in more detail in Chapter 11. Therefore, for the present discussion, we will limit ourselves to an examination of the most critical aspect from the perspective of the perpetrator—that is, his emotional need to have total control over another human being. In this regard, it is informative to look closely at stalking behavior, a particular type of domestic violence that has far-reaching implications (13 [pp 265–289], 29 [pp 53–77]).

Simple obsession stalking is so intimately related to domestic violence that the two are virtually inseparable—different extensions of the same controlling, dominating behavior. Like love obsession stalkers who begin by obsessing from a distance and often focus on celebrities, the time during which the offender's emotional dependence blossoms into a full-blown obsession can range from years down to weeks—or even just a few dates. And dangerousness can escalate remarkably quickly.

In cases where there has been a long-term relationship between victim and stalker, the history of the offender's abusive behavior makes him all the more menacing. He knows his victim in a way that celebrity or love obsession stalkers cannot; he knows which emotional buttons to push. He knows his victim's vulnerabilities. Even more frightening and dangerous, his past relationship with his victim has given him the intelligence he needs. He already knows her patterns, her schedule, where she keeps her money, who her doctor is, and whom she would count on and where she would go in an emergency.

There are warning signs but, unfortunately, they are often not revealed until the victim is already somewhat involved with the potential offender, which is why intelligent, otherwise self-protective women can find themselves in this type of situation. These offenders can be quite charming at first, creating a favorable initial impression. However, as time goes by, they reveal their true nature. They do not believe that ordinary social rules apply to them and therefore have no problem lying, cheating, or breaking the law to get what they want.

It is a common misperception that stalkers, indeed domestic violence abusers in general, are typically undereducated, unemployed, or hold menial jobs and live close to the poverty level. In fact, this is yet another crime where anybody can be an offender or a victim—people of all races and socioeconomic backgrounds and of either gender. According to one assessment, approximately one-third of men undergoing counseling for physically abusing a wife or girlfriend held respectable, professional occupations and often enjoyed high status in their community as executives, doctors, or even ministers (13 [pp 265–267]).

Whether he is a successful businessman who stalks his estranged wife or a high-school teen who cannot let go of his first serious girlfriend, the offender's criminal behavior grows out of a need to control and dominate his victim to boost his own self-esteem. This offender suffers from extreme insecurity and is often unable to develop and maintain personal and love relationships. Some may have psychological problems but, for the majority, the problem is a personality disorder that manifests as inappropriate behavior and impaired social skills. Such persons often feel powerless in everyday situations, which, coupled with their inadequacies, makes them invest their emotions and sense of self-worth in the relationship with the other person.

In a sense, these offenders operate in the world of fantasy relationships. Although they have had a relationship with their victim, what they are obsessed with is the feeling of power they got from the relationship, not the victim herself.

Before any physical and/or emotional abuse begins, the offender may appear very attentive, which is soon revealed to be possessiveness and jealousy rather than caring. He tries to control aspects of his mate's or girlfriend's life—from picking out her clothing, to trying to limit the time she spends away from him. An abusive husband or boyfriend may humiliate his victim, criticizing her appearance and downplaying her skills as a homemaker, mother, student, successful professional—whatever roles she holds within and outside their relationship that give her a sense of self-worth. He has more strength if he can keep her off balance.

His most successful gambit involves switching moods: loving and tender at one moment and angry and violent the next moment. His partner never knows with whom she is dealing, and although she fears and loathes one side of his behavior, she cares for the other and thrives under his attention.

To increase his control, the abuser tries to put his victim in a situation in which she is economically dependent on him. If there is a child involved, this makes it even easier for him to keep her under control because she may not feel capable of supporting herself and her child on her own. She may also be afraid that if she leaves he will get custody of—or outright kidnap—her children, and she will never see them or be able to protect them from him again. There have even been cases in which terrified mothers have escaped to a community "safe house," only to have the court force them to reveal their location when the abuser sued for visitation rights. Therefore, the same system to which a victim of domestic violence may turn for protection can also be used by her abuser/stalker to exercise further control over her and maintain his presence in her life even after she has physically fled their home. Sadly, it is easy to see why some victims, lacking the financial resources to fight what seems to them an endless legal war, either give up and return to face more abuse or disappear underground in desperation, giving up jobs, family, and friends.

As an abusive relationship continues, the offender grows increasingly critical of his victim's friends and family, and becomes more and more jealous, controlling the time she spends away from him. She may get to the point where she feels it is not worth the fight to see them and, if he has beaten her and the marks are visible, she may be too embarrassed to see them. There are cases where abusers force their victims to keep records of every minute of their day. Such abusers may check the mileage on the car or even count the change in the victim's purse, thereby micromanaging every aspect of the victim's life and wearing her down completely. Abusers do not acknowledge the true reason for their dependence on this relationship—or that they are in a position of dependence at all—but will project any blame for their actions on the victim. They may see their need to control as either their duty as a "good" husband or their right. In the offender's mind, violence occurs not because he is unable to cope with his emotions and lacks self-control, but because the victim did something wrong that set him off.

When a woman escapes such a relationship, the abuser may rationalize subsequent stalking behavior as efforts to win her back—often trying first the charm, flowers, and candy routine he used to win her the first time—or as the punishment she deserves for leaving him and treating him so unfairly.

The abuser's personality defects and pathologic rationalizations combine to make conditions extremely dangerous for a woman when she leaves such a man. Overwhelmed with his own inadequacy and impotence, his emotions at that point include rage over her rejection of him and her attempt to assert control, fear that he has been abandoned, and the drive for revenge. Threatened with losing the only aspect of his life that makes him feel powerful and in control, the abuser grows desperate. The stock phrase is, "If I can't have her, nobody will." As the stalker grows more frustrated by what he perceives as his victim's unwillingness to give him what he needs, he becomes increasingly harassing and threatening, in keeping with the abusive behavior he is accustomed to inflicting. If the victim tries to remove him permanently from her life at this stage, he may become violent in a last-ditch effort to reassert control over the relationship (30).

By the time a woman leaves an abuser, the two have often been through the cycle of courtship, intimidation, and violence more than once (29 [pp 63–65]). It is almost as if they are programmed in their roles. This is partly why it is so threatening to the abuser when the victim breaks the pattern. He does not like her to call any play changes—that is up to him—and he does not like the play she has called.

The offender's identity might be so tied up with his victim that he has no other means to possess her than to kill her. Once he has done that, there is nowhere else for him to go emotionally, which explains the frequency of murder–suicides.

Stalking is a terribly difficult crime for a victim to deal with because it can be long term and unpredictable. Unlike any other domestic crime, stalking can involve the perpetrator and victim for years rather than minutes, hours, or days. Imagine waking up every day for 20 years—or even 20 days—and having as your first thought, "Is this the day he gets me?" or "Is this the day he kills my kids?" Everywhere you go, you look around and expect to see him. Even if he is not standing outside the window, watching you make the kids' lunch, you know he is always somewhere out there. Every time the phone rings, you know who it could be. The mail could bring just bills and advertisements, or a photograph of you taken when you thought he was not around. Perhaps you secured a restraining order and police threatened to arrest him, so he has been quiet lately. That is no guarantee that he is not still watching and waiting. Statistically, overwhelmingly, he will be back.

Victims suffer all sorts of problems because of their experiences, ranging from depression, anxiety attacks, and physical ailments brought on by prolonged feelings of anger, stress, fear, and helplessness, to recurring nightmares and even posttraumatic stress disorder (29 [pp 115–131]). Just as some rape victims suffer from rape trauma syndrome, stalking survivors subjected to repeated and unpredictable acts of personal terrorism may go through life in a permanently stressed state, traumatized by their experiences.

The first step for any stalking victim who wants to stop the abuse should be to get in touch with someone local. Stalking laws vary from state to state, and what constitutes grounds for an arrest in one jurisdiction may be outside the arm of the law in another. In some cases—especially if the stalking behaviors cross jurisdictions or if threatening phone calls are made from one state to another—federal charges may apply under stalking and/or antiterrorism laws. Working alone, victims may be unaware of the procedures involved in filing a stalking or related complaint (31).

In many cases, early intervention is the key. David Beatty of the National Center for Victims of Crime (32) notes: "The potential positive outcomes at the early stages of a stalking case are far better than at the last stages. If someone is overtly threatening you with violence, the options are pretty narrow." By then, Beatty adds, probably the best that can be done is to press charges and get the offender locked up. But the chances are great that he will be back out again and even angrier for having spent some time in prison or suffering some other punishment.

In any domestic violence situation, the potential for continued or renewed violence does not abate until a means is found to keep the abuser permanently away from his victim. Even then, it is likely he will continue his abusive behavior in subsequent relationships.

CUES FOR EMERGENCY MEDICAL PERSONNEL

With regard to domestic offenders—be they abusers of children, spouses or partners, or the elderly—there is an important consideration for emergency medical personnel. Unlike other offenders, this type may show up with the victim when she or he is brought into the emergency department. Therefore, the staff should be sensitive to behavioral cues and other evidence from both parties.

One of the most suggestive indicators of a possible abuser is his or her unwillingness to leave nurses, physicians, or social workers alone with the patient. The abuser might also insist on telling what happened to the patient, such as a fall down the stairs. Clearly, the story should correlate with the physical findings of examination, particularly if there is a history of such "accidents." If there is any suspicion on the part of medical personnel, or if a story simply sounds "fishy," the patient should be evaluated carefully not only for injuries for which she was brought in, but also for evidence of older wounds, healed lacerations, or other evidence of a previous pattern of behavior. Particular attention should be directed to evidence of grabbing and attempts at physical control, such as abrasions on the neck or wrists.

Likewise, the behavior of the patient can be telling. Any child or adult who seems fearful, subdued, or unusually passive or accepting of her or his condition must be placed in a situation in which she or he feels comfortable in confiding with medical and/or legal personnel and assured of safety going forward.

Domestic abuse tends to escalate. So any possible opportunity for intervention should not be lost.

HOMICIDE

Behavior reflects personality. This is one of the guiding principles of criminal investigative analysis. It is equally true that behavior often reveals the true nature of the crime. To illustrate this point, let us consider the case of Linda Haney Dover in Cartersville, Georgia, who was murdered the day after Christmas in 1980 (2 [pp 284–287]).

The 27-year-old woman was separated from her husband, Larry, but remained on reasonably cordial terms with him. On the day of her murder, she was cleaning the house she used to share with her husband—a favor she did regularly—while Larry took their young son out for a day in the park. But when father and son returned from their outing, Linda was not there, and the bedroom appeared to have been ransacked. There were red stains on the carpet. When police arrived after Larry's frantic call, they found Linda's body wrapped in the comforter from the bedroom, with only her head exposed, in the crawl space under the house. As they unwrapped the body, they noted that her shirt and bra had been pushed up above her breasts, her jeans were around her knees, and her panties were pulled down to just below her pubic area. There was blunt-force trauma to the head and face and multiple stab wounds. The crime scene indicated that she had been assaulted initially in a bedroom and then her body had been moved outside. The presence of blood drops on her thighs indicated the killer had handled and positioned her.

The author (JED) was called in on the case in his capacity as profiler for the FBI. On the basis of crime scene photographs and information forwarded by the Cartersville Police Department, he stated that the unknown subject (UNSUB in law enforcement parlance) would be one of two types. Possibly, he would be a young and inexperienced, inadequate loner who lived nearby and essentially stumbled into this crime of opportunity while attempting a burglary. Police then mentioned problems with a neighborhood thug, of whom many of the residents were afraid.

But the crime had too many "staging" elements, which more strongly indicated the second type: someone who knew the victim well and therefore wanted to divert attention from himself. The only reason a killer would have felt the need to hide the body was what we classify as a "personal cause homicide." The trauma to the face and neck also seemed highly personal.

The author told police that he thought this UNSUB was intelligent, although only educated through high school, and had a job requiring physical strength. He would have a history of assaultive behavior and a low frustration level. He would be moody, unable to accept defeat, and was probably depressed at the time of the murder, most likely because of money problems.

The staging had its own internal logic and rationale. Whoever brutalized Ms. Dover did not want to leave her body in the open where another family member—particularly her son—might find it. That was why the UNSUB took the time to wrap her in a blanket and move her to the crawl space. He wanted to make it look like a sex crime—hence the raising of the bra and exposure of the genital area—although there was no forensic evidence of rape or sexual assault. He thought he had to do this but still felt uncomfortable with police seeing her bare genitals and breasts, so he covered them with the blanket. The behavior, therefore, suggested a domestic homicide disguised as a sex crime, pointing to the estranged husband, who fit the FBI profile in every significant aspect.

Unbeknown to the author, police had already arrested Dover for the murder and were using the profile to assure themselves that they were on the right track. In any event, justice was served. On September 3, 1981, Mr. Dover was convicted of the murder of Linda Haney Dover and sentenced to life imprisonment.

Let us compare this with a different type of homicide. Beginning in the summer of 1979, a number of victims—mostly women—disappeared while hiking and were subsequently found murdered in the area of Mount Tamalpais Park, north of San Francisco. The UNSUB was dubbed the Trailside Killer by the local media (2 [pp 152–159], 33,34).

In these cases, victims were stabbed and/or strangled and shot to death on remote park trails, which would, in the case of female victims, suggest an intention of sexual assault on the part of the offender. There were conflicting witness sightings of possible suspects, which is not unusual. The fact that each murder site was remote and heavily wooded, accessible only on foot, and involved a considerable hike suggested that the killer was local and intimately familiar with the area.

To the author, the multiple stabbings and blitz-style attacks from the rear indicated an asocial type who was withdrawn, unsure of himself, and incapable of engaging his victims in conversation with the intent of seducing or conning them. The victims were physically fit hikers, and the blitz attack was an indication that the only way he could control an intended victim was to devastate her before she could respond. In contrast to the previous case, these were not the crimes of someone who knew his victims. The sites were secluded and protected from view, which meant the killer essentially had as much time as he wanted to act out his fantasy with each victim. Yet he still felt the need for a blitz attack. There was handling of the bodies postmortem and probably masturbation in addition to any sexual assault. The victims represented a range of ages and physical types, indicating a nonpreferential killer. The profile concluded with the prediction that the killer would have a speech impediment. This was met with considerable skepticism by the investigating task force.

Yet when the suspect, David Carpenter, was apprehended after a complex investigation that included the tracing of eyeglass frames the killer had inadvertently left at one of the murder scenes, the 50-year-old industrial arts teacher did indeed have a stutter, which became pronounced under stress. The reason for including such an odd trait in the profile was that this subject clearly did not feel comfortable taking his time or striking up a conversation with his intended victim. Despite the unlikelihood of interference in so secluded a setting, he did not have confidence in his ability to control the victim through words and manner. This suggested that the killer was someone with a serious self-image/self-confidence problem. The most logical reason for this would be some sort of disfigurement or speech problem. Had there been disfigurement, it is likely that one or more witnesses would have made mention of a subject fitting this description. As none had, a speech impediment became the more likely factor.

Upon his arrest, Carpenter was found to be the product of a domineering and physically abusive mother and an at least emotionally abusive father. He was a child of well-above-average intelligence, who was picked on because of his severe stuttering. His childhood was also marked by chronic bed-wetting and cruelty to animals. In adult life, his anger and frustration turned into fits of unpredictable, violent rage. He had been convicted of a previous attack on a woman using a knife and hammer, which occurred following the birth of his child in an already strained marriage. The victim reported that during the brutal assault itself the terrible stutter had disappeared.

What we hope to emphasize with these two cases is that although violent perpetrators can be classified according to the type and manner of crime as well as the motive, it is critical to evaluate each incident and each offender on an individual basis, just as it is critical to thus evaluate and support each victim.

The *Crime Classification Manual* organizes homicide into four main groupings based on the motive (11 [pp 17–161]):

Criminal enterprise homicide is murder committed for material gain. This may include money, goods, territory, favors, or anything else perceived to have value to the individual. This category is further subdivided into contract (third-party) killing, gang-motivated murder, criminal competition homicide, kidnap murder, product tampering homicide, drug murder, insurance inheritance–related death (individual profit murder and commercial profit murder), and felony murder (indiscriminate felony murder and situational felony murder).

Personal cause homicide ensues from interpersonal aggression and results in death to a person or persons who may not be known to each other. This homicide is not motivated by material gain or sex and is not sanctioned by a group. It is the result of an underlying emotional conflict that propels the offender to kill. This category is divided into erotomania-motivated killing (i.e., growing out of a fantasy based on perceived idealized romantic involvement or spiritual union with the victim), domestic homicide (spontaneous domestic homicide and staged domestic homicide), argument/conflict murder, authority killing, revenge killing, non-specific motive killing, extremist homicide (political extremist homicide, religious homicide, and socio-economic extremist homicide), mercy/hero homicide, and hostage murder.

Sexual homicide involves a sexual element as the basis for the sequence of acts leading to murder and is distinguished from the aforementioned erotomania-motivated fantasy of an idealized relationship. Performance and meaning of this sexual element vary with the offender. The act may range from rape (either before or after death) to a symbolic sexual assault. This category is divided into organized sexual homicide, disorganized sexual homicide, mixed sexual homicide, and sadistic murder.

Group cause homicide pertains to two or more people with a common ideology that sanctions an act, committed by one or more of its members, that results in death. This category is divided into cult murder, extremist murder (paramilitary extremist murder and hostage extremist murder), and group excitement homicide such as a gang attack, fed by its own momentum and peer reinforcement, that escalates into murder.

According to this classification, we can see clearly that the Dover murder would be considered a personal cause, staged domestic homicide (11 [pp 80–85]). The Trailside murders would be mixed sexual homicides because (a) the sexual element is the motivating factor and (b) although planning and stalking of the victim are traits of an organized offender, the style of attack was a blitz and no attempt was made to conceal the bodies—traits of a disorganized offender.

For the purposes of this chapter, it is not necessary to delve into each of the homicide classifications and subgroupings; most are self-explanatory, and the overview itself is sufficient to give an understanding and insight for the emergency physician and health care worker. However, that understanding and insight can be enhanced through a brief look at the concept of organization versus disorganization of the perpetrator, which transcends individual crime classifications. This distinction was instituted as a result of research conducted under the auspices of the FBI in an attempt to get away from essentially psychiatrically based nomenclature and to come up with descriptive terminology that would be helpful to law enforcement personnel directly involved in solving cases.

As the author (JED) and his collaborators pointed out in the *Crime Classification Manual*, profiling is a form of retroclassification (classification that works backward). Typically, we classify a *known* entity into a discrete category, on the basis of the presenting characteristics that translate into criteria for assignment to that category. In the case of homicide investigation, we have neither the entity (e.g., the offender) nor the victim. It is therefore necessary to rely on the only source of information that typically is available: the crime scene. In essence, we are forced to "bootstrap," using crime scene–related data to make our classifications (11 [pp 21–22]).

Developmentally speaking, the *organized type* externalizes hurt, anger, and fear through aggressive, often senseless acts. He has a superior attitude and may be described by others as a troublemaker. He would generally have had multiple sex partners; is angry with himself, his family, and society in general; and begins acting out that anger in a manifest way in his teens or early twenties, through means such as cruelty to animals and serious arson (e.g., to occupied buildings or causing large monetary damage). He selects victims whom he can manipulate, dominate, and control.

This individual will be irresponsible and self-centered, methodical and cunning, and indifferent to the welfare of society, with a chameleon-like personality; that is, he fits well into a given society. He is likely to be above average in intelligence, is of middle class, with a neat appearance and good communication skills, but he has a history of sporadic employment. He possesses criminal sophistication, and his criminal history may include financial or property crimes. When his crimes escalate to murder, his choice of victims will be seemingly random; he will "cruise" for them, often many miles from where he lives or works.

The *disorganized type* internalizes hurt and anger and therefore becomes secluded and withdrawn. He rejects society, which he feels has rejected him, and therefore feels lonely. He is frequently described as shy, quiet, and cooperative, and he finds interpersonal relationships difficult. He is an underachiever with a poor self-image, emotional inadequacies, and/or physical ailments and disabilities. His appearance may be disheveled. He is unemployed or involved in some menial type of job. As a surrogate for normal sex, he substitutes such activities as voyeurism, fantasy drawings and writings, pornography, and theft of fetish items, such as underwear. His behavior may be masochistic and his crimes tend to be committed against those weaker or more helpless than himself, such as the young, the elderly, and animals. He might also indulge in arson, but his crimes will be more of a nuisance variety than those with serious human or monetary consequences.

When his crimes escalate to murder, he commits the crimes close to his home or some other zone of security. He lacks cunning and sophistication and is likely to kill in a frenzy. Unlike the organized type, who closely follows the media coverage of his crime and may actually change jobs or leave town, the disorganized type shows a minimal change in lifestyle after the crime (1 [pp 121–133]).

The crime scene itself gives us many clues to the perpetrator's level of organization. The organized offender may alter or stage the scene and will likely remove personal items belonging to the victim. He will use this souvenir to help him relive the crime in his own mind, or he may give it to a significant person in his life. This is common with jewelry. Because he has planned the crime, he will bring his weapon and other implements to the scene and not leave them behind. If it is an outdoor homicide, there will be a concerted effort to hide the corpse or an equally concerted effort to display the body in some sort of symbolic manner, depending on his motive. If the murder is the first or second one of this offender, the scene may be close to home. But as he refines his methods, he will move farther and farther from his zone of comfort so as to minimize the possibility of detection. By the same token, he might kill in one location, and then methodically move the corpse to another. He may cut up the body, amputate limbs, or remove clothing in an attempt to delay identification of the victim.

The disorganized offender's crime is more spontaneous. There is likely to be a blitz-style attack and little or no communication with the victim, whom he may have difficulty controlling. The weapon is one of opportunity, and there is little attempt to destroy evidence or conceal the corpse, with which he may engage in postmortem activity. Because he is unlikely to own a vehicle and relies on rides or public transportation, he will not move the body from the kill site to a dumpsite. If he takes a souvenir, it will be as a remembrance to help fuel a fantasy rather than to relive the crime, and he may later return it to the victim's grave or home.

The corpse may reflect a frenzy of uncontrolled stabbing or slashing, with postmortem bite marks on breasts, buttocks, neck, thighs, or abdomen. The offender might attempt to dissect the body after death or even once the victim has been rendered unconscious, as a matter of curiosity and exploration, not to obliterate evidence. This curiosity can extend to cannibalism and vampirism, where the perpetrator smears the victim's blood on himself or another surface, or inserts foreign objects into the anal or vaginal cavity. This last activity takes the place of penile penetration. The body may be left in a ritualistic or symbolic way, but the meaning will probably be obscure to all but the killer.

Following the crime, an organized offender changes his clothing and cleans himself and his car. He immediately establishes an alibi. We should note any difference in his demeanor and behavior,

including tension, insomnia, depression, episodes of explosive rage or anger, increased use of alcohol or drugs, renewed interest in religion, and a preoccupation with media. He may attend the funeral or burial of the victim and, if approached, will appear cooperative with investigators. Colleagues at work will notice a change in work habits, use of sick leave, irritability, perhaps resulting in quitting or being fired. He may return to the murder or disposal site and, if he feels police pressure, might seek a legitimate reason to leave the area.

The disorganized offender may also return to the scene or grave site, but it will be to engage in further mutilation or to "communicate" with the victim. He will become even more withdrawn, move or lose his job, and feel remorse over the victim being gone but not over his own act of killing. He may become fanatically religious and is far less likely to kill again than the organized offender.

We can see that there are some common elements between the two types of offenders, although often for different purposes. For example, both types may "experiment" with the victim, but the organized individual is more likely to do so before death whereas the disorganized will do so after death. Both may show rage in the evidence of overkill, but the organized killer's rage will be controlled, whereas the disorganized offender will be uncontrolled, random, and sloppy. Both may display a victim's body for symbolic purposes, but the organized offender may do so to degrade his victim, whereas the disorganized person does so for some arcane symbolism discernible only to himself.

It is possible for an organized killer to become disorganized at the scene. Factors for this transformation might include the youthfulness and inexperience of the offender, use of alcohol or drugs, the presence of more than one offender, an unexpected turn of events (such as another person showing up at the scene), or mental decompensation. However, it is extremely rare for the reverse transformation to occur and the scene to shift from the disorganized to the organized.

As mentioned with respect to the Trailside murders, human beings seldom fit neatly into rigid, predetermined niches. Therefore, we use the term "mixed" to describe a scene that has elements of both the organized and the disorganized perpetrator (11 [pp 133–136]). By weighing and evaluating the relative percentage of each type of behavior, we can go a long way toward describing the likely profile and behavior of the UNSUB.

MODUS OPERANDI AND SIGNATURE

One other behavioral indicator that is significant in evaluating the perpetrator of violent crime is the distinction between MO and signature. MO is learned behavior, which the perpetrator follows to commit the crime. It is dynamic, that is, it can change as the perpetrator progresses in his criminal career and realizes that one action or technique works better for him than another. Signature, on the other hand, although it may evolve, does not change radically. It is what the perpetrator has to do to fulfill himself. For example, a single bullet or other "clean kill" would be considered MO. A savage "overkill" would be a signature element.

This evaluation, however, must be made within the total context of the crime. An example would be two bank robbery cases in which the offenders forced their captives to undress. In one case, that was as far as it went. In the other, he posed them in sexual positions and photographed them. The first case would be deemed MO—the offender had his victims undress so they would be preoccupied and embarrassed rather than looking at him, rendering a positive identification difficult. In the second case, the posing and photographing is not helpful to the successful commission of the crime. In fact, it kept the offender on scene longer and therefore placed him in greater jeopardy of being caught. Yet having people under his control was something that clearly gave him satisfaction. The distinction between MO and signature can contribute to an understanding of the actions and motivation of a particular perpetrator.

SUMMARY

The forensic considerations of emergency physicians and practitioners dealing with the effects of violent crime will necessarily cut across a broad horizon of issues and procedures—from the physical and emotional treatment of victims, to gathering and handling evidence, to interacting with law enforcement authorities during the investigative process, to testifying in court. Although each of these activities requires its own special knowledge, talents, skills, and approach, the foundation and root cause of everything in forensic science harkens back to the perpetrator of the crime, because without his transgression there would be no need for the rest. For this reason, a basic understanding of the types and motivations of perpetrators is at the heart of all that we must do.

ACKNOWLEDGMENT

The authors gratefully acknowledge the contribution of Ann E. Hennigan to the preparation of this work.

REFERENCES

1. Ressler RK, Burgess AW, Douglas JE. *Sexual homicide: patterns and motives*. New York: Lexington Books, 1988.
2. Douglas J, Olshaker M. *Mindhunter: inside the FBI's elite serial crime unit*. New York: Scribner, 1995.
3. Newton M. *Hunting humans: an encyclopedia of modern serial killers*. Port Townsend, Washington, DC: Loompanics Unlimited, 1990.
4. Hegeman R. *Prosecutors to reveal evidence in BTK case*. Associated Press, April 15, 2005.
5. Douglas J, Olshaker M. *Unabomber: on the trail of America's most-wanted serial killer*. New York: Pocket Books, 1996:105–108.
6. Douglas J, Olshaker M. *The anatomy of motive*. New York: Scribner, 1999.
7. Bouton K. The prosecutor: Linda Fairstein vs. rape. *N Y Times Mag* 1990;25:21–23, 58–60.
8. Fairstein L. *Sexual violence*. New York: William Morrow, 1993:13–18.
9. Personal interview with Linda Fairstein, July 8, 1997.
10. Zeccardi JA. Medical exam of the live sexual assault victim. In: Hazelwood R, Burgess A, eds. *Practical aspects of rape investigation: a multidisciplinary approach*, 2nd ed. Boca Raton, Florida, FL: CRC Press, 1995:253–262.
11. Douglas JE, Burgess AW, Burgess AG, et al. *Crime classification manual*. New York: Lexington Books, 1992.
12. Burgess AG, Burgess AW, Hazelwood RR. Classifying rape and sexual assault. In: Hazelwood R, Burgess A, eds. *Practical aspects of rape investigation: a multidisciplinary approach*, 2nd ed. Boca Raton, Florida, FL: CRC Press, 1995.
13. Douglas J, Olshaker M. *Obsession*. New York: Scribner, 1998.
14. Hazelwood RR. Analyzing the rape and profiling the offender. In: Hazelwood R, Burgess A, eds. *Practical aspects of rape investigation: a multidisciplinary approach*, 2nd ed. Boca Raton, Florida, FL: CRC Press, 1995:155–160.
15. Hazelwood RR, Dietz PE, Warren JI. The criminal sexual sadist. In: Hazelwood R, Burgess A, eds. *Practical aspects of rape investigation: a multidisciplinary approach*, 2nd ed. Boca Raton: CRC Press, 1995:361–371.
16. Ressler RK, Burgess AW, Douglas JE. Rape and rape-murder: one offender and twelve victims. *Am J Psychiatry* 1983;140(1):36–40.
17. Yochelson S, Samenow SE. *The criminal personality*, Vol. I and II. New York: Jason Aronson, 1979.
18. Samenow SE. *Inside the criminal mind*. New York: Times Books, 1984:203–204.
19. Personal interview with Dr. Stanton E. Samenow, July 11, 1997.
20. Samenow SE. *Straight talk about criminals*. Northvale, NJ: Jason Aronson, 1998:155–168.
21. Lanning KV. *Child molesters: a behavioral analysis for law enforcement officers investigating cases of child sexual exploitation*, 3rd ed. Alexandria, Virginia: National Center for Missing and Exploited Children, December 1992.
22. Lanning KV. Child molestation: a law enforcement typology. In: Hazelwood R, Burgess A, eds. *Practical aspects of rape investigation: a multidisciplinary approach*, 2nd ed. Boca Raton: CRC Press, 1995.
23. Finkelhor D, Dziuba-Leatherman J. Victimization of children. *Am Psychol* 1994;49(3):173–183.
24. Meegan S. *Kids and company: together for safety, teacher's guide—a comprehensive manual for grades K–5/6*, 4th rev. ed. Alexandria, Virginia: National Center for Missing and Exploited Children, 1988:18–19.
25. Douglas J, Olshaker M. *Journey into darkness*. New York: Scribner, 1997:178–186.

26. Dietz PE. Sex offenses: behavioral aspects. In: Kadish SH, ed. *Encyclopedia of crime and justice*. New York: Free Press, 1983.

27. Lanning KV. Investigative analysis and summary of teaching points. In: Lanning KV, Burgess AW, eds. *Child molesters who abduct: summary of the case in point series*. Alexandria, Virginia: National Center for Missing and Exploited Children, 1995.

28. Personal interview with Peter D. Banks, July 8, 1996.

29. Schaum M, Parrish K. *Stalked: breaking the silence on the crime of stalking in America*. New York: Pocket Books, 1995:30.

30. *Stalking Questions and Answers*. Washington, DC: The National Center for Victims of Crime, 1995. Available at http://www.ncvc.org/src/main.aspx?dbID=DB_Questions_and_Answers109. Accessed on January 5, 2006.

31. *Stalking Safety Plan Guidelines*. Washington, DC, The National Center for Victims of Crime, 1997. Available at http://www.ncvc.org/ncvc/main.aspx?dbName=DocumentViewer&DocumentID=32460. Accessed on January 5, 2006.

32. Personal interview with David Beatty, July 22, 1997.

33. Graysmith R. *The sleeping lady—the trailside murders above the golden gate*. New York: Penguin Books, 1991.

34. Newton M. *Hunting humans: an encyclopedia of modern serial killers*. Port Townsend, Washington, DC: Loompanics Unlimited, 1990:52–54.

THE VICTIMS OF VIOLENCE

2

CARROLL ANN ELLIS ■

There is not a day that goes by that I do not see the evil face of violence that destroyed the me that was.
— *A Victim Survivor*

Victims of violence know full well the pain and disruption caused in their lives by the criminal and vile acts committed against them. They are forced to deal with violence in an immediate and direct manner, which sets the stage for law enforcement, prosecutors, judges, victim advocates, criminal justice agents, medical professionals, mental health specialists, and criminologists to deal with all the devastating dimensions of violence. When these professionals and their systems work, they represent a powerful response to the often incomprehensible problems posed by violence. The true experts on violence are its victims, who *help the helpers* gain the knowledge and understanding needed to create effective programs to support victims and ensure the effectiveness of systems for holding criminals accountable for their acts. It is from the victims that we are able to discern the medical, physical, psychological, and financial impact of criminal behavior. Victims often need medical care, emotional support, and financial help for injuries serious enough to be life threatening, mutilating, or disabling. In the aftermath of violence, medical professionals, as key responders to the pervasive problem of violence, are called upon to invoke their power, strength, and compassion; utilize developments in science and technology; and have direct contact with victims.

Victims are individuals who experience the physical, mental, emotional, and financial anguish

of crime; individuals who witness the crime episode; and the community left reeling with fear and disgust in the wake of criminal behavior. Violent crime must be considered in relationship to its impact on not only the tens of thousands of victims who suffer from the willful acts of violence but also the agents of the medical profession and the criminal justice system, and all other responsible agents and systems, including the community at large.

This chapter discusses sexual assault, domestic violence (violence inflicted by one intimate partner on another, including adolescents), family violence (any violence within a family unit), stalking, human trafficking, elder abuse, and child victimization in the context of the vital role of helping professionals and health care workers. Practical strategies for the care of victims will be offered as a general guideline on their rights, needs, and desires as human beings. Crime victims need to be informed about their rights as victims, as guaranteed by law, in terms, words, and ways they are able to understand. They also need to be informed about the services available to address their needs. They must be provided with access to these services to utilize them. They need help in understanding the criminal justice system and the physical, emotional, and mental reactions they may experience as a result of the crimes committed against them. And certainly, they have a need for safety, which can come only when well-constructed and well-orchestrated processes are in place. The needs of victims are fundamental: the ability to obtain help and support, some assurance of protection from any further harm at the hands of the offender and other forms of revictimization, knowledge and information about the criminal justice process and their ability to participate in it, and the expectation that the offender will be held accountable for the crime. Crime victims in every category need to know that the individual or individuals responsible for their victimization are being held accountable for their crimes by a competent criminal justice system. They also need to know that medical professionals are knowledgeable about the victim's experience and will respond accordingly. Finally, victims need to know that they and their experiences are valued in helping to ensure that others are not subjected to the same kind of criminal events or to the failures of the systems intended to help and protect.

Violent acts can occur suddenly and unexpectedly and are traumatizing to the victim. Chronic, insidious acts inflicted over a long period, which leave the victims with feelings of intense fear, helplessness, and loss of control, trust, and hope, are just as damaging. Aphrodite Matsakis, PhD, said, "Just as the body can be traumatized, so can the psyche. On the psychological and mental levels, trauma refers to the wounding of your emotions, your spirit, your will to live, your beliefs about yourself and the world, your dignity, and your sense of security" (1). Understanding the trauma associated with criminal victimization is the first step in addressing the special needs of victims. The neurobiology of trauma—the connection between the body and the mind and trauma—explains the behavior and reactions of victims who struggle to cope with their encounter(s) with violent acts committed against them. This chapter is about victims—individuals who become the targets of violent behavior—who experience trauma. This chapter offers information to health care providers who are the gateway to treatment and are skilled in giving comfort, support, and relief to victims of crime. Medical professionals must be equipped with information about victim issues and be knowledgeable about the effective programs, strategies, and resources available to address the special needs of victims. Further, medical professionals must continue in their efforts to act in collaboration with allied professionals, criminal justice agents, and advocates on behalf of the victims of violence.

THE VICTIM'S EXPERIENCE

Like one who seeks to warn the city of a pending flood, but speaks another language . . . so do we come forward and report that evil has been done to us.
—*Bertolt Brecht, German poet and playwright,*
1898–1956

I provide supportive services to victims of crime, from the vantage of a Victim Services Unit within the Criminal Investigations Bureau of a large police department. The painful, chilling, and humiliating abuse of the human body and spirit is a major element of my daily journey. I have witnessed firsthand the pollution that violent crime leaves in its wake. I often feel as though I am trapped in the belly of the whale—some large, powerful animal that thrashes about—so large, in fact, that it encompasses every aspect of the criminal justice system from the moment the crime occurs throughout its aftermath—while trying to help small fish swim out into safe waters. Through police-based victim service programs, victim advocates provide immediate and direct services and possible solutions to a victim's conflict. Working from within the system, one sees what victims of crime—most of them solid citizens, ordinary people living each day, just like you and me—encounter when faced with traumatic situations. For unsuspecting victims, crime is an ugly reality of circumstance that landed them in their own personal chamber of horror.

Imagine what a victim of sexual violence experiences when being forced by a rapist to submit to a physical act so degrading and abusive that it causes a disconnection from all previous coping techniques for survival. The criminal act is animalistic, nauseating, frightening, controlling, injurious, and painful. Victims of sexual violence experience the criminal act on several levels: the rapist not only invades and destroys the victim's innermost privacy, body parts, and concept of self but is also a robber who damages and steals property. And the criminal act is only the beginning. If the truth is to be known to the system, then rape victims must report the crime. For many victims, the decision to report the crime is overshadowed by their fear of revictimization at the hands of the system. Rape victims, for instance, must submit to an investigation that is not always sensitive and often begins with being told not to wash, shower, rinse, urinate, or remove their clothing until their body (which is evidence) and their clothing (which is evidence) can be "processed." Injury, disease, and pregnancy are immediate concerns and all too often become reality for some victims. The rape victim, regardless of age or gender, is again forced to submit, this time to an examination, which generally includes consenting to the photographing of intimate body areas. The victim is made aware that the photographs may be used as evidence in a court of law. A rape victim must submit to being touched by a medical examiner in places the rapist defiled and degraded. This early medical procedure is the victim's introduction to the legalities of the criminal justice system. Victims become aware that they are "cases" requiring study, examination, and analysis. All these procedures must occur before the victim can finally retreat to the privacy of a shower stall or bathtub to wash away the ravage of the event and the strain and stress of the examination. This process is taxing and dehumanizing; yet it is also a necessary component of the total response to the victims of sexual violence, and it should be conducted with sensitivity and expertise. Medical professionals are trained and skilled in helping victims withstand the process. Still, there is no preparation, planning, or training for the victim, who is at the center of the process and of all subsequent system responses.

It is not enough to deal with the trauma of physical injury from violence. Victims must also cope with the aftermath of the experience, and effective systems must work together to intervene with support, solution, and justice. Victims of crime experience extended trauma, which must be recognized as an area for scientific study, leading to a systematic approach that will enhance our current methods of addressing the needs of victims. Medical systems provide sensitive and expert assistance to sexual assault victims. Victims report they are being helped through medical examinations with compassion and discernible explanations of the procedure and the necessary aftercare.

Victims of domestic violence withstand bodily injury in the form of bruises, lacerations, broken noses, loss of eyesight, burns, broken limbs, punctured eardrums, and other disfigurements. The victims of this type of crime are seen most often in emergency departments, by family doctors, and in health clinics. Yet, too many physicians treat only the illnesses and injuries associated with the violence; in some cases, physicians fail to identify the violence. Even when violence has been recognized, too many physicians do not have adequate training or education that enables them to respond appropriately to the insidious problem of violent relationships. The victim is sometimes unable to share information with the physician because the batterer may be present. The victim may be unaware of the principle of patient confidentiality and is probably operating under the batterer's constant threat to life.

Domestic violence victims are often caught up in a complex relationship, in which abuse occurs on several levels: violent behavior, emotional cruelty, psychological threats to the victim and other family members, and financial/economic abuse. Although there are numerous theoretic explanations for the causes of domestic violence, no one theory is generally agreed on because of the dynamics involved in each abusive relationship. Victims suffer from feelings of shame and humiliation; as a consequence, they are frequently reluctant to discuss the abuse in some instances, particularly with a physician whose efforts they believe are directed toward mending the wound and not necessarily its cause.

One of the most tragic examples of system failure involved a woman who was tortured over a number of years by her husband. He inserted objects into her vagina and pulled large chunks of her hair from her head. He punched, kicked, and slapped her, particularly in the lower back area, and she was often treated for what they both described as her tendency to fall due to clumsiness. This victim was treated for kidney problems and other complaints over a 2-year period without any inquiry about domestic violence. The victim finally left her abuser, who resorted to stalking her in an attempt to regain the control that he needed. As she entered the parking lot at her place of employment one morning, her husband inflicted a fatal stab wound to her abdomen.

After deciding to leave the abusive situation, this woman had sought help from local authorities, used the system for protective orders, discussed her fractures with her doctor, informed her place of employment about her husband's behavior, and even developed safety plans. Despite the abuser's intent to destroy her, this victim might have been saved through early detection of danger, recognition of indicators, appropriate system intervention to address the abuser's behavior, and effective safety support strategies that included collaborative efforts by allied professionals. This case also represents a system that failed to remove the abuser from the home, recognize his behavior as being criminal, and support the victim's attempts to escape the situation. All too often, such abuse is undetected by the system until it reaches monumental proportions.

Coupled with domestic violence is the sinister crime of stalking, which involves conduct and behavior by the stalker directed at a person with the intent of having the person fear for his or her safety and/or that of family members. Stalking is the act of repeatedly following, viewing, telephoning, writing letters, and indulging in other types of threatening behaviors intended to control, create fear in, and "possess" the victim. Domestic stalking, or the stalking of domestic violence victims, generally occurs after the victim has ended the relationship with the stalker. The victim is stalked as if for revenge for having left the offender.

Victims of domestic violence seek help from medical professionals more often than from any other type of support and care. Health care professionals are in a prime position to identify the dynamics of domestic violence through careful examination of certain symptoms, reactions, and indications, which will alert them not only to physical violence but also to emotional and sexual abuse. Recognizing that medical illness and physical injury can result from domestic violence and that proper medical intervention can prevent further violence and its consequences, the American College of Emergency Physicians encourages emergency personnel to screen patients for domestic violence and offer contact information about local shelters, advocacy groups, and legal assistance to patients who are or may be experiencing domestic violence (2).

The health care approach of prevention, prevention/intervention during the early stages of a medical condition, followed by treatment/prevention is now being applied successfully to combat the global problem of domestic violence. To this end, great strides have been made in educating the public about the gravity of this form of criminal behavior. Special programs have been developed to meet the needs of victims of domestic/family violence, yet more effort is needed to overcome the centuries of acceptance of violent behavior toward women. The goal is to permeate and saturate cultural thinking to a state of intolerance to violent behavior of any sort. The enormous problem of domestic/family violence is still fueled by its cultural entrenchment (attitudes that foster and perpetrate violence toward women) and the lack of consistent response to the violence. Consistent health care responses by professionals along with all other responding agents (including protocols, procedures, and policies for victim care) must be in place throughout the nation.

The elderly are victims of crime less often than other age-groups. When they are abused, they are subjected to a dehumanizing denial of dignity as they strive to adjust to the aftermath of crime. They can suffer from different forms of exploitation coupled with physical and sexual abuse and neglect imposed by caregivers, who are frequently family members. Is there a greater insult than to live a long life with an expectation of peace, safety, contentment, and integrity in the final stages of life, only to have these longings destroyed by callous, violent behavior? Erikson's identification of the core crisis of the elderly—integrity versus despair—takes on a greater dimension in the face of crimes against this age-group. Those who feel few regrets achieve ego integrity; they have lived productive and worthwhile lives and have coped with their failures and their successes (3). The failure to achieve integrity leads to feelings of despair, hopelessness, guilt, resentment, and self-disgust. In the aftermath of violent crimes, elderly victims can experience intense feelings of isolation, be hampered in their ability to care for their spouse, face reduced income, and feel increasingly dependent on others.

Recognition of elderly crime victims and interventions for their care have increased; as a result, the specific problems of this group of victims are now being addressed. Domestic violence, sexual assault, and even murder are still often overlooked because of factors commonly associated with age. The medical profession must lead in the effort to ensure that the elderly population is understood. Elderly victims may be forced to live with family members or in respite care following victimization. For the elderly, such major life changes can affect their independence and concept of self. Diminished physical abilities, frailty, decreased financial resources, and loss of mobility are all issues to be considered when treating elderly victims.

Children also are victims of physical assault, sexual assault, neglect, and emotional trauma. They suffer abuse at the hands of parents (male and female), relatives, caregivers, and strangers. Witnessing violent episodes in the home among family members/household members imposes a tremendous psychological toll on children and increases their risk for behavior problems as they develop and grow into adulthood. Without therapeutic intervention, many abused children will grow up to become abusers or candidates for serious revictimization (4). It is intolerable that so many children witness sexual violence, physical assault, domestic violence, and even murder. Their lives are affected by what they see, and, unless intervention occurs at an early stage, the effects can be long lasting.

One of the pioneers in bringing the tragic world of child abuse to the attention of pediatricians in particular and the medical community in general is Martin Finkel, founder of the Camden County Coalition Against the Sexual Abuse of Children (in New Jersey). For more than 20 years, Dr. Finkel has aimed to improve the "system" through research and the provision of direct services to abused children (5). His staff of clinical psychologists, pediatricians, researchers, support staff, and outreach personnel work together to address the immediate problems of each child while providing help that can avoid the predictable outcomes of child sexual abuse.

The Aftermath of Crime

> I died in Auchwitz but no one knew it.
> —*Charlotte Delbo*

For victims, crime is a process endured from its inception throughout its execution and eventual aftermath, which is often a continuum of reverberating pain and anguish. Individuals who endure criminal insult often develop certain health conditions, which can be directly linked to the stress associated with the crime event. The insult of crime extends to the financial inconvenience of replacing stolen and destroyed items, living with continuous pain and discomfort, and being forced to readjust one's life to accommodate the havoc and stigma caused by the offender.

At the moment of the crime event, a relationship erupts between the offender and the victim—the victim/offender dyad. Experiences, interactions, reactions, feelings, injuries, and events born of the dyad constitute the core of both the injury and insult to the human body and spirit. This relationship forms the experience of and is in essence the victim episode. It is vital to the healing of crime victims to have their experience receive sensitivity, validation, and support from people charged with the responsibility for responding to their special needs. Responders must recognize the effects of crime on victims, be aware of the victim's tremendous needs in the aftermath of the crime, and take measures that will address those needs.

Services for Victims

Although the world is full of suffering, it is also full of the overcoming of it.

—*Helen Keller*

There are still pockets in this nation where victim services are ineffective. Even more amazing is that in areas where services to victims can be interlocked, customized, and guaranteed, the major components and agencies have failed to adopt a multidisciplinary, collaborative approach that would ensure the provision of vital services. Health care, mental health, religious, and social service agencies must work closely with police officers and detectives, prosecutors, judges, court personnel, correction professionals, and victim assistance providers to create a holistic approach to the many needs of victims. In the past, these professionals have not necessarily shared the same goals, nor were they necessarily amenable to working together. Turf issues, lack of knowledge and understanding of each other's roles and responsibilities, and limited knowledge about victims' issues and concerns were all responsible for inadequate systems. Law enforcement, criminal justice agencies, and allied professionals are working together more than ever before to cooperate and understand the separate but equally important roles that each must play in the overall response to victims. During meetings of stakeholders in child advocacy centers, it can be difficult to distinguish the police from the social workers and the medical professionals. This represents the ideal relationship of concerned, enlightened, and skilled professionals working with one accord as they address the needs of victimized children.

The victim episode, in many instances translated and recounted by the victims themselves, serves as a guide for developing specialized programs, fostering collaboration, and ensuring professional association in a system response to the victims of crime. As stated by Schornstein, "Doctors must treat the injuries and address the cause. Otherwise, the treatment is superficial and ineffective to prevent future injury" (6). Whether from medical expertise required in legal or criminal investigation, treatment, education, medical science, or research and technology, there is an overriding need for the health care community to provide frontline services for victims of crime. McAfee (7) emphasized the role of physicians in this effort:

> The AMA can bring its organizational resources to bear on a national agenda [of violence prevention through publications and advocacy] . . . . However, the true success of our commitment will come when we as physicians, treating patients one at time, make a difference by breaking the cycle of violence that engulfs people's lives.

There is increasing evidence that crime-related trauma takes a toll on the long-term physical health of victims. Crime victims have higher rates of health care utilization than people who have not been victimized (8). Compared with nonvictims, female victims have higher rates of several behavioral problems that jeopardize well-being: heavy alcohol and drug use, drunk driving, smoking, bulimia, and obesity.

Victimology

The attention given to crime victims, their issues and concerns, and the responsibility of our institutions and agencies, including legislation that guarantees rights for victims, has given birth to *victimology*, the study of the victims of crime. Victimology examines the relationships experienced by victims as a result of encounters with systems and agencies during the aftermath of crime. Victimology is concerned with family; community; criminal justice; legal, mental, and health care systems; the media; and defender relationships, which are the core of the victim episode. It is now a recognized discipline, conducting exciting research and holding great promise for improved support of the victims of crime.

Victim Assistance

Victim assistance is help and support for victims and witnesses of crime, emanating from a prosecutor's office, police department, judicial program, or corrections and from nonprofit victim groups. Through victim assistance organizations, victim specialists and advocates trained to reach out to victims provide special services based on legislated victims' rights in each state.

THE VIOLENCE PARADOX

> Violence "speaks" of an intolerable condition of human shame and rage, a blinding rage that speaks through the body.
>
> —*James Gilligan, MD* (9)

In their book *The Anatomy of Motive*, Douglas and Olshaker proclaim that every crime is a mystery story with a motive at heart, which can often explain violent sociopathic behavior (10). They expose the devious nature of violence and the irreversible harm it causes to the recipients. In their discussion of predatory behavior, they conclude that criminals, despite family background, intelligence, or emotional stability, choose to commit their acts of violence. Certainly, deviant behavior, as a choice that results in abuse and injury, is as old as recorded history. The magnitude of these choices continues to be grave, complicated, distressing, and of tremendous concern to society. Human violence remains the same: a manifestation of senseless, bizarre, incomprehensible acts inflicted on people who become victims of heinous crimes. From a historical perspective, most societies developed basic response systems for the management of violent behavior. However, early response systems were never adequate to address the length and breadth of violence in any society. Today, because of the combined efforts of criminal justice agencies, medical and mental health professionals, and members of the faith, business, educational, and legal communities, our response systems are making a difference in the lives of crime victims.

Violence, even as a means to achieve socially acceptable ends, is destructive, deprecating, dominating, painful, and, most importantly, unnecessary in any context. Criminologists, forensic psychiatrists, and correctional professionals can help us understand violence, but they often view the problem from their own field, which tends to preclude awareness of the lasting effect of violence on its victims. Dr. James Gilligan, former medical director of Bridgewater State Hospital for the Criminally Insane, believes that different forms of violence are motivated by shame. The purpose of violence is to diminish the intensity of the perpetrator's shame and replace it with the opposite feeling, pride (9). Conversely, victims of violence frequently experience feelings of shame, anger, rage, low self-esteem, helplessness, and defeat as a result of the perpetrators' efforts to eliminate their own uncomfortable feelings at the expense of the victim. For victims, the exposure creates a lasting relationship with perpetrators and their deeds. Such an injustice is not singular but is perpetrated on the entire society and is, quite simply, an outrage. Further outrage is that for every reported case of violence there are countless numbers of cases and instances of violent crimes in these categories and others that are not reported through the established gates of entry for help. The medical profession should be the gatekeeper for those victims who out of necessity seek medical help. Early detection of abuse, particularly in children, will diminish the number of children forced to live

with the pathology of criminal behavior. The insult of victimization demands not only moral and legal consideration but also response to the causes of violence, treatment of the causes, and utilization of this knowledge to prevent further violence.

SEXUAL ASSAULT

[Sexual assault] is a metamorphosis. Although the event is external, it is quickly incorporated into the mind, where it replicates itself, like a virus. There is no defense. And yet life goes on.

—*Nancy Venable Raine* (11)

Consider

By the age of 34, Karen had undergone a mastectomy and reconstruction breast surgery, earned a law degree, and was balancing a successful career. She was raped in her home by a 19-year-old man. He entered her garden apartment through an open window around 2 AM and subjected her to 3 hours of physical, emotional, and psychological torture engineered through painful and humiliating acts. He raged and tormented her, calling her unspeakable names and demanding that she "shut up." He defiled and destroyed her apartment while demanding that she give him cash. He ripped the earrings from her ears and hurled items about the room in search of money. His sexual violence was engineered through vaginal penetration and forced anal and oral sodomy. She sustained vaginal tearing and anal injury. She had facial and neck bruises and swelling from slaps, blows, and choking. Her back and buttocks were scratched, and she had multiple superficial stab wounds on her upper torso. Her front tooth was chipped when her head was banged against the edge of the bathtub. Karen was kicked repeatedly in the lower back and side. She underwent extensive surgery to repair the damage to her spine and kidneys. In addition, her hands bore the cuts and slashes from the knife used to force her into submission. Karen still bears the scars of her upper chest stab wounds. She was beaten and threatened with death if she reported the incident. Before fleeing Karen's apartment, the rapist promised to return. When Karen finally received help, the rapist kept his promise and returned to Karen's apartment, in the early hours of a subsequent morning, expecting to continue his rampage of violence. When he returned, he was arrested, and Karen underwent nearly 2 years of court trials before the rapist was finally sentenced to a prison term of 65 years. Part of his conviction was based on the effective collection of evidence by a sexual assault nurse examiner (SANE).

After several surgeries and ongoing medical attention, Karen describes her life today as having been derailed from its former track; she has disconnected from previous relationships, and her activities have diminished in scope. No longer living alone, she describes her fear of being left alone in her parents' large house, "I cannot sleep until everyone is in the house. My windows must be closed at all times and I am afraid of the dark. I still wake up in the night terrified that I will be attacked again and no one will hear my cries for help. I avoid men, particularly young men." Karen is no longer with a law firm but is now working as a sales clerk in a bookstore. She is quick to offer that she considers herself lucky to be alive and is grateful for encounters with a criminal justice system and allied professionals who were knowledgeable about the "victim episode."

The physical injuries sustained during Karen's fateful ordeal have long since healed. What remains is the insult of injury; it is an infestation of conflict. One of the major residuals of violence for victims is the stigma associated with the crime. Karen's residuals are manifested by her vow of celibacy, inability to resume her former career, medical expenses, financial needs, lingering legal matters, and safety issues. Karen's needs were addressed by a continuum of care and support, which began from the moment her call for help was received by police emergency services. The call set into motion a response system that included criminal justice agencies and trained allied professions working together to achieve common goals. After 5 years, Karen is entering therapy.

The system of response worked for Karen. She was interviewed by knowledgeable detectives and treated at the hospital emergency department by sensitive medical professionals. A medical examination was conducted promptly, procedures were explained, and hospital protocol was followed. Karen received a nonjudgmental approach from examining practitioners, which helped reduce her anxiety and support her empowerment. She received individual care and treatment, which took into consideration her physical history with all its complications. During the initial phase of Karen's aftercare, a victim service provider arrived at the hospital to ensure that Karen was receiving psychological support, to serve as a liaison with family and friends, and to provide information about victims' rights, the criminal justice system, and available services. Karen received a complete explanation of all procedures, as well as reasons for and protocols associated with evidence collection. The examination was conducted, and Karen was referred for physician evaluation and treatment for her other injuries. However, this interaction with the health care system was only the beginning.

Victims' Reactions to Rape

Professor Ann Burgess, a psychiatric nurse, and Lynda Lytle Holmstrom, a sociologist, first described the reactions of rape victims as *rape trauma syndrome* (12). The short-term effects include denial, shock, disbelief, disruption, and feelings of guilt, shame, blame, and hostility. The long-term effects may be more deeply rooted, causing phobias and sexual problems and affecting the victim's ability to "function."

Rape victims have very specific concerns (13):

- Safety of self
- Safety of children
- Mistrust of men/husband/dating
- Frustration with impaired sexuality
- Frustration with impaired emotional intimacy
- Loss of self-esteem, self-respect, and level of functioning
- Perceptual distortion
- Marriage/dating problems
- Divorce
- Concern about the rapist being released and looking for them
- Fear of being revictimized

In addition, subsequent events occur in the lives of many rape victims that lead to additional emotional trauma and financial expense. These constitute secondary victimizations:

- Divorce
- Loss of sexual desire
- Cost of home safety equipment
- Cost of self-defense classes
- Cost of counseling (both victimization and marriage/family)
- Change of job
- Lack of information about legal procedures
- Fear of acquired immunodeficiency syndrome

Definition of Sexual Assault

Each crime category has its distinct markings. Rape is a violent crime engineered through sexual acts that are forced and degrading. The idea is to control, humiliate, force, harm, and overpower the victim. We have long since moved beyond the old myths surrounding rape and sexual assault as being invited, confined only to women, stranger motivated, and uncommon. Sexual assault does not always transpire between a female victim and a stranger lurking in the dark. Rape occurs between acquaintances, which makes the act no less disgusting and degrading. Rape defies age and gender. Victims are children, elderly people, people with physical or mental disabilities, and anyone who falls prey to the predator. Women are the victims of rape and sexual assault most often, but men are also raped.

Current definitions of rape include male and female children and adolescents, as well as men and women, as victims. Rape by acquaintance and forced oral or anal sex are also considered to be rape and sexual assault. These more recent expansions have come about after years of definitions that have varied widely from state to state. The Illinois Criminal Sexual Assault Statute is considered the national model for a broad definition of rape (14,15). It has the following characteristics:

- Rape is defined as "gender neutral," which broadens earlier definitions of rape so that it now includes men and women.
- It includes acts of sexual penetration other than vaginal penetration by a penis.
- It distinguishes types of sexual abuse on the basis of the degree of force or threat of force, similar to the "aggravated" versus "simple" distinction of physical assaults.
- It recognizes threat and overt force as a means of overpowering the victim.
- It introduces a new category of rape: taking advantage of an incapacitated victim. These victims include the mentally ill and people under the influence of drugs or alcohol. (Some states require that the perpetrator had to give the victim the intoxicant in order to obtain sexual access.)

Most states do not define "rape" as broadly as that set forth in the Illinois statute.

At the federal level, a 1986 statute (Federal Criminal Code, Title 18, Chapter 109A, Sections 2241–2243) defines two types of sexual assault (14):

- *Sexual abuse*: causing another person to engage in a sexual activity by threatening or placing that person in fear or engaging in a sexual act if that person is incapable of declining participation in or communicating unwillingness to engage in that sexual act.
- *Aggravated sexual abuse*: when a person "knowingly causes another person to engage in a sexual act . . . or attempts to do so by using force against that person, or by threatening or placing that person in fear that the person will be subjected to death, serious bodily injury, or kidnapping; when a person knowingly renders another person unconscious and thereby engages in a sexual act with that person, or administers to another person by force or threat of force, or without the knowledge or permission of that person, a drug, intoxicant, or other similar substance and thereby substantially impairs the ability of that person to appraise or control conduct and then engages in a sexual act with that person."

Male Rape

Sexual assault and abuse are not restricted to women and children; men are also sexually assaulted and therefore require services designed to meet their specific needs arising from sexual assault and domestic violence. Male victims also experience the debilitating aftermath, with the added dimension of myths, gender stereotyping, and the stigma associated with male vulnerability to victimization (16). Men and boys are reluctant to report the crime of rape; as a consequence, male rape is grossly underreported and undertreated (17).

Many state codes do not recognize male rape unless the man has been raped by a woman. The more commonly used term for *male rape* by another man is *sodomy* (forced anal or oral sex).

Most male rape victims are raped by other men, in the sense that they are forced to submit to anal intercourse, oral sex, mutual masturbation, masturbation of the offender, or other sex acts. Fear of bodily harm can cause a man to have an erection; therefore, a man can be raped by either a man or a woman. In addition, men can be raped by women in that they can be coerced or intimidated into sexual behavior they do not desire. Furthermore, a percentage of sexual abuse is perpetrated by adult females on young boys. It is a myth that only gay men are raped. Most male rape victims do not report their assaults, nor do they receive medical attention or counseling. Male victims suffer from feelings of shame and a sense of guilt, associated with the stigma of sexual contact with another male.

Data on the reactions to and specifics of male sexual assault are limited; however, it is believed that the shock of sexual assault is greater in male rape victims than in female victims because of societal conditioning, which prepares a female for the possibility of rape. Male victims may be led to question their sexual orientation on the basis of being subjected to what is considered a nonmasculine episode. Male victims may suffer sexual malfunctions because of sexual assault. They are often isolated, and their needs for victim services go unmet because of the lack of information about the problem, reluctance of providers to commit to services, lack of trained and skilled personnel to adequately address their needs, and system's insensitivity to male victims of sexual assault. Medical sensitivity, public education, and training of professionals who deal with the victims constitute a start toward greater initiatives in treatment, research, and program development.

Rape

Stranger rape is among the most feared of all crimes. It is a rape executed by a person or persons who have had no previous contact with the victim. However, most rape victims (approximately 75%) know their assailants, perhaps only casually (18–22). Acquaintance rape occurs among college students more than any other age-group (23). They may have a close relationship, may have dated steadily, and may even have been sexual partners. Nonstranger rapes are commonly not reported because of the difficulty in prosecution, the stigma, and the lack of information about the right to receive victim services (24). Many victims of rape do not label their experience of being forced to have sex as "sexual assault." However, the fact that a gun or knife was not used does not eliminate the trauma experienced by the victim. The shame of rape in any context is so overwhelming that the victims may not report it, particularly in non-stranger rape; they wonder who will believe them. In giving voice to their experience, victims are sometimes met with telling reactions from the listener, which mirror shame to victims. Victims of acquaintance rape are often blamed for the incident, thereby placing the responsibility for the rape on the victim. Nonstranger rape may account for most rapes committed each year, but its incidence cannot be measured because of the failure of victims to report it.

Rape in which a more defined relationship exists between the individuals at the time of the event is underreported, difficult to prosecute, and extremely prevalent. These types of rapes are made more complex by dating norms and the extent of the relationship between the people involved. Victims may take responsibility for the event because they chose to date the offending individual. They experience the additional burdens of betrayal, self-accusation, and personal failure in being able to select dating partners. Like other types of acquaintance rape, date rape is common and difficult to prosecute. Dating behavior is defined by dating expectations. Men may expect that sex will be part of the dating experience; women may want a sense of commitment before they become intimate in a relationship.

Marital Rape

Recognition of a woman's right to say no to sex within the state of marriage is responsible for the term *marital rape*. The legal definition of rape varies, but many states have adopted a proactive stance on this underreported type of sexual assault. In Virginia, for example, a person is guilty of rape if he or she has sexual intercourse with his or her spouse against the spouse's will, by force, threat, or intimidation. To make a charge of marital forced sodomy, or marital object sexual penetration, a victim must be living apart from her spouse or have suffered bodily injury when the husband forced the wife to have oral or anal sex or penetrated the wife's vagina or anus with an object or forced her to penetrate

herself with an object against her will. If the victim is residing with her husband and has not suffered serious physical injury, the husband is still guilty of marital sexual assault if he has, through force, threat, or intimidation, sexual intercourse, oral sex or anal sex with his wife against her will, penetrates his wife's vagina or anus with an object, or forces his wife to penetrate herself with an object.

In relationships in which violence is a common and recurring process, sexual assault is considered an appendix of the violence. Approximately 40% to 45% of physically abused women are also forced into having sex (25–27). Forced rape is seldom reported and is often used by the spouse rapist as punishment, retaliation, or bargaining tool in custody issues. Sexual assault is tied to patterns of abusive behaviors associated with domestic violence. This type of forced sex is connected to the belief still held by some that a woman is obligated to submit to her husband on demand.

Reporting Sexual Assault

> The effects of rape are far-ranging, far-reaching, long-lasting, and late-arising.
> —*Cynthia Carosella* (28)

Most sexual assaults are never reported to law enforcement; consequently, there is no apprehension of many perpetrators for prosecution and incarceration. The rapist remains at large, free to assault again. In many instances, victims of rape are young, unsuspecting, frightened girls. They become prey to dates, employers, customers, relatives, and strangers. In surveys that asked victims why they did not report the rape, they gave the following reasons: shame; embarrassment; fear of rejection, exposure, or ridicule; fear of the rapist; distrust of the system; and lack of information about victims' rights.

Very often, when cases are reported to law enforcement, the report comes from some source other than the victim. A victim who arrives at an emergency department for help after a sexual assault is asked whether she wants to report the crime to law enforcement. In most states the victim is allowed to make the decision but is encouraged to cooperate with the police investigation. It is generally believed that the best interest of the victim is served through her ability to make decisions. Victims who at least reach an emergency department have a chance of being examined by a medical professional, informed about pregnancy and disease prevention, and treated for injury. Sexual assault victims who require medical attention and fail to receive it are left with unattended issues of great magnitude.

We will never know how many of those who have been raped lost their jobs, ended relationships, or experienced sexual dysfunction, addictions, eating disorders, procrastination, or loss of hope as the effects of being raped. These effects range from subtle to extreme and can be both physical and emotional. They are seen in the male victim who cannot bear to be spoken to in a certain way by his boss because it reminds him of his rapist's demanding voice and in the woman who cannot bear to lose the protective covering of the weight that she gained after she was raped (28).

A Measure of the Problem

Obtaining accurate measurements of the incidence of rape and other types of sexual assault poses many challenges. The number of reported rapes and other types of sexual assault reflects how these crimes are defined and measured. The following statistics are derived from different sources, which often measure different factors using different methodologies.

- In 1996, the National Crime Victimization Survey found that more than two thirds of rapes/sexual assaults committed in the nation remained unreported (29).
- Using a definition of rape that includes forced vaginal, oral, and anal sex, the National Violence Against Women Survey found that 1 of 6 US women and 1 of 33 US men experienced an attempted or completed rape as a child and/or adult (30).
- Approximately 14.8% of women and 2.8% of men in the United States are victims of rape; an additional 2.1% of women and 0.9% of men are victims of attempted rape (30).
- More than 52% of rape/sexual assault victims are females younger than 25 years (31).
- The National Violence Against Women Survey found that "rape in America is a tragedy of youth" because most rapes occur during childhood and adolescence (30).
- Of first or only rapes experienced by women, 21.6% occurred before the victim was 12 years old.
- Of all rapes, 20.8% were committed against girls between the ages of 15 and 16.

Underserved Populations

Special attention and programs must address the needs of victims who have been overlooked in the past. The programs must include screening, diagnosis, treatment, evaluations, and psychological, as well as case service assistance, which take into consideration the special needs of each group.

The Elderly

Older people are often the target of sexual assault. Women with impaired functioning are particularly at risk. Health care professionals who are not aware of the signs may fail to respond to the problem. The elderly are sometimes assaulted in health care facilities, where they are unable to resist or escape their predators. Care and attention must be given to this special population (see Chapter 10).

People with Disability

A person with a disability has a physical or mental impairment that substantially limits one or more major life activities, has a record of such an impairment, or is regarded as having such an impairment (32). Special programs with skilled and trained staff must be available throughout the continuum of care (including the criminal justice system) to meet the needs of individuals with impairments, whether the needs are medically based or the result of mental illness. More than 49 million Americans have disabilities with a vast array of impairments. Persons with disabilities are devalued when programs and systems are not formulated with their special needs in mind. Basic information about the hearing impaired and individuals with speech impairments (such as their preferred means of communicating) must be considered. Victims with visual impairment or blindness may not be able to identify their assailant or visually describe the events of their victimization; nevertheless, through other senses that are heightened, the victim will be able to provide extensive information. Every device and effort should be used to ensure that these victims have access to resources that address their needs. Sexual assault victims with mental disabilities, mental retardation, or mental illness require special protocols for criminal justice participation and aftercare.

Gay Men, Lesbians, Bisexuals, and Transgendered People

The gay, lesbian, bisexual, and transgendered community is an "invisible minority" because its members do not look different from others in their respective ethnic groups. Approximately 2% of Americans—approximately 6 million people—are gay (33). Gay and lesbian victims of sexual assault tend to refrain from reporting their victimization because they fear the response will be insensitive and inadequate. Some victims do not wish to disclose their sexual orientation because they fear that such disclosures will jeopardize their jobs, family relations, and other vital aspects of their lives.

Non–English-Speaking, Ethnic Minority, and Foreign-Born Victims

When considering the aftercare of victims from culturally diverse backgrounds, myriad issues emerge. Language and culture are primary in setting up protocols for response. Victims of sexual assault will view the rape dynamic from its occurrence throughout the aftermath on the basis of their cultural experience. They must be assisted in special ways that eliminate barriers to information and make the available services tailored to their needs.

Refugees and Resettlement Victims of Sexual Assault

Many women have been displaced from their countries for political or other reasons, such as war and natural disaster. They may be resettled in refugee camps, where they are sometimes forced into prostitution, forced to trade sex for food for their children, and/or brutalized by systematic rape. Victims who have experienced gang rape and repeated rapes often fail to report the crimes and blame themselves because of their relegated submissive roles and religious and cultural mores.

The Aftermath of Sexual Assault

> Forensics is the silent witness ... it does not speak for or against the victim. It merely speaks the truth.
> —*Detective Jeffrey Miller, Forensic Expert, Fairfax, Virginia*

The rape victim deserves the best evidentiary examination possible through a program designed for the gathering, collection and documentation of that evidence for the court system.
> —*Sue Brown, Sexual Assault Nursing Examiner, Fairfax, Virginia*

In sexual assault cases, the victim's body is the primary "crime scene," and the forensic medical examination is an extremely important part of evidence collection (8). Emergency medical care, especially the collection of evidence through a forensic examination, is critical both for the victim and for protecting the evidence for prosecution. Trained medical professionals must meet the rape victim's medical and emotional needs and must collect evidence to be used in a legal proceeding. When victims are made a part of this process as a stakeholder, their cooperation increases and the procedures are not as difficult and prolonged. The local protocol, which may include agreements and cooperation among participating agencies, should be explained to victims. They need information about the process—what, how, why, and when—with simple direct explanations that can be understood even in the midst of conflict.

A comprehensive medical protocol to be used in the aftermath of rape includes the following components:

- Evidentiary examination (the patient has the right to refuse an examination for this purpose)
- Police report
- Gynecologic examination
- Consent for the taking of photographs
- For minors, parental notification
- Directions for taking medication to prevent pregnancy; side effects of drugs
- Referrals to anonymous human immunodeficiency virus (HIV) antibody testing facilities
- Counseling referrals
- Information about victim services for information on legislation, court proceedings, and civil suits

Sexual Assault Response Team

A sexual assault response team is a designated group of professionals available to respond on demand when a sexual assault has occurred. The team consists of a law enforcement officer, a sexual assault advocate, a nurse examiner, a SANE, and a physician when necessary.

Collection of Forensic Evidence

Examination of a rape victim includes the following:

- An internal examination
- Pubic hair combings
- Nail scrapings
- Saliva samples
- Deoxyribonucleic acid (DNA) swabbings
- Hair sampling
- Medical history
- Medical care and treatment of injuries
- Diagnosis and treatment of sexually transmitted diseases (STDs)
- Pregnancy test
- Collection of clothing

Recommendations for Health Care Providers

1. Create a sensitive environment in which patients are encouraged to express their feelings, concerns, and needs related to the assault.
2. Be responsive to questions and concerns about procedures and treatment and involve patients in decision making on follow-up care and notification of family members.
3. Comply with the global challenge recommendation in *New Directions from the Field: Victims' Rights and Services for the 21st Century* (34) to institute victimology in the curriculum in medical schools, nursing schools, and schools of social work.
4. Ensure that policies, procedures, and protocols are in place for identifying sexual assault, obtaining medical histories from victims, treating victims, reporting the assault, and performing follow-up evaluation.

5. Ensure that culturally appropriate information is available to victims of sexual assault. They should be able to read and understand medical information, which will help in their recovery process. In addition, when language is a barrier, ensure that interpreters are available to help in dispensing services.

6. Engage in campaigns to heighten public awareness on sexual assault as a preventive measure and to garner support for victims.

7. If forensic evidence has been collected, ensure that expert testimony is available for court cases.

8. Create programs that train personnel as a SANE, sexual assault nurse clinician, or sexual assault/forensic examiner to offer sensitive outreach to adult and child victims of sexual assault in a nonthreatening environment. These programs employ highly trained and skilled medical professionals who are contacted immediately by law enforcement to respond to victims. They are present in the emergency department to address the injuries, initiate the process of evidence collection for prosecution, and provide special counseling to victims to allay their fears of infection and pregnancy. Medical professionals are the only agents qualified to make careful diagnosis, dispense treatment, and prescribe medications for victims of sexual assault. Additional help from other agents is satellite to the physical and mental issues set in motion by an emergency response to the problem.

The National Victim Assistance Academy (14) offers a "Promising Practices" segment that outlines innovative programs and approaches to working with victims. A few of these exceptional programs are described in the subsequent text:

■ The Rape Treatment Center (RTC) at Santa Monica-UCLA Medical Center (www.911rape. org), established in 1974, has provided care for more than 24,000 sexual assault victims. In April 1999, the RTC created a state-of-the-art clinic to enhance the treatment of victims immediately after a sexual assault. In the past, rape victims received emergency services in hospital emergency departments. In these facilities, victims are often subjected to long waits and a chaotic environment, and, as a result, the victim's trauma may be compounded and critical evidence can deteriorate. In contrast, the RTC's new clinic is located in a safe, private, therapeutic hospital environment. The 24-hour facility is dedicated exclusively to the care of sexual assault victims. It is staffed by advanced practice nurse practitioners and professional therapists, who use advanced forensic equipment and technologies. In addition to medical and evidentiary services, victims receive crisis intervention and other advocacy and support services. They also receive special health-related educational materials; all services are free. In the development of the clinic, and in its ongoing operations, the clinic has collaborated with law enforcement agencies, crime labs, and other victim service providers.

■ In Montgomery County, Maryland, rape counselors have developed a rape crisis videotape in Spanish. The 12-minute video, produced with $30,000 of state grant money, was introduced during the 1999 National Crime Victims' Rights Week. It features Spanish-speaking people (a police officer, prosecutor, and rape counselor, among others) explaining the legal process that follows the reporting of a sexual assault.

■ The Anonymous and Confidential Internet Support Counseling Service was launched in March 1997 by the Brazos County Rape Crisis Center (www.rapecrisisbv.org) in Bryan, Texas. It offers anonymous support counseling to victims/survivors of sexual abuse or assault, their friends, and their family members. Victims/survivors anywhere in the world can access this technology and service. Users can write to the center electronically at any time (24 hours a day, 7 days a week) to request information or seek help. Through the secure server, the user's identity and location are protected and kept confidential. It allows users to tell or talk about their sexual abuse/assault without the fear of someone knowing who they are or from where they are calling.

DOMESTIC VIOLENCE

What's love got to do with it?

—Tina Turner

The human heart is a strange mystery.

—Alexandre Dumas

Consider

Angela, a state department employee, and Tom, an insurance claims adjuster, were married for 3 months before the indicators of violence became apparent. Angela recalls that what she once considered Tom's love was in fact a mean, sinister obsession with every aspect of her life. He monitored her phone calls, her mail, and her relationship with coworkers and family. He demanded control of her income and portioned out a limited allowance for incidentals only. He required special meals and formal eating arrangements. Tom always explained his actions as manifestations of his love, protection, and concern for Angela. He called himself a perfectionist who had found the perfect wife for the perfect family and life. He explained that his aggression was intended to guard and protect their perfect life.

By the end of their first year of marriage, Angela had become the victim of Tom's physical, verbal, sexual, and emotional abuse. The first attack was swift and harsh. Tom confronted Angela when she arrived home after working late on a Friday night. As she exited the car, Tom struck her with such force that she fell to the ground, scraping her face and fracturing her right cheekbone and several bones in her right foot. She was knocked unconscious and remembers awaking to Tom's concerned face as he applied ice to her bloody and rapidly swelling face, forehead, and hands. She was baffled and confused. Tom was remorseful and loving. He vowed never to hurt her again. He begged for forgiveness and promised that his newly acquired habit of drinking every night would stop. Angela was subsequently treated at the emergency department of a local hospital. Tom explained her "fall" as a nasty accident. This initial incident was the beginning of 8 years of beatings, sexual abuse, drinking bouts, rages, fear, embarrassment, shame, stalking, and threats, as well as attempts by Angela to conceal the effects of abuse and many attempts to escape the situation. After the birth of two children and three miscarriages (caused by severe beatings), Angela finally received safe passage to a new life, with the support of the criminal justice system and legal, health, and mental health service agencies.

On the basis of a literature review, Gazmararian et al. calculated that the prevalence of violence during pregnancy ranges from 1% to 20% (35). Several complications of pregnancy—including low birth weight, insufficient weight gain, substance abuse, inadequate prenatal care, and premature delivery—have also been associated with abuse (36). Connections between abuse during pregnancy and miscarriages are strongly suspected (37).

Angela found asylum from years of pain and the threat of death from a husband determined to possess her on his own terms. She endured broken limbs; severe injuries to her eardrums, ribs, nose, fingers, and throat; frequent black eyes and broken teeth; and a spinal cord injury. She had also been forced to participate in painful and humiliating sexual acts. Conviction of Tom for his crimes against Angela and her eventual escape did not come swiftly or easily. It took years, starting with Angela's process of leaving a destructive relationship. Time after time she left and sought help through family and friends. Each time she tried to leave him, Tom was able to convince her that life would be different and he would change.

Over the years, the beatings became more severe and the psychological/emotional abuse became more intense. The children were exposed to Tom's drinking bouts and irrational behavior, and Angela feared for their physical safety and her own. After regaining consciousness following one of Tom's choking episodes, Angela finally resolved that he would never change and that she had to escape or die. Years of being locked in a violent and destructive relationship resulted in Angela engaging in whatever Tom wanted or needed, including criminal activities such as fraud and theft. She describes her self-loathing and shame in having engaged in certain behavior. Her physician, who documented his findings and followed through with his suspicions of the reason for her frequent injuries, asked Angela the right questions. It was this informed physician who identified and recognized that Angela was the victim of recurring violence in her home. The same physician was responsible for recognizing and reporting the emotional and psychological abuse of Angela's two children. The end of Angela's ordeal with Tom came as a result of medical intervention, not the workings of the criminal justice system. Her cries for help to law enforcement were minimized, overlooked, and in several cases denied. When police were called in, they encouraged the couple to work it out. When she attempted to obtain orders of protection, the system denied them on the basis of the assumption that they were not needed to stem the situation. Tom has long since served his brief term in jail for assault. Angela has relocated and seemingly moved on with her life. Her children have grown into teenagers without the presence of their father in the home. To her knowledge, Tom is unaware of their location. For Angela, the years of violence still dominate her life. She confesses that she is never free from her fear that Tom will find her and kill her.

The intense concerns of victims of domestic violence were summarized by Brown (13):

- Physical safety of self and children
- Fear of the abuser locating them
- Concern about how they will survive
- Not having a safe place to stay away from the abuser
- Not having money, a job, or work skills
- Having no transportation

Additional problems emerge as aspects of secondary victimization:

- Lack of protection from law enforcement agencies
- Lack of services available to help with transition
- Lack of training, money, and information about how to increase work skills
- Stigmatization by being labeled a "spouse abuse victim"

Definition of Domestic Violence

All aspects of abuse (physical, sexual, and controlling behavior, including emotional degradation) are important to the resultant effects on women's health and opportunities for interventions in the health care system.

—*Jacquelyn C. Campbell* (38)

Angela's story is a typical example of the cycle of violence. Confusion, imbalance of power, isolation, appeasement, secrecy, separations/reunions, and alcohol and drug use all reflect this complex and insidious practice of violence. Domestic violence is defined as a systematic pattern of abusive behaviors that, over a period, may become more frequent and severe and are carried out for the purpose of control, domination, and/or coercion. Such behavior may include verbal abuse and threats; physical, psychological, and sexual abuse; and destruction of property and pets. The batterer frequently accomplishes the abuses in an environment of his own creation that ultimately traps the victim in a state of fear, isolation, deprivation, and confusion.

Domestic violence episodes are not random acts of violence or incidents of mere loss of temper. Rather, such episodes are part of a complex, continuing pattern of behavior, of which the violence is but one dynamic (6). A general definition of domestic violence is any assault, battery, sexual assault, sexual battery, or criminal offense resulting in personal injury or death of a family or household member caused by another, who is or was residing in the same dwelling unit. Generally speaking, "family or household member" means spouse, former spouse, persons related by blood or by marriage, persons who are presently residing together as a family, those who have resided together in the past as a family, and persons who have a child in common regardless of whether they have been married or have resided together at any time.

We are knowledgeable about the cycle of violence; we know about power and control. We understand the drama and tragedy of abuse. We even have a long list of why women stay in abusive relationships, but what we fail to talk about is the power of love often inherent in these destructive relationships. Love being battered and tortured . . . no way; love and longing for the battering partner to change his behavior . . . absolutely. Most women are initially shocked and confused by the battering behavior perpetrated by the men they love and trust. Such violence usually appears after a bond of commitment develops. The victim is caught unaware and is soon caught in a web, with the belief that the batterer's behavior will change. Domestic violence victims generally return to their violent situations six to eight times before finally leaving the relationship. They usually return because they do not want to separate their children from their father, because they love their partner, and/or because they have no other options of making a living. During the process of leaving, the victim is in greatest danger when the batterer realizes the leaving is final. During this period, he may increase his attacks, stalk the victim, vandalize, assault, rape, kidnap her and/or the children, and threaten and even attempt to kill them. Separating and returning only reinforces the batterer's violence, and he becomes convinced that his aggression accomplishes the goal of keeping his partner under control.

Working with battered women is especially difficult, requiring great patience on the part of listening parties. Women who are victims of domestic violence typically establish a history with law enforcement, child protective services, and the courts. When women have been in a violent situation for a long time and it is perceived that they are reluctant to leave, they need help from sensitive sources who understand that leaving is a process. Just as the cycle of violence progresses as a process, so does the eventual leaving. It sometimes takes years before the woman is able to finally accomplish this goal. Battered women are sometimes assumed to be weak and ineffectual, but the opposite is true. There is strength in the ability to withstand and endure the amount of abuse that is inflicted in violent relationships.

Battered women can develop symptoms of posttraumatic stress disorder (PTSD) (39), which is defined as a cluster of symptoms that almost anyone subjected to trauma outside the range of usual human experience would develop. These include, but are not limited to, intrusive recollection of the trauma(s), psychic numbing of emotions, flashbacks, appetite and/or sleep disturbance, hypervigilance, exaggerated startle response, disturbance in concentration, unpredictable irritability or anger, anxiety, and depression. Victims of domestic violence may also experience symptoms of learned helplessness, passivity, indecisiveness, and chronic physical illnesses that range from frequent colds, flu, and allergies to chronic urinary, vaginal, and gastrointestinal problems. In the most serious cases, ulcers and eating disorders have also been related to abuse (40). According to research conducted by Kilpatrick et al. (8), "victims of violent crime may suffer undiagnosed PTSD for many years, at great cost to their health and the health care system."

Children Who Witness Violence

Children who witness violence in their homes are affected by the experience in various ways. The immediate negative effects appear to translate into low self-esteem, behavioral problems, reduced social ability, depression, and anxiety (41). Children who experience violence in the home as victims or observers are at risk for continuing the cycle of violence in their lives as adults (42). Men and women who report being hit by their parents are more likely to hit their own children (43).

A Measure of the Problem

■ In 1996, women experienced an estimated 840,000 rapes, sexual assaults, robberies, aggravated assaults, and simple victimization at the hands of an intimate (30).

■ Intimate violence is primarily a crime against women. In 1996, females were the victims of three of every four murders of intimates and approximately 85% of the victims of nonlethal intimate violence (9).

■ Data from the National Violence Against Women Survey (30), the first national study on stalking, sponsored jointly by the National Institute of Justice and the Centers for Disease Control and Prevention, confirm previous reports that violence against women is predominantly intimate-partner violence. Of the women who reported being raped and/or physically assaulted since the age of 18, three fourths were victimized by a current or former husband, cohabiting partner, date, or boyfriend.

■ Women are significantly more likely than men to report being raped or physically assaulted by a current or former intimate partner, whether the time frame considered was the person's lifetime or the 12 months preceding the survey. Moreover, when raped or physically assaulted by a current or former intimate partner, women are significantly more likely than men to sustain injuries (30).

■ Women of all races are about equally vulnerable to violence by an intimate partner (29).

■ Women aged between 19 and 29 and women in families with incomes below $10,000 are more likely than other women to be victims of violence by an intimate partner (29).

■ Among victims of violence committed by an intimate partner, the victimization rate of women separated from their husbands is approximately three times higher than that of divorced women and approximately 25 times higher than that of married women (29).

■ Females are more likely to be victimized at a private home (their own or that of a neighbor, friend, or relative) than in any other place (18,29). Males are most likely to be victimized in public places such as businesses, parking lots, and open spaces (29).

■ Approximately four of ten inmates serving time in jail for intimate violence had a criminal justice status—on probation or parole or under a restraining order—at the time of the violent attack on the intimate (29).

■ Approximately one of four convicted violent offenders confined in local jails had committed the crime against an intimate; approximately 7% of state prisoners serving time for violence had an intimate victim (29).

Recommendations for Health Care Providers

Be aware of the dynamics of domestic violence; be clear that no one should ever have to submit to violence. Domestic assaults can involve pushing, shoving, kicking, grabbing, throwing things at the victim, strangulation, beatings, punching, and emotional/verbal abuse, including threats of violence.

Be familiar with local and national resources for victims. For example:

■ Children's Hospital in Boston had the nation's first program to offer advocacy and support to abused mothers at the same time that the hospital offered protection to abused children. Advocacy for Women and Kids in Emergencies (AWAKE) (44) was formed to broaden the child abuse program to include intervention on behalf of battered women and to coordinate services that were often offered separately, and in conflict, to women and to children (45).

■ The American Academy of Facial Plastic and Reconstructive Surgery, in partnership with the National Coalition Against Domestic Violence (the umbrella group for most domestic violence shelters in the United States), provides free consultation and surgery to victims of domestic abuse (45).

Design a set of questions that will detect violence in the home. Be specific and ask directly about violence. The following set of questions was compiled by Salber and Taliaferro (46):

1. You have a number of bruises. How did they happen?
2. What happens when your spouse loses his temper?
3. Are you in a relationship in which you are being hurt?
4. Has your partner ever harmed or threatened to harm someone or something you love?
5. Does your spouse use drugs or alcohol? How does your spouse behave toward you when he is drinking or using drugs?
6. Do you have children? Are they living in a safe environment?

It is imperative to ask these questions when the patient is alone and not in the presence of anyone who accompanied her to the appointment. She will most likely refrain from any admissions or discussions until she feels that the information can be imparted to an empathetic listener.

Physicians should specifically look for evidence of domestic violence. In *The Physician's Guide to Domestic Violence*, Salber and Taliaferro (46) suggest that clues to the presence of domestic violence can be ascertained from the history and physical examination:

- The reported history of the incident is not consistent with the kind of injury.
- There is a time delay between injuries and presentation.
- The patient has a history of being "accident prone".
- The patient has attempted suicide or experienced depression.
- The patient has had repeated psychosomatic complaints.

Further actions to be taken by health care professionals are as follows:

1. Develop multidisciplinary approaches to working with domestic violence victims. Ensure that medical personnel join coalitions, boards, and committees whose task is to provide service to domestic violence victims.
2. Develop threat assessment protocols to ensure the safety of victims.
3. Provide emergency department security for victims of domestic violence.
4. Develop a protocol for questioning patients when domestic abuse is suspected.
5. Ensure continuity of services to victims through coordination with all agents of the care continuum.
6. Document the patient's condition in medical records.
7. Educate patients about domestic violence.
8. Participate in public health campaigns to educate the public about domestic violence on the basis of research.
9. Optimize technology to inform victims about the medical aspects of domestic violence.
10. Develop a multicultural approach to deal with victims of domestic violence in an attempt to help overcome ethnic, cultural, and religious barriers to provide help and healing.
11. Provide educational resources for health care personnel:
    - *Family Violence: An Intervention Model for Dental Professionals* is a training program funded by the Office for Victims of Crime

for dentists and dental ancillary staff, which presents information about the dynamics of family violence and appropriate interventions by dental professionals (47).
- The American College of Obstetricians and Gynecologists (ACOG) offers a number of publications and lectures on domestic violence, including violence during pregnancy and that directed against the elderly (48). Domestic violence is one of many topics covered in the ACOG-sponsored book *Special Issues in Women's Health* (49).

STALKING

Stalking, that is, unwanted pursuit, following, contacting, or harassment, is closely related to domestic violence. Stalking is recognized as criminal victimization rather than simply a nuisance behavior. Stalkers are likely to follow their targets, monitor their activities, bombard them with telephone calls, and spy on them using binoculars, telescopes, microphones, and cameras to achieve their end, which is to exert control and create fear. They will use any means to connect with their victims. Stalking behavior is obsessive, can escalate in intensity, and can be extremely dangerous because it inflicts emotional distress, injury, and, in some instances, death. Before 1990, when the first antistalking statute was established, stalking was not considered illegal. The exploration of this strange and insidious crime is new, and data are developing on a daily basis about its psychological nature.

The 1998 National Violence Against Women Survey (30) documented that 1 in 12 women and 1 in 45 men will be stalked during their lifetime. The stalker is known to 77% of female and 64% of male victims. Most (87%) stalkers are men.

In the national survey, victims of stalking provided the first glimpse into the tactics to which they were most often subjected (30,50):

- Being followed or spied on from outside their home or place of work (82%)
- Receiving unwanted phone calls (61%)
- Receiving unwanted letters or items (30%)
- Having property vandalized (30%)
- Having pet threatened or killed (9%)

The number and nature of these behaviors, and the context in which they occur, communicate a threat. It is this element of threat to the safety of another that makes the stalker's conduct a crime. Most legal definitions of stalking specifically address the presence of an element of threat (30).

Categories of Stalking

1. Simple obsession stalking represents 60% of all stalking cases, including those arising from previous personal relationships (e.g., those between husbands/wives, girlfriends, domestic partners). Many simple obsession cases are actually extensions of a previous pattern of domestic violence and psychological abuse. The exercise of power and control over their victims gives stalkers a sense of power and self-esteem that they otherwise lack. These individuals often relentlessly pursue and are fixated on the object of their affection. They imagine that their feelings are reciprocated. The psychological disorder erotomania is defined as this type of obsessive preoccupation with another, very often a celebrity figure, who becomes the object of the stalking behavior. Erotomaniacs are delusional and virtually all of them suffer from mental disorders—often schizophrenia.
2. Vengeance/terrorism stalking is fundamentally different from the other types of stalking. Vengeance stalkers do not seek a personal relationship with their targets. Rather, they attempt to elicit a particular response or a change of behavior from their victims. Although vengeance is their primary motive, these stalkers seek to punish their victims for some wrong they perceive the victims have caused them.
3. Love obsession stalking involves stalkers who seek to establish a personal relationship with the object of their obsession—contrary to the wishes of their victims. Love obsession stalkers tend to have low self-esteem and often target victims they perceive to have exceptional qualities and high social standing. These stalkers seek to raise their own self-esteem by associating with those whom they hold in high regard (9).

Victims who are pursued and harassed by stalkers experience a wide range of reactions, including loss of sleep, weight loss, depression, anxiety, and difficulty concentrating. Stalking victims represent a category that deserves not only study but also programs that offer safety and relief from this menacing criminal behavior.

ELDERLY CRIME VICTIMS

Winter is on my head, but eternal Spring is in my heart: I breathe at this hour the fragrance of the lilacs and violets, as at twenty years ago. The nearer I approach the end the plainer I hear around me the immortal symphonies of the heavenly chorus that waits to welcome me.

—*Victor Hugo, French novelist, 1802–1885*

Old age is often thought of as a time of loss and separation. Physical abilities, eyesight, hearing, agility, memory, and health can become diminished or lost. Loss also occurs through the death of friends, the abandonment of activities, and physical limitations. Pipher (51) likened being elderly to living in another country, where the terrain and the language are different, a country that provides little escape from violence and crime. Old age brings almost a natural reliance on support from others in new and different ways. Roles become reversed: children become parents, and parents become childlike in their need for protection and care.

Victimization of the elderly includes sexual assault, domestic violence, physical assault, homicide, burglary, and fraud. Elderly victims are particularly vulnerable in their limited ability to endure the aftermath of the crime if they do indeed survive the crime event. Their vulnerability is not only the result of physical and mental considerations but also the result of living in a time and place where beliefs and values were vastly different from those of the present day.

People born early in the 20th century were taught to keep their feelings to themselves. For example, most World War II veterans do not talk about their wartime experiences. They were shell shocked and did not necessarily understand their own psychological states. They also thought that their friends and families would not want to hear the truth (51). The importance placed on privacy and independence by elderly people, as well as their attitudes toward gender roles and sexual relations, is sometimes evident in their response to victimization. Sexual assault victims in particular are extremely reluctant to report the assault, and most express strong reluctance about family members being made aware of the nature of the assault. They need help in understanding the ramifications of the crime and in accepting the help that is available.

Victims of fraud admit shame and humiliation at being "taken in" at their age by unscrupulous criminals. When marriages/relationships between elders become violent for the first time, the victim is fearful of both the violence and the discovery of the violence by their children or other intervening agents. This fear is often predicated on retaliation by the abuser, loss of support, or loss of the relationship with the abuser. When the abuser is the child of the elderly victim, the parent may feel shame and guilt at having raised an abusive child. An elderly relative of a homicide victim can be greatly affected by the crime. The typical reactions to death by homicide are magnified for the elderly. Their attempts to comprehend the criminal justice process, media attention on the crime, limited support systems, and resulting physical, emotional, behavioral, and cognitive reactions combine to create an overwhelming circumstance for the elderly relative of a homicide victim.

The elderly have more exposure to the medical profession than do younger people. Theirs is a world of frequent medical considerations, balancing doctor appointments and securing prescriptions. Members of the elderly population tend to regard physicians highly and may not likely admit to abuse for fear of judgment. On the other hand, some patients may be willing to disclose on the basis of trust. Whatever the circumstances, abuse must be differentiated from the normal aging process. For example, the elderly are naturally more likely to lose their balance and fall, more likely to suffer skeletal fractures and bleed, and more likely to experience poor vision, mental confusion, bruising, and stiffness. These conditions can also be indications of abuse. The health care provider is crucial in the recognition of abuse and can therefore make a significant difference in the quality of life for elderly victims of crime.

Consider

Ruth, a 79-year-old retired teacher, was recovering from a stroke that left her partially paralyzed. After making excellent progress and regaining some normal functioning of her legs and speech, Ruth was released from the hospital and moved in with her daughter, Jane, a registered nurse. Jane was skilled in balancing her career with caring for her mother. She engaged a number of family members, friends, and home companions to help with Ruth's care. After years of independent living, driving her own vehicle, and managing her own affairs, Ruth was now totally reliant on Jane. But she was spirited and anxious to recover, and Jane's roster of helpers worked well. Frank, Ruth's nephew, volunteered to sit with her on Tuesday nights while Jane attended choir rehearsal. During those evenings, Frank began to sexually assault Ruth. It started with inappropriate touching under the guise of helping her get in and out of bed. He put sleeping pills in her nightly drink. After she was asleep, he removed her clothing and engaged in fondling and masturbation. When Jane returned home, her mother was always sleeping soundly. Jane assumed that all was well and proclaimed the offending nephew as her best sitter.

Three months later, Jane became aware of the abuse. Ruth became withdrawn and depressed. In contrast to her early enthusiasm to regain her physical functioning, she now had little to no interest in her therapy. She was tearful and frightened when Jane was away from the house and became hysterical when Jane was preparing to leave on Tuesday nights. At the same time,

Jane was becoming concerned about the deep sleeping episodes, which transpired only after Frank's watch. Jane questioned Ruth about Frank's visits and discovered that Ruth had some awareness of his activities but was afraid to address the issue with her daughter. She was able to tell Jane that she was not entirely asleep on occasion and was aware that Frank was touching her body and himself. Ruth also expressed how concerned she was that Frank's behavior be kept a secret. Jane promptly dismissed Frank without explanation. Ruth's excessive sleeping ceased. Jane did not confront Frank directly; however, she did consult Adult Protective Services and Victim Services about her discoveries. The situation ended with Frank's banishment from the family; Jane was not willing to follow through with any real investigation of the behavior. She has become an advocate for the elderly and tells her story to help others become aware of exploitation and victimization.

The Aftermath of Domestic Violence Against the Elderly

All too often, as with crimes against children, crimes against the elderly are underreported and, even when there are convictions, the sentences are light. Elderly victims have extreme difficulty in recovering from the disruptiveness of a crime. When the crime involves a family member, the burden is magnified by the betrayal. Elderly victims sometimes have limited mobility and require special transportation. Their financial resources tend to be limited, which influences their ability to recover from the ravages of victimization. Most elderly people spend a great deal of time in their homes, which is where they are most often victimized by exploitation, caregiver abuse, or sexual assault. Elderly victims may not have the opportunity to engage in the criminal justice process because of their diminished capacities.

Brown (13) summarized the concerns held by elderly people who have become increasingly dependent on others and who are threatened with or have become victims of abuse:

- Fear of retaliation (applies to abuse by a relative or an institution)
- Fear of relocation
- Fear of senility
- Fear of death
- Fear of becoming a burden
- Embarrassment about being abused by a relative/child
- Fear of having to go to court
- Fear of institutionalization
- Fear of further abuse or death
- Fear of having food or medication withheld

Forms of Domestic Violence Against the Elderly

The following definitions of abuse, neglect, and exploitation pertain to elders living in domestic settings (where most crimes against the elder transpire):

Physical abuse is the use of force that may result in bodily injury, physical pain, or impairment. It may include striking (with or without an object), hitting, beating, pushing, shoving, shaking, slapping, kicking, pinching, and burning. The inappropriate use of drugs and physical restraints, force feeding, and physical punishment of any kind are also examples of physical abuse.

Signs and symptoms of physical abuse include the following:

- Bruises, black eyes, welts, lacerations, and rope marks
- Bone and skull fractures
- Open wounds, cuts, punctures, and untreated injuries; injuries in various stages of healing
- Sprains, dislocations, and internal injuries
- Broken eyeglasses, physical signs of punishment, and signs of being restrained
- Laboratory findings of medication overdose or underutilization of prescribed drugs
- An elder's report of being hit, slapped, kicked, or mistreated
- An elder's sudden change in behavior
- The caregiver's refusal to allow visitors to see an elder

Sexual abuse is nonconsensual sexual contact of any kind. Sexual contact with a person incapable of giving consent is also considered sexual abuse. It includes unwanted touching, all types of sexual assault or battery such as rape and sodomy, coerced nudity, and sexually explicit photographing.

Signs and symptoms of sexual abuse include the following:

- Bruises around the breasts or genital area
- Unexplained venereal disease or genital infections
- Unexplained vaginal or anal bleeding
- Torn, stained, or bloody underclothing
- An elder's report of being sexually assaulted or raped

Emotional or psychological abuse refers to the infliction of anguish, pain, or distress through verbal or nonverbal acts. Emotional/psychological abuse includes verbal insults, threats, intimidation, humiliations, and harassment. Other examples are treating an older person like an infant; isolating an elderly person from his or her family, friends, or regular activities; giving an older person the "silent treatment"; and enforcing social isolation.

Signs and symptoms of emotional/psychological abuse may manifest in the following ways in an elderly person:

- Being emotionally upset or agitated
- Being extremely withdrawn, noncommunicative, or nonresponsive
- Exhibiting unusual behavior associated with dementia, such as sucking, biting, and rocking
- Reporting verbal or emotional mistreatment

Neglect refers to the refusal or failure to fulfill any part of a person's obligation or duties to the elder. Neglect may also involve a person who has a fiduciary responsibility to provide care to an elder (e.g., not paying for necessary home care services). Neglect typically means the refusal or failure to provide an elderly person with necessities such as food, water, clothing, shelter, personal hygiene, medicine, comfort, and safety.

The following are signs and symptoms of neglect:

- Dehydration, malnutrition, untreated bedsores, and poor personal hygiene
- Unattended or untreated health problems
- Hazardous or unsafe living conditions/arrangements (e.g., improper wiring, no heat, no running water)
- Unsanitary and unclean living conditions (e.g., dirt, fleas, lice, soiled bedding, fecal/urine smell, inadequate clothing)
- An elder's report of being mistreated

Financial or material exploitation refers to the illegal or improper use of an elder's funds, property, or assets. Examples include cashing an elderly person's checks without authorization or permission, forging an older person's signature, misusing or stealing an older person's money or possessions, coercing or deceiving an older person into signing any document (e.g., a contract or will), and improper use of guardianship or power of attorney.

Elderly Victims of Domestic Violence

Much of what is known about the older battered woman is anecdotal or drawn from practical wisdom. There are several patterns of domestic violence among the elderly:

- *"Spouse abuse grown old"*: the victims have been abused for most of their adult lives.
- *"Late-onset" cases*: the abuse begins late in life by partners who had not previously been abusive. This type of abuse seems to be associated with age-related conditions or stresses, including retirement, dependency, changing patterns in relationships, or sexual dysfunction.

■ *Entering abusive relationships late in life*: the abuser is frequently the victim's second or third spouse or intimate partner. In many instances, financial gain through financial abuse accompanies the physical abuse.

■ Situations in which elderly women who were battered earlier in their lives by their husbands (or who abused their children) are battered by their sons and daughters (9).

Many situations of abuse are unreported as a result of elderly victims being unable to ask for help or having no one to tell because of isolation. Health care providers are the gateway to ending the neglect and abuse of our oldest citizens.

Recommendations for Health Care Providers

1. Make the identification of elder abuse and neglect a priority. Work with other community agents to ensure that communication and understanding are paramount in terms of the health and safety of the elderly. Participate in partnerships, coalitions, and boards to facilitate support, understanding, and knowledge about issues and concerns related to the elderly. Familiarize yourself with Triad, Association for the Advancement of Retired Persons, Adult Protective Services, Area Agency on Aging, and other organizations that assist the elderly.
2. Provide public education on guidelines for detecting symptoms of abuse and neglect, as well as diagnosis, treatment, referral, and reporting for health and safety purposes.
3. Create specialized units to establish protocols for early detection of abuse in order to ensure patient safety as well as aid in the active investigation and prosecution of the abuser.
4. Provide scientific and medical evidence to help in the prosecution of the perpetrators of crimes against the elderly.
5. Ensure that health care professionals are knowledgeable about local and national resources that provide services to the elderly.
6. Establish reciprocal referral systems among victim service providers, social service counselors, mental health professionals, and criminal justice agents.
7. Establish training in the cultural diversity of elderly victims; stress the importance of awareness of ethnic and cultural differences.
8. Ensure that the elderly are assessed routinely for indications of abuse and neglect and that any signs or symptoms are documented in their medical records.

9. Provide continuing education about the consequences of victimization to the health care providers in the community who come into contact with elderly victims.
10. The health care community should provide specific training to victim service providers in the important role they can play in assisting victims.

CHILD VICTIMS

Just when I think I've outdistanced "it," the runner catches up again and comes alongside me to let me know that it has enough wind to keep on running and can overtake me anytime it wants to. It takes the time to rest and recharge, but I just keep on running.
—*An adult who was sexually abused as a child*
You are a child of the universe no less than the trees and the stars; you have a right to be here.
—*Max Ehrmann*, Desiderata, *1927*

Perhaps our nation's greatest scourge is the victimization of our most vulnerable population. Children are sexually abused, beaten, and murdered by their own family members at an alarming rate each year. When children are subjected to emotional abuse and neglect, experience the trauma associated with domestic violence, and deal with physical and sexual assault, they are forced to engage in a difficult, complex psychological aftermath. The same disturbing reactions of humiliation, shame, anger, low self-esteem, blame, and confusion as experienced by adult victims become a part of the child victim's world. Children should not have to cope with the magnitude of such emotions, particularly those related to sexual issues. Little girls and boys are not supposed to have venereal diseases. They are not supposed to satisfy the crazed need of a demented mind. Children should not have to endure the pain of blows, kicks, choking, and burns. They should never have to be hungry, dirty, or maltreated in any context. Children are not supposed to grapple with devastating long-term effects, which continue to haunt their dreams.

The maltreatment of children has its origins in the historical premise that children were the property of their parents. As property, children could be sold into bondage, abused, married off at any age and to anyone the parents selected, abandoned, or murdered. There were no legal repercussions to offending parents. Sadly, this type of thinking and behavior remains in some cultures. However, all states have laws that require certain persons (i.e., teachers, doctors, social workers, police officers, and others) to report suspected abuse or neglect of children and adolescents.

Forms of Child Abuse

The National Victim Assistance Academy (4) defines the following types of child victimization:

Physical abuse is most often classified as a nonaccidental injury inflicted by a parent or caregiver to a child younger than 18. This type of abuse occurs when a parent willfully injures a child or allows a child to be injured, tortured, or maimed out of cruelty or as excessive punishment.

Mental health professionals recognize *emotional abuse* and *emotional neglect* as two forms of emotional maltreatment of children. The former consists of a chronic pattern of behavior in which the child is typically belittled, denied love to promote specific behavior, marginalized from siblings, or subjected to extreme and inappropriate punishments. The latter is characterized by the failure to provide a child with appropriate support, attention, and affection. Occurring alone or coupled with other forms of abuse, emotional maltreatment can impair the psychological growth and the emotional development of the child.

Acquaintance perpetrators, such as family friends, neighbors, teachers, coaches, religious leaders, and peers, will normally win the confidence of the child through affiliation with the family or community. They tend to prey on children with low self-esteem and those who are unsupervised. Perpetrators who command positions of respect because of their positions in community affairs, such as church, and civic and business affiliations, are more likely to intimidate or threaten the child once sexual abuse has occurred. There has been a marked increase in the number of juvenile perpetrators committing sexual abuse.

Sexual abuse is the exploitation of a child or adolescent for another person's sexual and psychological gratification. Family members, trusted friends, acquaintances, community program personnel, day care workers, and other paid caregivers, as well as strangers are known perpetrators. Child sexual abuse ranges from oral and genital stimulation and penetration to voyeurism and the involvement of a child in prostitution or the production of pornography.

Intrafamilial sexual abuse is committed most often by an individual known to the child. The abuser can be a blood relative who is part of the nuclear family or a surrogate parent such as a live-in companion or stepparent. Older siblings are frequently responsible for child sexual abuse. The family will likely be dysfunctional in other areas and may have been destabilized by alcohol and substance abuse or severe spousal discord with a history of physical violence.

Stranger sexual abuse, frequently referred to as pedophilia (although the term describes any individual who has a sexual preference for children), is by far the most publicized form of child sexual abuse but constitutes only 10% of all reported cases. There is no evidence that perpetrators choose child victims on the basis of race, but there is increased victimization of children of lower socioeconomic groups.

On-line sexual predators, a new breed of child abusers, have entered the picture as a result of children's increased and often unsupervised recreational use of the Internet. Investigations of computer sex offenders demonstrate that on-line sexual predators roam chat rooms and post sexually explicit material on the Internet to make contact with young children and teenagers. Victimization may be indirect and limited to showing a child pornographic sites to initiate sexually overt conversation in a chat room, by e-mail, or by instant messages.

Consider

Kelley is 40 now, but she can still hear Uncle Bruce pleading to her when she was 8 years old. He was left in charge of Kelley and her baby sister, Katy, when their parents made occasional trips away from home. Uncle Bruce was single and only 21 years old, but to Kelley he seemed ancient. It started with Uncle Bruce bouncing her on his knee and tickling her until she nearly wet her pants. It was so much fun, and even her parents enjoyed watching Uncle Bruce entertain Kelley. One day while bouncing on Bruce's knee, Kelley felt his hands touch her between her legs. She was not sure she had felt that sudden shift in his attention to her body, but when the touch returned, she knew. She also knew there was something different, dark, but pleasant about the touch. It was compelling and then it stopped as abruptly as it started. Uncle Bruce left and Kelley did not see him for a while, but when he returned Kelley was anxious to start the games and curious about the strange touch. It came again, but this time it was more directed and rhythmic. Uncle Bruce was stroking her between her legs and telling her how wonderful it was and how he thought she was the most beautiful little girl in the world. Although the abuse ended when Kelley reached 13, the secret is still alive.

The Aftermath of Child Abuse

The concerns of abused children have been summarized by Brown (13):

- Inability to trust others
- Removal from home or removal of offender
- Guilt, shame, and stigma

- Disclosure
- Loss of family/friends
- Healing from physical/sexual injuries
- Misunderstanding of what is happening emotionally
- Helplessness, lack of control

When adults betray children by shepherding them into negative behavior, the children suffer long-term reactions to the experience. Guilt and shame coupled with humiliation are feelings that seem to accompany this type of victimization. The child can be overwhelmed by feelings of anger, generally self-directed. In addition, sexually abused children may sexually abuse younger children. When there is no avenue for disclosing the abuse, children are forced to compartmentalize the event. Sometimes they become preoccupied with sexual activities and engage in sexual acting out. Young children who become victims of sexual abuse are vulnerable and have little or no knowledge about STDs. They may recognize that the sexual behavior is inappropriate but have difficulty in processing the magnitude of the episode. The sexual arousal can be pleasant yet embedded in a blanket of ill feelings that cling, confuse, and harm them. Sexually abused children may experience nightmares, hostile behavior, changes in eating habits, and changes in school performance, including radical improvement in grades (overachieving) (13). Medical systems must be positioned to recognize the symptoms of child sexual assault.

Recommendations for Health Care Providers

Many of the following recommendations from *New Directions from the Field: Victims' Rights and Services for the 21st Century* (34) are now in effect throughout the nation. The information presented in *New Directions*, representing the collective thinking of several programs, is offered here in broad terms to serve as a guide for instituting programs and protocols for action:

1. Communities should establish children's advocacy centers to provide child-friendly locations where abused children can receive the services they need to heal and to provide information for the evaluation and investigation of their cases. To ensure the highest quality of intervention, training should be provided to professionals in conducting forensic interviews, to medical professionals in conducting child abuse examinations, and to mental health professionals in employing abuse-specific treatment approaches.

2. Children who witness violence should be given the same level of victim assistance and special protections within the criminal and juvenile systems as child victims.
3. To ensure that child abuse cases are recognized and reported as early as possible, training in the identification of signs of abuse, as well as the impact of child victimization, should be provided to all professionals who come into contact with child victims.
4. There should be improved governmental response to the problem of missing, abducted, and sexually exploited children.
5. All jurisdictions should establish or support "court preparation" programs to educate child victims and witnesses about the court process.
6. States should enact legislation to allow access to criminal history records, and they should adopt regulations and policies necessary to meet the requirements of the National Child Protection Act.
7. Early intervention programs, such as Head Start and Healthy Start, should be implemented nationwide. The staff of these programs must be trained in how to recognize the signs of child abuse, how to report abuse to appropriate authorities, and how to provide referrals for victims and their families.
8. Specially trained lawyers and court-appointed special advocates should be provided to children in all civil child protection and other abuse-related proceedings.
9. All states should consider alternatives to live in-court testimony for children younger than 18 years.
10. Federal and state governments should support the significant additional research that is needed to document effective treatments for child victims, especially victims of child sexual and physical abuse and children who witness violence.

Recommendations Specific to the Health Care Community

1. All professional schools that educate future health care professionals, including schools of medicine, nursing, social work, rehabilitation, hospital administration, and public health, should incorporate victim issues into their curricula.
2. All patients should be assessed routinely for indications of domestic abuse or other

history of violence. Any signs or symptoms of abuse should be documented in their medical records.

3. Hospitals should establish training programs and protocols for all hospital personnel about the rights and needs of victims of crime.

4. Medical facilities, including hospitals and rehabilitation and trauma centers, should serve as gateways to assist victims of crime. Response staff should be available in these settings to provide on-site crisis counseling and follow-up to patients and to serve as links to in-house and community resources.

5. Victims of sexual assault should be given emergency medical care, forensic examinations, and testing for HIV and STDs at no out-of-pocket cost and in a supportive setting. More hospitals should consider establishing SANE programs to respond sensitively to the needs of sexual assault victims.

6. Cultural competency guidelines should be developed to help health care providers improve screening and intervention services for victims from diverse backgrounds.

7. Medical personnel should be knowledgeable about statutory privacy protections and have policies that ensure that statutory privacy protections are applied to medical records, abuse reporting forms, and medicolegal evidence. They should respect the confidentiality and privacy needs of all victims of crime and assist them in dealing with unwanted media attention, especially in cases of sexual assault and assaults on children.

8. Counseling and prevention programs and/or a referral system to such programs should be established in medical facilities that treat violence-related injury, including gunshot victims, to address the broad spectrum of needs of these victims.

9. Protocols for appropriate security and safety procedures should be developed to assist hospital personnel in responding to gang, family, and other violence that might result in staff victimization.

10. Pediatricians, emergency physicians, family practitioners, internists, and other health care professionals treating young children should be educated about the effects that witnessing domestic violence and violence in the community will have on children.

11. Technology should be utilized to improve medical services to crime victims, especially in underserved and rural areas.

12. All health care professionals should be educated about sensitive techniques for notification of death.

13. Statutes and policies should be adopted to prevent insurance companies from discriminating against victims of crime by denying and/or canceling coverage or by charging higher premiums for such coverage.

14. Victims with catastrophic physical injuries, including survivors of assaults and crashes caused by drunk drivers, should receive specialized neuropsychologic evaluation in health care facilities.

Major challenges have been placed on our response systems through recommendations from the field, as outlined in *New Directions from the Field: Victims' Rights and Services for the 21st Century* (34). This excellent compilation of data collected from the field of victim service provision over a 20-year period offers five global challenges from the field of victim assistance to our total response systems:

1. To enact and enforce consistent, fundamental rights for crime victims in federal, state, juvenile, military, and tribal justice systems and administrative proceedings.

2. To provide crime victims with access to comprehensive, high-quality services regardless of the nature of their victimization, age, race, religion, gender, ethnicity, sexual orientation, capability, or geographic location.

3. To integrate crime victims' issues into all levels of the nation's educational system to ensure that justice and allied professionals and other service providers receive comprehensive training in victims' issues as part of their academic education and continuing training in the field.

4. To support, improve, and replicate promising practices in victims' rights and services built on sound research, advanced technology, and multidisciplinary partnerships.

5. To ensure that the voices of victims of crime play a central role in the nation's response to violence and those victimized by crime.

Implicit in each of the challenges is the need for the health care community to emerge as the frontline player.

ACKNOWLEDGMENT

The author thanks Connie J. Kirkland, MA, Director of Sexual Assault Services at George Mason University in Fairfax, Virginia, for reviewing the manuscript and providing valuable insights and updates.

REFERENCES

1. Matsakis A. *I can't get over it: a handbook for trauma survivors.* Oakland, CA: Harbinger Publications, 1996:17.

2. American College of Emergency Physicians. *Domestic violence fact sheet*. Dallas, TX: American College of Emergency Physicians, June 2003. Available at www.acep.org/webportal/PatientsConsumers/HealthSubjectsByTopic/Violence/FactSheetDomesticViolence.htm. Accessed on February 17, 2006.

3. Corey G. *Theory and practice of counseling and psychotherapy*. Belmount, CA: Brooks/Cole, 1991:110.

4. Whitcomb D, Hook M, Alexander E. Child victimization. In: Seymour A, Morray M, Sigmon J, et al. eds. *National victim assistance academy*, Chapter 11. Washington, DC: U.S. Department of Justice, Office for Victims of Crime, 2002.

5. Finkel MA. Technical conduct of the child sexual abuse medical examination. *Child Abuse Negl* 1998;22(6):555–566.

6. Schornstein S. *Domestic violence and health care: what every professional needs to know*. Thousand Oaks, CA: Sage Publications, 1997.

7. McAfee RE. Physicians and domestic violence. Can we make a difference? [editorial]. *JAMA* 1995;273(22):1790–1791.

8. Kilpatrick DG, Resnick HS, Saunders BE. Rape, other violence against women, and posttraumatic stress disorder: critical issues in assessing the adversity—stress—psychopathology relationship In: Dohrenwend BP, ed. *Adversity, stress, and psychopathology*. New York: Oxford University Press, 1998:161–176.

9. Gilligan J. *Violence: reflections on a national epidemic*. New York: Vintage Books, 1997.

10. Douglas J, Olshaker M. *The anatomy of motive*. New York: Scribner, 1999.

11. Raine NV. *After silence: rape and my journey back*. New York: Crown Publishers, 1998.

12. Burgess AW, Holmstrom LL. Rape trauma syndrome. *Am J Psychiatry* 1974;131(9):981–986.

13. Brown SL. *Counseling victims of violence*. Alexandria, VA: American Association for Counseling and Development, 1991.

14. Kilpatrick DG, Whalley A, Edmunds C. Sexual assault. In: Seymour A, Morray M, Sigmon J, et al., eds. *National victim assistance academy*, chapter 10. Washington, DC: U.S. Department of Justice, Office for Victims of Crime, 2002.

15. Epstein J, Langenbahn S. *The criminal justice and community response to rape*. Washington, DC: U.S. Department of Justice, National Institute of Justice, 1994.

16. Rentoul L, Appleboom N. Understanding the psychological impact of rape and serious sexual assault of men: a literature review. *J Psychiatr Ment Health Nurs* 1997;4(4):267–274.

17. Walker J, Archer J, Davies M. Effects of rape on men: a descriptive analysis. *Arch Sex Behav* 2005;34(1):69–80.

18. Read KM, Kufera JA, Jackson MC, et al. Population-based study of police-reported sexual assault in Baltimore, Maryland. *Am J Emerg Med* 2005;23(3):273–278.

19. Sugar NF, Fine DN, Eckert LO. Physical injury after sexual assault: findings of a large case series. *Am J Obstet Gynecol* 2004;190(1):71–76.

20. National Institute of Justice. *Extent, Nature, and Consequences of Rape Victimization: Findings from the National Violence Against Women Survey*. Special Report from the National Institute of Justice., Washington, DC: U.S. Department of Justice, Office of Justice Programs, January 2006.

21. Kilpatrick DJ, Edmunds CN, Seymour A. *Rape in America: a report to the nation*. Arlington, VA: National Victim Center, 1992.

22. Sexual Assault Crisis Centers in Virginia. *Annual summary of services*. Charlottesville, VA: Virginians Aligned Against Sexual Assault, 2002.

23. Virginia Department of Health. *Prevalence of sexual assault in Virginia*. Richmond, VA: Virginia Department of Health, 2003.

24. Fisher B, Cullen F, Turner M. *Sexual victimization of college women (NCJ 182369)*. Washington, DC: U.S. Department of Justice, Office of Justice Programs, 2000.

25. VAASA Fact Sheet. *Marital sexual assault: the law and your rights*. Charlottesville, VA: Virginians Aligned Against Sexual Assault, 2006. Available at http://www.vaasa.org/MaritalSA.pdf. Accessed on March 2, 2006.

26. Russell DEH. *Rape in a marriage*. Indianapolis: Indiana University Press, 1990.

27. Campbell JC. Women's responses to sexual abuse in intimate relationships. *Health Care Women Int* 1989;10:335–346.

28. Carosella C. *Who's afraid of the dark? a forum of truth, support, and assurance for those affected by rape*. New York: HarperCollins, 1995.

29. Ringel C. *Criminal victimization in 1996, changes 1995–1996 with trends 1993–1996*. Washington, DC: U.S. Department of Justice, Bureau of Justice Statistics, 1997.

30. Tjaden P, Thoennes N. Prevalence, incidence, and consequences of violence against women: findings from the National Violence Against Women Survey. In: *Research in brief*. Washington, DC: U.S. Department of Justice, National Institute of Justice, November 1998.

31. Perkins C. *Age patterns of victims of serious crimes*. Washington, DC: U.S. Department of Justice, Bureau of Justice Statistics, September 1997.

32. Ruffino NC. *Managing diversity: people skills for a multicultural workplace*. Lawrence, KY: Thomson Executive Press, 1995.

33. National Survey of Family Growth. *Sexual behavior and selected health measures: men and women 15–44 years of age, United States, 2002*. Hyattsville, MD: Centers for Disease Control and Prevention, 2002. Available at http://www.cdc.gov/nchs/nsfg.htm. Accessed on January 10, 2006.

34. Office for Victims of Crime. *New directions from the field: victims' rights and services for the 21st century*. Washington, DC: U.S. Department of Justice, 1999.

35. Gazmararian JA, Lazorick S, Spitz AM, et al. Prevalence of violence against pregnant women. *JAMA* 1996;275(24):1915–1920.

36. Parker B, McFarlane J, Soeken K. Abuse during pregnancy: effects on maternal complications and birth weight in adult and teenage women. *Obstet Gynecol* 1994;84(3):323–328.

37. Campbell JC, Pugh LC, Campbell D, et al. The influence of abuse on pregnancy intention. *Women's Health Issues* 1995;5(4):214–223.

38. Campbell JC, Humphreys J. *Nursing care of survivors of family violence*. St. Louis: Mosby, 1993.

39. American Psychiatric Association. *Diagnostic and statistical manual of mental disorders: DSM-IV*. Washington, DC: American Psychiatric Association, 1994.

40. Snipe B, Hall EJ. *I am not your victim*. Thousand Oaks, CA: Sage Publications, 1996.

41. Carlson B. Adolescent observers of marital violence. *J Fam Violence* 1990;5:285–299.

42. Stark E, Flitcraft A. Woman-battering, child abuse and social heredity: what is the relationship? In: Johnson N, ed. *Marital violence*, London: Routledge and Kegan, 1985.

43. Cappell C, Heiner RB. The intergenerational transmission of family aggression. *J Fam Violence* 1990;5:135–152.

44. Advocacy for Women and Kids in Emergencies. Available at http://www.child-protection.org/CPT/Providers/AWAKE.pdf. Accessed on January 11, 2006.

45. Wallace H, Seymour A. Domestic violence In: Coleman G, Gaboury M, Murray M, et al., eds. *National victim assistance academy*, Chapter 8. Washington, DC: U.S. Department of Justice, Office for Victims of Crime, 1999.

46. Salber PR, Taliaferro E. *The physician's guide to domestic violence*. Volcano, CA: Volcano Press, 1995.

47. Littel K. *Family violence: an intervention model for dental professionals*. OVC Bulletin, December 2004. Available at http://www.ovc.gov/publications/bulletins/dentalproviders/ncj204004.pdf. Accessed on January 11, 2006.

48. The American College of Obstetricians and Gynecologists. *Women's issues*. Washington, DC: The American College of Obstetricians and Gynecologists, Available at www.org/navbar/current/womensIssues.cfm. Accessed on January 11, 2006.

49. The American College of Obstetricians and Gynecologists. Special Issues in *Women's health*. Washington, DC: The American College of Obstetricians and Gynecologists, 2006.

50. Tjaden P, Thoennes N. *Extent, nature, and consequences of intimate partner violence*. Washington, DC: U.S. Department of Justice, National Institute of Justice, NCJ 181867, July 2000. Available at http://www.ncjrs.gov/pdffiles1/nij/181867.pdf. Accessed on January 11, 2006.

51. Pipher M. *Another country: navigating the emotional terrain of our elders*. New York: Penguin Putnam, 1999.

3

■ PEGGY L. JOHNSON
■ JOHN S. O'BRIEN, II

FORENSIC MEDICAL INTERVIEWING

Medical interviewing serves as the cornerstone for the performance of medical evaluations and the formulation of treatment plans. The patient's medical history serves as the background and context within which the presenting clinical complaints have arisen. When undertaken in a thorough and comprehensive fashion, the history provides a rich source of clinical information that can be of major assistance in the diagnosis and treatment of medical, surgical, and psychiatric conditions. The medical interview and history, correlated with findings on examination, assist with the diagnostic process and often serve as the primary factor in the formulation of directions for further clinical workup. This combined information is also useful for following a patient's clinical response to treatment.

The format of medical interviewing and general medical history taking is directly applicable to evaluations occurring in emergency departments and in forensic contexts. The overall format includes documentation of the patient's clinical complaint, usually in his or her own language, followed by a history of present illness, a review of medical history, family and social history, and a review of systems. An overview of general medical interviewing and history taking appears in Table 3-1. This structure is always useful as the basic outline for case assessment, documentation, and case presentation in emergency departments and all other clinical/medical settings. It serves as a structured approach to data gathering, focusing on a chief complaint for the purposes of diagnosis and treatment. It is also useful for documentation in medicolegal contexts. In the clinical/medical context, clear and structured documentation is useful to carry out the essential function of medical records—serving as a communications device that summarizes clinically relevant information that permits subsequent caregivers, who may not have direct contact with one another, to collaborate efficiently and effectively. In a medicolegal context, structured, thorough documentation is useful for the documentation of clinical presentation, diagnosis, and management; demonstration explicitly or implicitly of the rationale underlying clinical conclusions and diagnoses; and the recording of therapeutic interventions undertaken in response to the clinical conclusions and diagnoses, as well as the patient's response to them.

Medical interviewing or history taking in an emergency department is essentially the same as general medical interviewing and history taking, except that it is more focused on the chief complaint and the patient's immediate needs for evaluation and treatment. Documentation tends to focus primarily on pertinent positives and negatives, both historically and on examination. The interview and documentation are oriented around an evaluation of the patient's urgent clinical needs and the initiation of lifesaving and/or immediate appropriate treatment. An additional purpose is triage of patients for referral for outpatient follow-up or subspecialty evaluation and further treatment. Clinical/medical documentation in the emergency department is essential for communication about

TABLE 3-1

MEDICAL INTERVIEWING AND HISTORY TAKING

1. General medical interviewing—history taking
2. Chief or presenting complaint—"patient's own words"
3. History of present illness
4. Medical history
   a. Medical
   b. Surgical
   c. Psychiatric
   d. Substance abuse
   e. Trauma
5. Family history
   a. Medical
   b. Surgical
   c. Psychiatric
   d. Substance abuse
6. Social history
   a. Life circumstances
   b. Habits, for example, drugs or alcohol (see medical history)
7. Risk exposure
   a. Interpersonal
   b. Vocational
   c. Avocational/recreational
8. Review of systems

the patient's chief complaint, pertinent history, and clinical presentation to subsequent clinicians for the purpose of facilitating further evaluation and management. These clinicians either function as part of the emergency care team or provide care for the patient following treatment and release from the emergency department. Medicolegally, the emergency department record is a useful retrospective source of information that summarizes the patient's history and clinical presentation, the diagnoses or conclusions drawn about the patient, and the treatment initiated or triage undertaken for further evaluation and follow-up. Retrospective medicolegal assessment of the record often focuses on the conclusions drawn, the treatment provided, and the rationale for both and seeks to legally establish "facts" based on what is documented in the record. It also allows assessment of the appropriateness of clinical conclusions drawn and of subsequent treatment sought by the patient after emergency department evaluation.

Forensic medical interviewing/history taking is essentially the same as general medical interviewing/history taking. It includes the consideration of clinical and legal issues defined by the context in which the interview or history is taken and the nature of the legal issues being considered. Such interviewing and history taking has a variety of purposes, such as evaluating the patient's clinical presentation; arriving at a diagnosis or an explanation of the presentation; recommending treatment; establishing a record of the evaluation and the conclusions drawn as future evidence, which may be useful in a legal proceeding; and preserving observations and findings for future reference in legal contexts.

Perhaps the most significant difference between forensic medical interviewing/history taking and general medical or emergency medical interviewing/history taking is the attention to documentation that is necessary. The documentation must be as objective and detailed as possible, including observations of and conversations with the patient. It should be primarily data oriented and include only those conclusions or explanations that are based soundly on the data collected both historically and clinically. Forensic medical records should also be written in a way that avoids rendering legal conclusions or definitive opinions that are the province of a legal fact finder. The clinician should thoroughly document the patient's history, general observations of the patient, and the results of the clinical examination. The clinician can draw clinical conclusions and can express an opinion that those conclusions are consistent with a particular cause, without arriving at a conclusion with factual certainty. This approach allows the cause to be determined factually in a legal context later, following consideration of all the evidence, which is often not known or understood by the clinician at the time of the evaluation. The clinician may also make appropriate referrals for follow-up treatment and other support services based on clinical conclusions consistent with a particular cause, without arriving at a definitive conclusion about the cause of the clinical presentation.

Treating patients in emergency departments often involves an evaluation of clinical complaints that have medicolegal significance, either at the time of presentation or later. Most patients who present as victims of violence or abuse have immediate medicolegal involvement, and patients who were injured in accidents may be involved in subsequent litigation focusing on the injuries they sustained. Therefore, a large proportion of cases seen in emergency departments may ultimately have medicolegal significance. Preparation of the emergency department record with an awareness of its medicolegal significance may be extremely helpful to the patient, who may be involved in litigation later, and to the clinician, who may be called on to testify retrospectively and who may need to rely on the record as the primary source of information during the testimony. Frequently, this testimony is requested after a significant time has passed since the emergency visit.

Although there may appear to be tension between the necessity to evaluate, treat, and triage patients in an emergency department and to document that process efficiently and the necessity to generate a comprehensive and informative medical record for medicolegal purposes, the two necessities are not incompatible. The approach to documentation must be flexible enough to permit the addition of more extensive information when it is both clinically and medicolegally indicated. In this manner, the patient's narrative and/or the clinician's observations of the patient's demeanor and behavior, and other potentially relevant medicolegal information, can be included in the emergency department documentation to assist a fact finder in assessing the clinical presentation and determining its cause in subsequent legal proceedings.

Underlying the process of performing clinical interviews and obtaining medical histories are interview techniques oriented to eliciting information from the patient for the purposes of diagnosis, treatment, and medicolegal documentation. Generally, medical interviewing techniques commence with open-ended or broad questioning and proceed to more focused or narrower questioning. The clinician attempts to elicit the patient's history in the patient's own narrative, which is very useful in the clinical evaluation of the presenting complaint and especially helpful in forensic contexts. Some patients are not communicative, for a variety of reasons, so the clinical history must be obtained from collateral sources. Those sources should be documented in the record in terms of both identity and content. If a patient is not communicative about his or her own history, the record should reflect that fact and should contain observations of the patient and an assessment of any clinical reasons for the inability to communicate. Furthermore, if the patient is conscious and alert but not communicative, collateral history is most appropriately obtained outside the patient's presence and documented as such to reduce the possibility that any subsequent communication by the patient was prompted or suggested by the collateral source. This is especially necessary if the patient is an awake but reticent or mute young child who may be developmentally susceptible to prompting, which can result in an inaccurate history.

A mental status examination or cognitive capacity screening examination should be done as part of the assessment of the potential clinical reasons for the patient's uncommunicativeness. These exams may also have clinical importance for the assessment of the patient's clinical presentation, diagnosis, and initiation of further workup, or appropriate treatment. When evaluating noncommunicative patients, observations of their behavior must be documented as thoroughly as possible. Such patients may never provide information regarding their history or circumstances, so behavioral observations and clinical findings documented in the record may be all that will be available for clinical evaluation and treatment and for future use in medicolegal contexts.

Victims of violence and abuse represent a variable but significant percentage of the patients who present to physicians' offices and emergency departments for clinical evaluation. As many as 3 million children have been reported to state agencies as victims of child abuse or neglect in single calendar years and approximately 900,000 of those referrals are substantiated (1). Approximately 10% to 15% of cases of child abuse are first reported by medical care providers (2).

Victims of violence and abuse presenting to emergency departments can be divided into four categories by age and by virtue of whether they are directly and reliably communicative: child noncommunicative, child communicative, adult noncommunicative, adult communicative. For communicative individuals, both children and adults, interviewing and history taking are largely based on the patient's narrative. Very young children (younger than 4 or 5 years) represent a special population whose narratives may not be credible or reliable. The narratives of very young children should be recorded and documented; however, historical information may also need to be derived from collateral sources, outside the presence of the child, to evaluate the young child's presenting complaint more thoroughly. For noncommunicative patients, information must be obtained from collateral sources. These sources should be identified in the record, along with careful observations of the patient and thorough documentation of the results of mental status or cognitive capacity screening examination for noncommunicativeness.

INTERVIEWING CHILDREN

Interviewing or obtaining a medical history from a communicative child relies largely on the patient's own description of his or her history and chief presenting complaints. A potentially significant issue when talking with a child is assessing credibility and reliability. Although definitions of child competency, as contained in statute and case law, vary somewhat among jurisdictions, reference to a general definition may be beneficial. Generally, competency consists of the ability to understand and answer questions intelligently and accurately; to provide truthful versions of an experience; and to understand the difference between right and wrong and truth and falsehood. Studies of child credibility focus on the influence of childhood development, on the content of the information provided, on the relationship between the content and the context in which the event occurred, and on subsequent statements about the event (3). One measure of a child's credibility is the stability of information provided and its unchanging nature over time. The stability of information must be placed in the psychological context of the child who provides it (4). In a study of children receiving therapy for sexual abuse, 75% initially denied the abuse and 22% recanted previous disclosures, whereas other studies indicate that most children maintain their claims of abuse and never deny them to officials once they are questioned (5). One clinically observed pattern of disclosure is that the child is initially silent, but allegations emerge once an adult becomes suspicious and questions the child. Upon questioning, the child may at first deny the allegations, but he or she subsequently discloses details because of weariness of the abuse or fear that something worse may happen. However, children will often not disclose the information because of shame, fear, or embarrassment or because they do not want to get into trouble (6).

There appears to be a general agreement that children younger than 3 years cannot be competent witnesses and that there is significant variability of competency among children between the ages of 3 and 5 years (7). The older the children, the more likely they will discuss child abuse and be reliable informants. Children older than 4 years make more disclosures of abuse than nondisclosures or inconclusive disclosures, in comparison with 2- and 3-year-olds. Some studies suggest that allegation-blind interviewing techniques, requiring more patience and attentiveness to the child and fostering the development of better rapport, facilitate disclosure by the child (8). These techniques also appear to yield higher disclosure rates of abuse by children to interviewers unknown to them.

When interviewing a communicative child, it is best to begin with open-ended questions such as, "Why are you here today?" This type of questioning is not suggestive and thus allows the child to provide his or her own information instead of responding to prompts (2). However, some children do not respond to open-ended questioning. Younger children provide less information spontaneously during free recall or in response to open-ended prompts. At some point, directed questioning usually becomes necessary to elicit information about body touching, the circumstances of the abuse, and the identity of the abuser (9). Sternberg and colleagues showed that open-ended questions yielded longer and richer responses from child witnesses than direct, leading, or suggestive questions. An explanation for this difference is that open-ended questions probe recall memory, whereas focused questions probe recognition memory, which is more likely to elicit erroneous responses. Open-ended questions also yield more relevant and detailed information from children who have reported multiple incidents of abuse than from children who reported only one act of abuse (10). Some studies suggest that open-ended questions used in the introductory or report-building phase of the evaluation help the child become comfortable with the interviewer and with the interviewer's expectations of the child (11).

It may be necessary to pose two types of specific questions to children: questions that request particular information and questions that require only yes/no answers to confirm or disconfirm information posed to the child (12). Questions intended to elicit particular information do not suggest a predetermined answer, whereas yes/no questions provide the child with adult-generated information with which the child must agree or disagree. Questions requesting particular information are preferable, except for very young children, most of whom do not yet have the syntactic ability to form appropriate responses (12).

Some studies have examined the influence of leading and misleading questions on the accuracy of child reports about an event. For all age-groups, responses to leading questions were very accurate, but responses to misleading questions were less accurate (and extremely inaccurate from very young children) (13). Older children are more resistant to misleading questions. Younger children tend to agree with misleading questions, possibly because of their desire to comply with the authority figure asking the question. Furthermore, children presented with misleading information are more suggestible when a stranger provides the information. Children not presented with misleading questions are more likely to disclose both accurate and inaccurate information to their parents, as opposed to strangers. Children tend to be more suggestible when they perceive the interviewer to be authoritarian, intimidating, or unfriendly. They tend to comply with the interviewer when their knowledge of the event is limited, assuming the interviewer to be more knowledgeable (14). At a threshold age of about $4\frac{1}{2}$ years, childhood suggestibility decreases. Developmental advances in the ability of children to understand conflicting mental representations are accompanied by age-related declines in suggestibility among 3- to 5-year-olds. However, there appears to be some disagreement about the reasons for changes in the reliability of reporting between ages 3 and 5 years: some investigators point to developmental linguistic capability (15), whereas others attribute unreliability to feelings of discomfort about an emotional or painful situation, not to limited vocabulary or linguistic ability (16).

In general, the literature supports interviewing children in a minimally suggestive manner and in a setting that is comfortable and informal. Furthermore, it appears that allegation-blind interviewers fare better in terms of establishing rapport with children and minimizing the likelihood of leading or misleading with information obtained from collateral sources. There may, therefore, be clinical and forensic benefit to interviewing the communicative child first and then obtaining collateral information afterward, again preferably not in the child's presence. A child's suggestibility may also be reduced if the interviewer clarifies expectations and emphasizes the importance of telling the truth and admitting confusion over guessing. Furthermore, telling a child that repeated questions do not imply that the initial response was incorrect may minimize the child's tendency to change an answer (14).

Evaluating noncommunicative children presents significant challenges to the emergency department physician. Documentation of collateral information and of observations about the child during the physical examination is essential. Assessment of the reasons for the lack of communicativeness is clinically, and maybe forensically, appropriate and necessary. Mental retardation should be documented, as should the results of a cognitive capacity screening and/or mental status examination, if conducted. Intellectually or cognitively deficient children who may be victims of violence or abuse can be evaluated if they are not regarded as incompetent in a legal sense, and documentation of any history provided by them should be undertaken (17). A patient's silence during the interview may be completely unrelated to any mental disease or defect. A child may be attempting to collect his or her thoughts or decide whether or not to trust the interviewer. A child may fall silent because of the interviewer's insensitivity (18). Children with specific impairments of speech or hearing may require an evaluation utilizing nonverbal interview techniques, such as playing, drawing, or painting. Such approaches are usually the province of specialists trained in evaluating children with those deficiencies. Severely depressed children may not speak during interviews; however, they may become communicative later, after effective treatment has been initiated (19). If a child is exhibiting elective mutism, there is no universally successful method for eliciting verbal responses. The record may have to reflect observations of the child's appearance, demeanor, and behavior, as well as the results of the examination, and can document the child's mutism and the fact that all the history was obtained from collateral sources. Referral of the patient to a specialist trained in child interviewing may be necessary to conduct as thorough an examination as possible and avoid inappropriate and unproductive utilization of emergency department personnel.

Documentation of the evaluation of a noncommunicative child in an emergency department should include observations of the child and any clinically relevant information regarding the lack of communication, along with the physical examination. Collateral information obtained outside the child's presence should be documented, and observations made regarding the interaction of the child with the collateral source. The collateral source can be called on to comfort the child or to facilitate conversation between the clinician and the child if the child is communicative in the presence of the other person; however, the physician and the collateral source should be careful to avoid leading or prompting the child. Documentation should reflect the presence of the source and any observable effect that it has on the child.

INTERVIEWING ADULTS

Adult victims of violence can also be communicative or noncommunicative. A communicative adult is evaluated using his or her own narrative, relying on techniques that elicit a general medical history. The information should be documented, with consideration given to the medicolegal importance of the record generated. Open-ended interview techniques are generally favored; however, reticence can create a barrier to the free flow of information, particularly in situations of spousal abuse or other forms of intrafamilial violence. These circumstances may prompt the patient to avoid discussion or misrepresent the history underlying physical injuries. The patient's behavior and demeanor should be documented and correlated with the reported history of injury and the actual physical findings. It may be necessary to point out discrepancies between the verbal representation and the clinical findings as a means of sympathetically eliciting greater disclosure. However, such efforts may be met with resistance and might not be successful. In those instances, merely documenting the discrepancies between the patient's account and the physical findings and providing the patient with appropriate resources to discuss the possibility of familial violence may be all that is possible in an emergency department setting.

Some adults may appear to be communicative, but their communication is unreliable as a result of another clinical condition. Patients with delirium as a result of substance abuse or withdrawal and those with dementia may appear communicative but, on further questioning, are revealed to be incapable of providing accurate or useful information or clinical data. Again, the discrepancy between the patient's verbal report and any injuries or physical problems should be identified in the record, along with the clinician's observations of the individual and his or her performance on mental status or cognitive capacity screening examination. As with children, some noncommunicative adults whose mental status examination reveals depression may become more communicative after the initiation of treatment for the underlying depression.

More than 4 million Americans suffer from Alzheimer's disease, with variable but at times highly significant impairment in mental processing, comprehension, and communication. This group is at high risk for neglect and abuse. Some studies suggest that closed-ended questions are easier for this type of patient to answer [20], but other studies reveal no significant difference in the proportion of relevant responses among open, closed, and mixed types of questioning [21]. As patients' cognitive capacity screening examination scores decrease, the number of questions necessary to elicit a response increases and the proportion of relevant responses to open-ended questions decreases [21]. This highlights the need to further characterize the basis for impairment in communication with clinical examination and mental status and cognitive capacity screening examinations. The findings available from such examinations have diagnostic importance and help the clinician choose an interview strategy that will be most likely to elicit reliable information. In the emergency department, documentation of observations of the patient, objective data regarding his or her cognitive capabilities, as well as findings on physical examination may be all that can be accomplished in the evaluation of patients suspected to have been victims of violence or abuse. These patients should be referred to appropriate agencies for further evaluation and follow-up.

Patients with delusional ideations as part of their symptoms represent another particularly challenging group to assess for abuse. Their communication may be metaphoric or vague. Their description of violence or abuse may be part of a systematic delusional framework potentially leading to a tendency to dismiss the complaint. In the interview, neither challenging a delusion for its truthfulness nor pretending to believe delusional ideations is recommended. A more useful approach is to indicate that the interviewer understands the patient believes the delusion to be true [22]. As with any patient for whom there are questions regarding reliability, the acquisition and documentation of collateral information and objective findings on the physical exam are crucial.

SUMMARY

Clinical interviewing and history taking is a skill applicable in all clinical settings. Approaching

patients with a genuine sense of interest, and in a manner indicating they are being listened to, is highly beneficial to the establishment of trust and rapport. The subsequent elicitation of information about the patient is an invaluable tool for the evaluation, diagnosis, and initial clinical management and subsequent referral for treatment. Victims of violence or abuse require the same care and attention as other patients but may need additional intervention to soothe emotional upset and establish rapport and trust. The challenge for emergency department personnel is to undertake this process effectively in as time-efficient a manner as possible, but also in a manner that makes the patient feel as comfortable and as communicative as possible, given his or her age, emotional state, and concurrent medical, mental, or neurocognitive conditions.

A significant percentage of emergency medical intervention may have medicolegal significance in the future. Integral to the forensic aspects of emergency medical practice are patient interviews, the elicitation of medical and event histories, accurate and thorough documentation of that information, behavioral observations, and physical findings. Approaching the patient with an open mind, listening, documenting what is said, observing the patient, and documenting those observations are essential. Some patients present specific challenges. This chapter has suggested approaches intended to elicit as much reliable information as possible for the purposes of clinical assessment and forensic documentation. The goal is to generate a medical record that accurately and thoroughly reflects the patient's clinical presentation, emergency evaluation, and treatment, for future reference by other clinicians, and documents a descriptive snapshot of the patient for future reference and consideration during fact-finding in a legal context.

REFERENCES

1. National Clearinghouse on Child Abuse and Neglect Information. *Child maltreatment 2003: summary of key findings*. Washington, DC: National Clearinghouse on Child Abuse and Neglect Information, 2005. Available at http://nccanch.acf.hhs.gov/general/stats/index.cfm. Accessed on November 7, 2005.
2. Monk M. Interviewing suspected victims of child maltreatment in the emergency department. *J Emerg Nurs* 1998;24(2):31–34.
3. Von Klitzing K. Credibility examinations of children and adolescents on the question of sexual abuse. *Acta Paedopsychiatr* 1990;53:181–190.
4. Jáskiewicz-Obydzinska T, Czerederecka A. Psychological evaluation of changes in testimony given by sexually abused juveniles. In: Davies G, Wilson C, Lloyd-Bostock S, et al. eds. *Psychology, law, and criminal justice: international developments in research and practice*. Berlin, Germany: Walter de Gruyter, 1995:160–169.

5. Bruck M, Ceci SJ. The suggestibility of children's memory. *Annu Rev Psychol* 1999;50:419–439.

6. Kellogg ND, Hoffman TJ. Child sexual revictimization by multiple perpetrators. *Child Abuse Negl* 1997;21(10):953–964.

7. Lamb ME, Sternberg KJ, Esplin PW. Making children into competent witnesses: reaction to the amicus brief in re Michaels. *Psychol Public Policy Law* 1995;1(2):438–449.

8. Cantlon J, Payne G, Erbaugh C. Outcome-based practice: disclosure rates of child sexual abuse comparing allegation blind and allegation informed structured interviews. *Child Abuse Negl* 1996;20(11):1113–1120.

9. Faller KC. Interviewing children who may have been abused: a historical perspective and overview of controversies. *Child Maltreat* 1996;1(2):83–95.

10. Sternberg KJ, Lamb ME, Hershkowitz I, et al. The relation between investigative utterance types and the informativeness of child witnesses. *J Appl Dev Psychol* 1996;17:439–451.

11. Jones DPH. The influence of introductory style on children's ability to relay information in forensic interviews [editorial]. *Child Abuse Negl* 1997;21(11):1131–1132.

12. Peterson C, Biggs M. Interviewing children about trauma: problems with "specific" questions. *J Trauma Stress* 1997;10(2):279–290.

13. Greenstock J, Pipe M-E. Interviewing children about past events: the influence of peer support and misleading questions. *Child Abuse Negl* 1996;20(1):69–80.

14. Reed LD. Findings from research on children's suggestibility and implications for conducting child interviews. *Child Maltreat* 1996;1(2):105–120.

15. Aldridge M, Wood J. Talking about feelings: young children's ability to express emotions. *Child Abuse Negl* 1997;21(12):1221–1233.

16. Harris PL, Jones DPH. Commentary on "Talking about feelings" (Aldridge and Wood, 1997). *Child Abuse Negl* 1997;21(12):1217–1220.

17. Quinn KM. Competency to be a witness: a major child forensic issue. *Bull Am Acad Psychiatry Law* 1986;14(4):311–321.

18. Bates B. *A guide to physical examination and history taking*, 8th ed. Philadelphia, PA: JB Lippincott, 1991.

19. Baker P. *Clinical interviews with children and adolescents*. New York: WW Norton, 1990.

20. Tappen RM. Alzheimer's disease: communication techniques to facilitate perioperative care. *AORN J* 1991;54(6):1279–1286.

21. Tappen RM, Williams-Burgess C, Edelstein J, et al. Communicating with individuals with Alzheimer's disease: examination of recommended strategies. *Arch Psychiatry Nurse* 1997;11(5):249–256.

22. Kaplan HI, Sadock BJ. *Synopsis of psychiatry: behavioral science clinical psychiatry*, 9th ed. Baltimore, MD: Lippincott Williams & Wilkins, 2002:240–274.

FORENSIC EMERGENCY MEDICINE: PENETRATING TRAUMA

4

WILLIAM S. SMOCK ■

Forensic emergency medicine is the application of forensic medical knowledge and appropriate techniques to living patients in the emergency department. Patients with penetrating trauma will seek care in the emergency department; they are usually not victims of happenstance or accident, but of malice and intent at the hands of assailants. This phenomenon reflects a major change in our society's interactional dynamics. Given this new reality of our patient population, physicians must practice medicine—trauma medicine, in particular—in a new way, with attention to details heretofore overlooked. What was once considered confounding clutter that gets in the way of patient care (such as clothing and surface dirt) takes on a whole new significance when recognized for what it really is—evidence.

Traditionally, emergency physicians and nurses have been trained in the provision of emergency medical care without regard for forensic issues. In the process of providing patient care, critical evidence can be lost, discarded, or inadvertently washed away (1–12). Victims then lose access to information that can be of critical significance when criminal or civil proceedings arise secondary to their injuries (13,14).

ACKNOWLEDGING THE VOID

The earliest references in the US medical literature to the practice of forensic medicine on living patients in our country decry its absence (1,15). These articles were written by two forensic pathologists and pioneers in clinical forensic medicine, John Smialek, MD, and William Eckert, MD. In 1986, Cyril Wecht, MD, JD, former president of the American College of Legal Medicine, stated

> It's a great shame and a source of much puzzlement why a group similar to police surgeons hasn't developed here. Even within our adversarial judicial system and with our guaranteed civil rights—which are much greater than in many of the countries where forensic clinicians are commonly found—I believe those persons with both medical and forensic training could remove much of the guesswork, speculation, and hypotheses from the disposition of accident or assault cases involving living persons (10).

FILLING THE VOID

The first postgraduate training program for emergency physicians dealing with clinical forensic medicine was a 2-day seminar in Chicago in 1990, sponsored by the Illinois chapter of the American College of Emergency Physicians. This program was suspended after its first year. An annual postgraduate clinical forensic medicine training seminar was subsequently established in Louisville in 1994 by the Kentucky chapter of the American College of Emergency Physicians. This program continued through 1998.

The Department of Emergency Medicine at the University of Louisville School of Medicine and the Kentucky Medical Examiner's Office established the first formal clinical forensic medicine training program for residents in the United States in 1991 (3,4,9,11,16). Two years later, the first fellowship in clinical forensic medicine was created, also in Louisville. Concomitantly, the first formal clinical forensic medicine consultation service in the United States was established (3,4,9,11). In 1996, Dr. David Wells, in cooperation with the Australian College of Emergency Medicine and the Victorian Institute for Forensic Medicine, established a 6-month fellowship in clinical forensic medicine for emergency physicians (17).

UTILITY OF FORENSIC EMERGENCY MEDICINE

Emergency physicians and nurses, by design and default, evaluate and treat people with gunshot and stab wounds and victims of physical assault, sexual abuse and assault, domestic violence, and motor vehicle crashes. All of these patients have injuries or conditions that have criminal or civil forensic medical implications and the prospect or specter of courtroom sequelae (2). A patient's emergency medical evaluation must be detailed and the documentation comprehensive. Comprehensive documentation ideally contains three components: narrative, diagrammatic, and photographic. The failure to document clinical findings comprehensively may have far-ranging consequences for a patient, an accused suspect, and, potentially, the treating physician (1,2,5,6,8,9,11–14,17–21). In a review of 100 charts of patients who presented to a level I trauma center in California, Carmona and Prince reported poor, improper, or inadequate documentation in 70% of cases (2). In 38% of these cases, potential evidence was improperly secured, improperly documented, or inadvertently discarded (2).

The forensically *untrained* emergency physician or nurse may easily overlook and inadvertently destroy evidence, both gross and trace, in the course of providing patient care. The emergency care provider may misinterpret physical injuries and evidence, and form an inaccurate opinion as to their cause (1–8,10–14,17–21). Such opinions, when recorded in the patient's emergency department chart, may pose a considerable problem for the patient, the court, and the emergency physician if circumstances progress to legal proceedings.

If forensically untrained physicians and nurses can make mistakes that may haunt them and others in court, forensically trained physicians and nurses

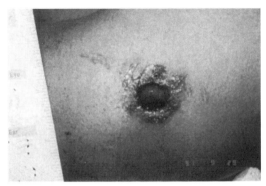

FIG. 4.1 The presence of soot and seared wound margins is indicative of a loose-contact wound. The patient stated he was shot from a distance of 30 ft. The physical evidence does not support the history given by the patient.

may be able to preclude the courtroom consequence entirely. One example of such avoidance is seen in a case involving a 20-year-old man who presented to a level I trauma center with a perforating gunshot wound to the left shoulder (4,11). The patient stated that he had been shot from a distance of 30 ft and that he knew the assailant's name. When the police arrived in the emergency department, the patient requested that the assailant be arrested immediately, as he felt his life was in danger. Examination of the wound revealed soot surrounding the larger anterior wound, as well as soot on the patient's shirt (Fig. 4.1). The examining emergency physician was aware that the presence of soot was indicative of a close range of fire and that the physical evidence did not support the history given. When the patient was confronted with this information, he recanted his story and admitted the wounds were self-inflicted in an attempt to "set up" the accused (4,11). The ability of the emergency physician to determine that the wound was consistent with having been inflicted at a close range prevented the accused from being arrested for a crime he did not commit. Traditionally, such wounds have been cleaned and debrided, removing all evidence in the process, including evidence that would distinguish entrance from exit and range of fire.

FORENSIC ASPECTS OF GUNSHOT WOUND MANAGEMENT

Emergency nurses and physicians treat more than 250,000 victims of gunshot wounds annually. Because they evaluate gunshot wounds before therapeutic or surgical intervention obscure the wound's appearance, they are in an ideal position to evaluate and document the injuries. Documentation of gunshot wounds in the medical record by the treating physician and nurse should include the number, location, size, shape, and characteristics of the wound(s). A precise description of a gunshot wound requires a basic understanding of wound ballistics and a familiarity with relevant forensic terminology (11).

Wound Ballistics

Wound ballistics is the study of the effect(s) of penetrating projectiles on the body (18–25). Several factors determine a bullet's potential for wounding (22–30): the bullet's velocity and weight, deformations/fragmentation upon impact with tissue, and the characteristics and location of the impacted tissue itself (22,23,26,27,31,32). The mechanism by which a bullet wounds is the transference of its kinetic energy to the relatively stationary tissue it hits. The severity of the wound inflicted is directly related to the amount of kinetic energy transferred to the tissue, rather than the total amount of kinetic energy possessed by the bullet itself (23–27). Bullets traveling at higher velocities have more kinetic energy and theoretically higher wounding potential; however, the physician should not assume that injuries associated with high-velocity projectiles from rifles will necessarily be more severe than those associated with low-velocity projectiles (Fig. 4.2). Wound severity is dictated by the interplay of several variables, not the bullet's velocity alone.

Crushing is the principal mechanism by which bullets from handguns impart damage to tissue. A bullet traveling through tissue generates two cavities. The first is a temporary one, lasting only 5 to 10 ms from its generation until its collapse. The second is the permanent one, the crushed

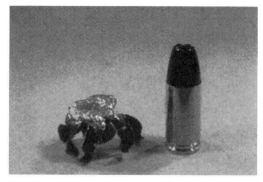

FIG. 4.3 Hollow-point ammunition, like this 9-mm "Black Talon" bullet, has the capacity to significantly increase its surface area upon impact with tissue.

tissue we observe. The size of the cavity remaining (i.e., the wound) varies with the size, shape, and configuration of the bullet. A hollow-point bullet that mushrooms upon impact can increase its diameter by as much as 2.5-fold (Fig. 4.3). The hollow-point bullet's capacity to change its shape increases the area of tissue crush it generates by 6.25 times that of a nondeformed bullet of a similar caliber (27).

Forensic Terminology Associated with Gunshot Wounds

Most misinterpretations of gunshot wounds made by nurses and physicians involve the distinction between entrance and exit wounds. The errors are invariably based on the fallacious assumption that an exit wound will be larger than its corresponding entrance wound. The first study to compare the interpretations of emergency physicians, trauma surgeons, and neurosurgeons at a level I trauma center with those of a forensic pathologist determined that fatal gunshot wounds were interpreted correctly by the clinical practitioners in only 47.8% of cases (18).

Five factors determine the size of gunshot wounds, both entrance and exit: the size, shape, configuration, and velocity of the bullet as it contacts tissue and the physical characteristics of the impacted tissue itself.

FORENSIC ASPECTS OF HANDGUN WOUNDS

Entrance Wounds

Range of fire is the distance between the gun muzzle and the victim. There are four categories of range of fire. Each has an entrance wound whose characteristics are unique to it. The entrance wounds

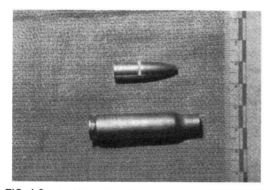

FIG. 4.2 A .308 caliber high-velocity rifle round. By virtue of their speed, high-velocity rounds have the potential to transfer large amounts of energy to body tissue.

bear the name of the range of fire from which they are inflicted: contact, near-contact or close range, intermediate or medium range, and indeterminate or distant range.

Contact Wounds

A contact wound is generated when the barrel or muzzle of the gun is in actual contact with the victim's skin or clothing. These wounds can be further divided into "tight contact," where the barrel is pushed hard against the skin, and "loose contact," where the barrel is incompletely or loosely held against the skin or clothing. Tight-contact wounds can vary in appearance from a small hole with seared blackened edges (Fig. 4.4) to a gaping stellate wound (Fig. 4.5). Large stellates wounds are caused by gases expanding under the skin and are often mistaken for an exit wound. The small tight-contact entrance wound's blackened edges are caused by the discharge of hot gases and an actual flame.

In tight-contact wounds, all materials—bullet, gases, soot, incompletely burned pieces of gunpowder, and metal fragments—are forced into the wound. When the wound occurs over thin or bony tissue, the hot gases cause the skin to expand to such an extent that the skin stretches and tears (Fig. 4.6). These tears generally have a triangular configuration, with the base of the triangle overlying the entrance wound. Large tears are usually associated with ammunition of .32 caliber or greater, or magnum loads (Fig. 4.7A–C).

However, stellate tears are not pathognomonic for contact wounds. Some exit wounds appear stellate, as do wounds associated with ricochet or tumbling bullets (Fig. 4.8A, B). Tangential wounds frequently appear stellate, also. One way to distinguish wounds

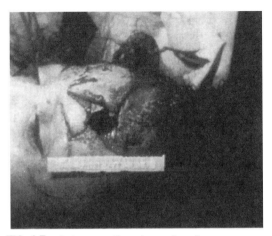

FIG. 4.5 A large stellate laceration from a contact wound with a .357 magnum handgun. The triangular lacerations are the result of the injection of gases. Emergency physicians should never base an opinion of entrance versus exit on the size of the wound.

that mimic the tight-contact wound from the tight-contact wound itself is the absence of soot and powder within and around the wound.

In some tight-contact wounds, a contusion that mirrors the muzzle can be seen. This pattern contusion results when the hot gases cause the skin to expand back against the muzzle tip (Fig. 4.9A, B). Patterns like these are helpful when establishing the type of weapon used (revolver vs. semiautomatic) and should be documented before debridement or surgery.

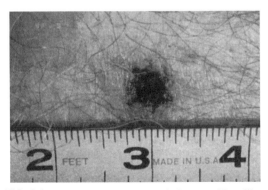

FIG. 4.4 A tight-contact wound from a .22 caliber handgun. The wound margins are seared and soot covered. Small, triangular-shaped tears are the result of tissue expansion from the injection of gases into the wound.

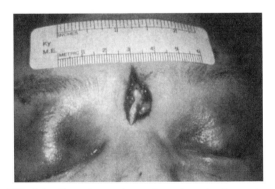

FIG. 4.6 Seared margins and a triangular laceration from a tight-contact wound inflicted by a .38 caliber revolver. The victim's husband stated that the wound was self-inflicted from a distance of approximately 14 in. On the basis of statements made to the treating physicians, which were inconsistent with the physical properties of the wound, the husband was charged with murder.

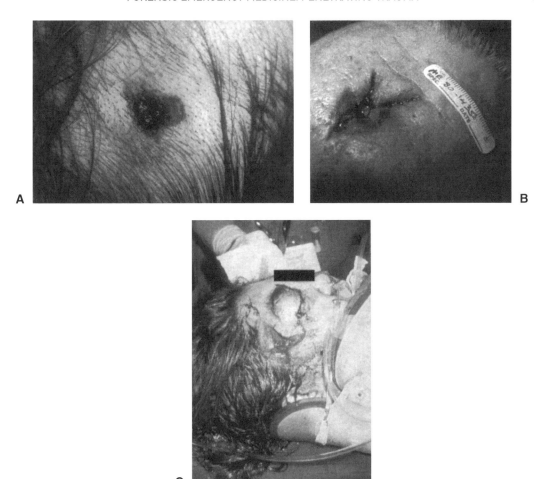

FIG. 4.7 **A:** A tight-contact wound from a .25 caliber handgun. The wound displays soot, seared margins, and a muzzle contusion at the 3 o'clock position. The muzzle contusion resulted from the forceful displacement of skin against the gun muzzle. **B:** Tight-contact wound with a muzzle contusion from a .38 caliber handgun. **C:** Large stellate lacerations from a tight-contact wound inflicted by a .380 semiautomatic handgun. The large wound is the result of tissue expansion from the injection of gas into the tissue.

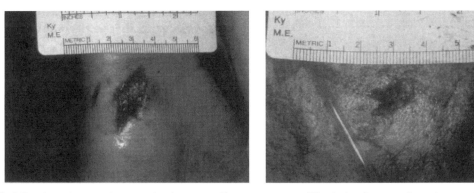

FIG. 4.8 **A:** Exit wounds may also have a stellate appearance. The lack of soot and searing on the wound margins can differentiate stellate-appearing exit wounds from contact wounds. **B:** Stellate exit wound from a .380 semiautomatic handgun.

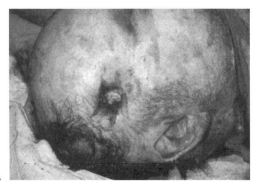 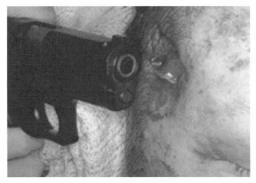

A   B

FIG. 4.9   **A:** A "muzzle contusion" or "muzzle abrasion" overlying the right temple, associated with a tight-contact wound. Close examination of contact wounds may reveal clues as to the type of handgun used (e.g., semiautomatic vs. revolver). **B:** Forceful expansion of the skin overlying the right temple resulted in a muzzle contusion from the barrel of a 9-mm semiautomatic handgun (see color insert).

Soot is a black, dusty by-product of combustion and will be observed within and around a contact wound in which the gun's muzzle was loosely contacting (incompletely contacting) or angled, relative to the skin (Fig. 4.10). The angle between the muzzle and the skin dictates the soot pattern observed. A perpendicular, loose-contact, or near-contact wound causes searing of the skin surrounding the wound, as well as the deposition of soot. A tangential, loose-contact, or near-contact wound results in searing and soot deposition elongated in shape, marking the path the bullet took at entry.

Close-Range Wounds

Close range is defined as the maximum range at which soot is deposited on the wound or clothing (Fig. 4.11A–C). This muzzle-to-target distance is usually less than 6 in. Soot has been noted on victims with a skin-to-muzzle distance of 12 in., but this is uncommon (26,27,31). Beyond 6 in., the soot usually falls away and does not reach the target. The concentration of soot varies inversely with the muzzle-to-target distance and is influenced by the type of gunpowder and ammunition, the barrel length, and the caliber and type of weapon. A precise range of fire, such as 1 cm versus 10 cm, cannot be determined from a soot pattern.

If the patient is stable and therapeutic manipulation of the wound can be delayed, the soot pattern should be described in detail and photographed before it is removed. Forensic crime laboratories can determine the range of fire of an assault by test-firing the offending weapon at a target at various distances until they succeed in reproducing the soot pattern observed on the patient. Of course, they must use a weapon and ammunition similar to those that caused the wound.

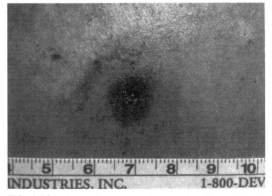

FIG. 4.10   Soot deposition is associated with both loose-contact and close-range gunshot wounds. This asymmetric soot pattern is produced when the handgun barrel-to-skin angle is less than 90 degrees when the weapon is discharged.

Intermediate-Range Wounds

"Tattooing" or "stippling" is caused by contact with partially burned and wholly unburned pieces of gunpowder. They appear as punctate abrasions and are pathognomonic for intermediate-range gunshot wounds (Fig. 4.12A–C). Therefore, the "medium or intermediate range" is sufficiently close to cause tattooing.

Tattooing is generally seen in wound-to-muzzle distances of 60 cm or less but has been reported as close as 1 cm and as far away as 1 m. The pattern and density of the tattooing are dictated by the muzzle-to-skin distance, the length of the gun's barrel, the type of ammunition used, the type of gunpowder used, and the presence of intermediate objects (such as clothing and hair).

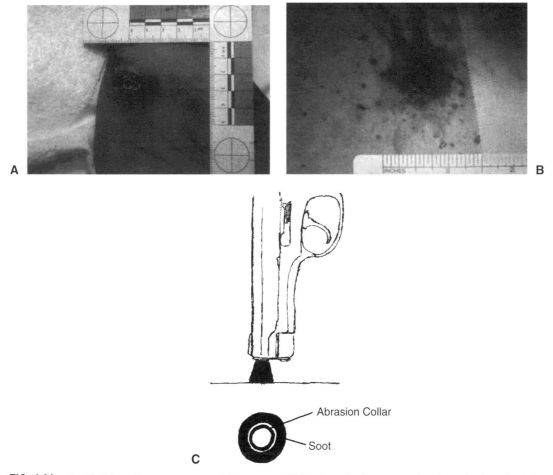

FIG. 4.11 **A:** Visible carbonaceous material or soot will be deposited on wounds when the barrel of the handgun is discharged within 6 in. The presence of soot defines a wound as "close range." **B:** Soot associated with the discharge of a 9-mm semiautomatic pistol from a distance of 1 in. **C:** Deposition of soot associated with the wound in (**B**).

Long-Range Wounds

The long-range or distant wound is inflicted from a range sufficiently far that only the bullet makes contact with the clothing and skin. No tattooing or soot is observed. As the bullet penetrates the skin, the skin is indented, resulting in the creation of an "abrasion collar," also called "abrasion margin," "abrasion rim," and "abrasion ring" (Fig. 4.13A, B). The collar is an abraded area of tissue that surrounds an entry wound and is caused by friction between the bullet and the epithelium, not by thermal changes associated with a hot projectile. The width of the abrasion collar will vary with the angle of impact (Fig. 4.12C). Almost all entrance wounds have abrasion collars. Some high-velocity handgun rounds, for example, .357 magnum, will produce very small abrasion collars, which can be seen only on examination of

the tissue (Fig. 4.14). Because of the inelasticity of the tissue on the palms of the hands and the soles of the feet, entrance wounds in these areas usually appear slit-like and lack abrasion collars (27).

Exit Wounds

Exit wounds are the result of a bullet pushing and stretching the skin from the inside out. The skin edges are generally everted, with sharp but irregular margins. True abrasion collars, soot, and tattooing are not associated with exit wounds.

Exit wounds can assume a variety of shapes and configurations and are not necessarily consistently larger than the entrance wounds that preceded them (Fig. 4.15A–C). The exit wound's size is principally dictated by the amount of energy that

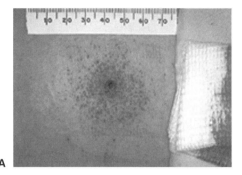
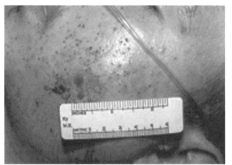

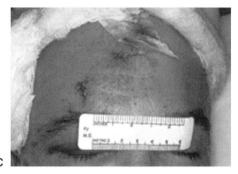

FIG. 4.12 **A:** "Tattooing" is the result of partially burned or unburned gunpowder making contact with the skin. The "tattoos" are punctate abrasions associated with an intermediate-range gunshot wound. Tattooing has been seen with wounds as close as 1 cm and as far away as 1 m. **B:** This patient stated he was shot with a .22 caliber handgun at a distance of 12 in. His cheek exhibited punctate abrasions or "tattooing" associated with intermediate-range gunshot wounds. **C:** Forehead "tattooing" from an intermediate-range gunshot wound. The patient reported he was shot with a .38 caliber revolver from a distance of 18 in. (see color insert).

the bullet possesses as it exits the skin. Other factors that affect wound size are the bullet's size and configuration. A bullet's configuration will change from its usual nose-first attitude on entering the skin, to tumbling and yawing after impact with tissue. A bullet with sufficient energy that exits the skin in a sideways configuration, or one that has increased its surface area by mushrooming, will have an exit wound larger than

its corresponding entrance wound (Fig. 4.16) (22, 26,27,31).

Atypical Exit Wounds

A "shored-exit" wound is one with a *false* abrasion collar. If the skin is forcibly pressed against or supported by a firm object or surface at the moment the bullet exits, the skin can be squeezed between the exiting bullet and the supporting surface

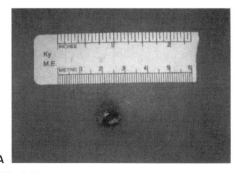
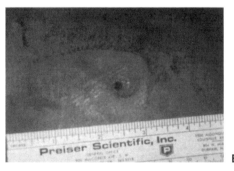

FIG. 4.13 **A:** An abrasion collar is the result of friction between a bullet and the skin. Abrasion collars are associated with gunshot wounds of entrance. **B:** An abrasion collar may also be called an "abrasion rim" or "abrasion ring." The width will vary with the angle of the bullet's impact.

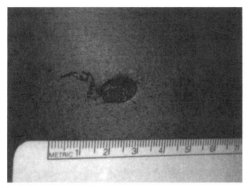

FIG. 4.14 An entrance wound associated with a high-velocity handgun round (.357 magnum). The abrasion collar can be seen only when the tissue is everted.

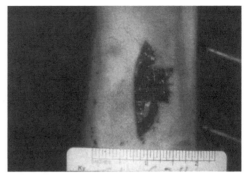

FIG. 4.16 A stellate exit wound of the forearm from a .22 caliber-long rifle bullet. The wound size and shape are the result of bone extrusion. The lack of soot and seared skin distinguishes this wound from a contact wound.

(Fig. 4.17A–C) (31,32). Examples of supporting structures include floors, walls, doors, chairs, and mattresses, as well as less flexible articles of clothing, such as belts or jewelry.

On rare occasions, soot may be present at an atypical exit wound site (28). If an entrance wound is located sufficiently close to it, soot may be propelled through the short wound track and appear faintly on the exit wound's surface.

Entrance Versus Exit

Emergency physicians, health professionals, and law enforcement officials will make grievous errors in

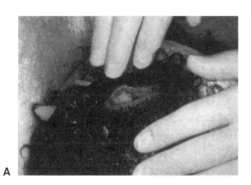

A

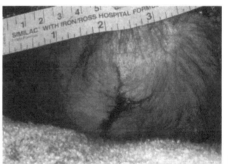

B

C

FIG. 4.15 **A:** An exit wound at the vertex of the skull associated with an intraoral entrance wound. Forceful extrusion of bone resulted in the enlargement of this exit wound. **B:** A triangular exit wound with irregular wound margins. Exit wounds may be larger or smaller than their associated entrance wounds. **C:** A slit-like exit wound on the lateral neck. The size of the exit wound depends on multiple variables, including bullet velocity and tissue elasticity.

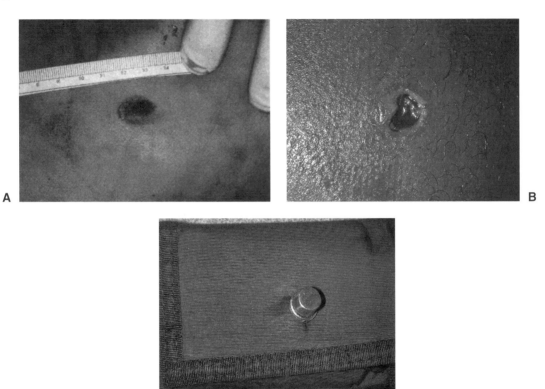

C

FIG. 4.17   **A:** A shored-exit wound. The "false" abrasion collar occurs when the exiting projectile pushes the skin against a supporting object. This wound resulted from a .357 magnum projectile exiting the patient's back when he was against a brick wall. **B** and **C:** A shored exit associated with impact with the victim's wallet.

the documentation and determination of entrance versus exit wounds if the diagnosis is based solely on the size of the wound (2,4,5,8,11,18,21). If emergency physicians and nurses receive adequate forensic training and have familiarity with the proper forensic terminology, then the distinction of entrance from exit wounds will not be difficult. When in doubt, the emergency care provider should refrain from placing statements regarding "entrance" and "exit" in the medical record. At such times, the patient and health care provider will be better served if the wound is measured, photographed, and accurately described using appropriate forensic terminology and tissue sent to the forensic pathologist for microscopic analysis.

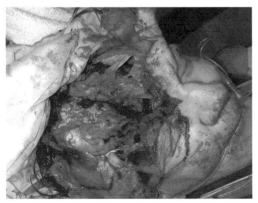

FIG. 4.18   Massive cranial injury from a high-velocity centerfire .30-30 rifle, the most popular hunting rifle in the United States (25).

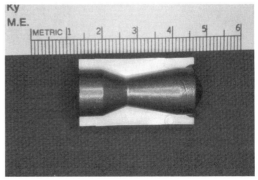

FIG. 4.19   Sabot 12-gauge shotgun slug weighing more than 500 g.

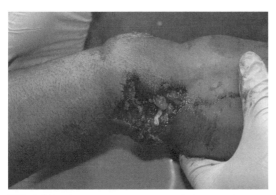

FIG. 4.20 Gaping entrance wound from a 12-gauge shotgun slug. No abrasion collar is appreciated. The wound is slightly larger than its associated exit wound (Figure 4.21).

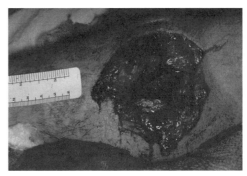

FIG. 4.22 Exit wound from a high-velocity .308 centerfire rifle round. The size of the wound is related to the energy transferred to the underlying bone and tissue.

Shotgun Slug and Centerfire High-Velocity Rifle Wounds

Projectiles discharged from centerfire rifles and slugs from shotguns have the potential to inflict massive tissue damage (Fig. 4.18). A bullet's wounding potential is based on the kinetic energy it possesses. The higher the velocity and mass of a projectile, the greater the potential to inflict tissue damage, based on the following formula:

$$\text{Kinetic energy} = \text{mass} \times \text{velocity}^2/g$$

Injuries will result from the transference of the kinetic energy from the projectile to organs and bony structures.

The caliber of a shotgun is defined by the term *gauge* and historically referred to "the number of lead balls of the given bore diameter that make up a pound," for example, 12-lead balls to make 1 pound (27). Shotgun slugs are single projectiles

that can weigh 200 times more than handgun ammunition, for example, a 12-gauge slug can weigh 547 g compared with a .22 long rifle bullet at 2.6 g (Fig. 4.19). The massive damage caused by slugs may obliterate the abrasion collar usually associated with entrance wounds (Fig. 4.20). Shotgun slugs will almost uniformly exit the body with large exit wounds (Fig. 4.21). The velocity of shotgun slugs is usually in the range of 1,500 to 1,800 ft per second.

The calibers of centerfire bullets, .223 to .308 in., are similar in diameter and weight to handgun ammunition, but their wounding potential is greatly enhanced by the velocity of the round (27,31). With high-velocity rounds (velocities >2,000 ft per second), a temporary cavity is formed along the wound tract. The temporary cavity may approach 11 or 12 times the diameter of the bullet and can result in tissue damage away from the physical tract taken by the projectile itself (27). Temporary cavitation, in combination with the direct tissue disruption and energy transfer from a fragmenting or yawing (turning sideways) projectile, is what

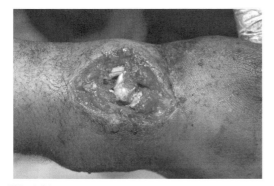

FIG. 4.21 Exit wound from a 12-gauge shotgun slug. Bone fragments are seen extruding from the wound. The wound is slightly smaller than its associated entrance wound (Figure 4.20).

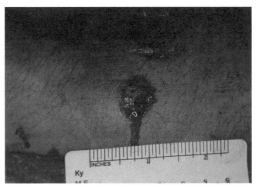

FIG. 4.23 Entrance wound from a high-velocity .308 centerfire rifle round. An abrasion collar is present.

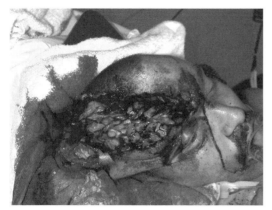

FIG. 4.24   Contact wound from a .223 centerfire rifle. Soot is visible on the bridge of the nose.

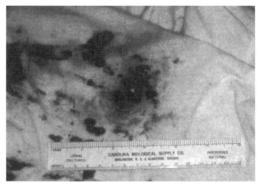

FIG. 4.26   Soot deposition is associated with a close range of fire. Examination of the patient's clothing by the emergency physician will assist in the determination of entrance versus exit wounds and the range of fire. Each article of clothing should be packaged separately in paper bags to avoid the transfer of residue between articles.

determines the size of the internal injury and that of the exit wound. Owing to the amount of energy possessed and transferred to the underlying tissue, exit wounds associated with centerfire rifles are generally, but not necessarily, larger than their corresponding entrance wounds, in contrast to those associated with handguns (Fig. 4.22) (11,27).

Entrance wounds associated with high-velocity centerfire projectiles do not significantly differ from those that are caused by handguns. Entrance wounds generally exhibit abrasion collars or microtears on the skin surface (Fig. 4.23). Contact wounds from centerfire rifles will have soot, triangle-shaped tears, and massive damage from the increased volume of gas and greater kinetic energy (Fig. 4.24). Close and intermediate-range wounds, like handgun wounds, will also have associated soot deposition and tattooing. Because of a number of variables, that is, muzzle length, the amount of power in a

given cartridge, muzzle configuration, and the type of gunpowder (ball vs. cylindrical), the range of fire associated with rifle wounds is not as clearly defined as in handgun wounds. An exact range of fire for rifles and shotguns is best determined through controlled testing performed by a firearms examiner at a crime laboratory.

High-velocity lead core and jacketed bullets generally break up into hundreds of fragments, called a *lead snowstorm*, upon entering tissues, creating significant tissue damage (Fig. 4.25) (11,27). In deep tissue and body cavities, the bullet fragments may fail to exit and be embedded within the victim. Therefore, it is possible to sustain an injury with a

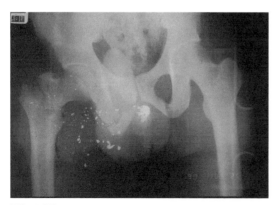

FIG. 4.25   "Lead snowstorm" from a high-velocity projectile. High-velocity lead rounds have a tendency to fragment into hundreds of particles on contact with bone.

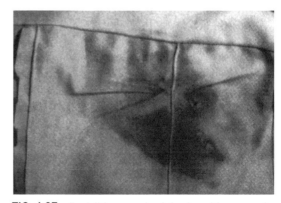

FIG. 4.27   Invisible vaporized lead residues can be visualized with colorimetric testing by the forensic crime laboratory. All clothing associated with victims of gunshot wounds should be preserved for crime lab testing, even if no visible residues are appreciated.

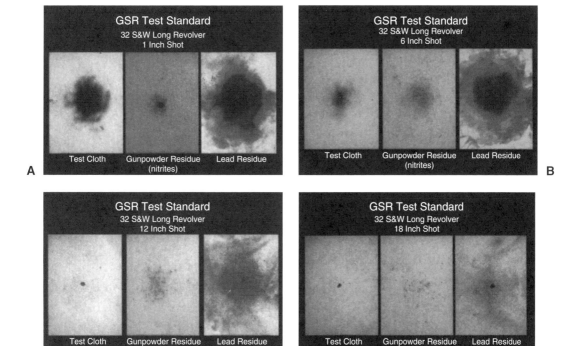

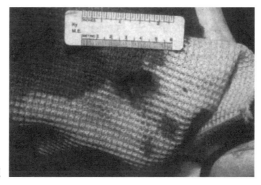

FIG. 4.28 Gunshot residue (GSR) testing of a .32 caliber handgun on cloth. The forensic crime laboratory will examine clothing for evidence of visible and invisible GSRs, including carbonaceous soot from the burning of gunpowder, nitrates from unburned gunpowder, and vaporized lead residue. Nitrates and lead residues are visible only with the application of specialized forensic testing. **A:** At the 1-in. range, heavy concentrations of soot, nitrates, and lead residues are deposited on the test cloth. **B:** At the 6-in. range, there is minimal soot with heavy concentrations of nitrates and lead residues. **C:** At the 12-in. range, there is no soot; heavy concentrations of nitrates and lead residues are present. **D:** At the 18-in. range, there are no visible residues. The concentrations of nitrates and lead residues are significantly reduced. **E:** At the 24-in. range, no residues are deposited on the test cloth.

high-velocity round and not exhibit an exit wound. High-velocity rounds with steel cores will almost uniformly exit intact and continue down-range. Both of these facts can confound the forensic investigator's efforts to find an adequate projectile sample to submit to the firearms examiner as evidence for ballistic analysis.

EVIDENCE

In the evaluation and treatment of patients who are victims of a gunshot wound, emergency physicians and nurses usually have the opportunity to preserve and collect short-lived evidence, but first they must recognize it as such. Carmona and Prince

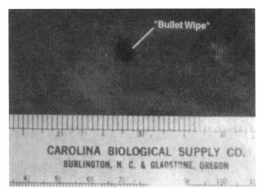

FIG. 4.29 "Bullet wipe" on clothing is the deposition of lead and lubricants by the projectile as it penetrates. This residue is best appreciated on white clothing, but it may be detected on dark clothing through forensic testing for lead residues.

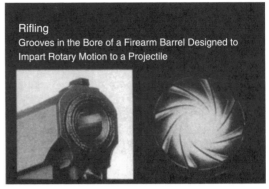

FIG. 4.31 Microscopic marks or "rifling impressions" are imparted to bullets as they travel down the gun barrel. The impressions are a mirror image of the marks left in the gun barrel during its manufacture. Like a fingerprint, the barrel etchings are unique to each barrel.

reported that trauma physicians "usually have little or no training in the forensic aspects of trauma care and therefore necessary evidence may often be overlooked, lost, inadvertently discarded, or its admissibility denied because of improper handling or documentation" (2).

In the case of gunshot wounds, the victim's clothing may yield information about the range of fire and help distinguish entrance from exit wounds (Figs. 4.26–4.28A–E) (1,7,11,26,27,31). Clothing fibers will deform in the direction of the passing projectile. Gunpowder residues and soot will deposit on clothing, just as they do on skin. Some of the residue will be invisible to the naked eye but can be detected using standard forensic laboratory staining techniques.

Bullet wipe is a lead and/or lubricant residue left on clothing through which a bullet has passed

(Fig. 4.29). When articles of clothing are removed from a wounded patient, they should be packaged separately (to avoid cross-contamination) and placed in a paper bag (to minimize the risk that static electricity will lift fragile evidence off their surface). Bloody clothing may be left in plastic bags for a short period of time, but should never be left in a location where they could mold and destroy forensic evidence.

A gunshot residue (GSR) test may determine whether a victim or suspect has been in a location where a weapon has been fired (24,25,27,33–40). The GSR test checks for the presence of invisible residues from the primer: barium nitrate, antimony sulfide, and lead peroxide. A positive test does not

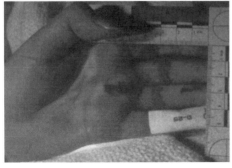

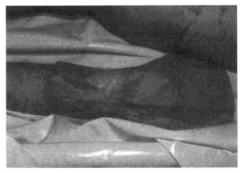

A   B

FIG. 4.30 A: Examination of the hands may reveal visible gunshot residues. The presence of soot indicates the patient's hand was within 6 in. of the weapon when it was discharged. This patient held a .32 caliber revolver in her left hand during her suicide. B: Placement of paper bags over the hands of a gunshot wound victim helps preserve gunshot or primer residues. *Never* cover the hands with plastic bags. Placement of plastic bags will result in the accumulation of moisture and result in the degradation and contamination of evidence.

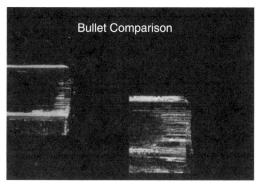

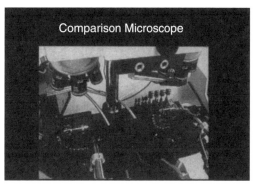

FIG. 4.32   A: Microscopic impressions are a unique fingerprint of the gun's barrel and can be examined with a comparison microscope. Care must be taken in the collection of bullets to avoid metal-to-metal contact from surgical instruments, such as hemostats, or damage from the dropping of projectiles into surgical pans. B: The comparison microscope is used to compare bullets collected from a patient with a known bullet standard.

indicate with certainty that the individual fired the weapon, as it is possible to transfer residues from a shooter's hand to someone else (25). The sensitivity of the test decreases with the passage of time, and law enforcement agents may not have access to a patient during the "golden hour" (21). Factors that affect the sensitivity include washing the skin with alcohol or povidone-iodine (Betadine), placing tape on the skin, rubbing the hands against clothing, and placing plastic bags over the patient's hands, which may cause moisture to develop on the skin. If a GSR test is to be performed, or if soot is noted on the patient's hand, paper bags should be placed over the hands early in the treatment (Fig. 4.30A, B).

Analysis of lead isotopes was recently added to the toolbag of the crime laboratory (40). Isotope analysis compares the chemical composition of firearms discharge residue (FDR) found within a specific gunshot wound with the FDR of a specific weapon. This investigative tool may assist crime laboratory personnel in determining which wounds were caused by which weapon in cases involving multiple shooters (40).

When a weapon is discharged, it imprints multiple unique microscopic marks on the side of a bullet (26,27). The bullet's markings result from its contact with the tool marks or "rifling"

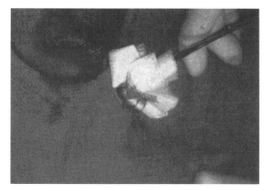

FIG. 4.33   To avoid damage from surgical instruments to the bullet's microscopic impressions, hemostats and pickups should be covered with gauze. Any metal-to-metal contact will destroy these microscopic marks and make the job of the forensic scientist more difficult.

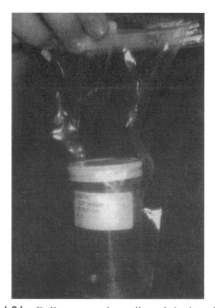

FIG. 4.34   Bullets must be collected in breathable containers (paper boxes or envelopes). Placement of bullets in airtight containers will result in contamination and degradation of the evidence from the collection of moisture and the proliferation of bacteria.

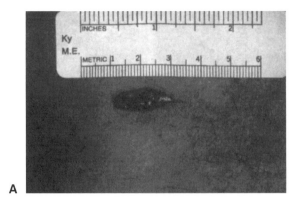

A

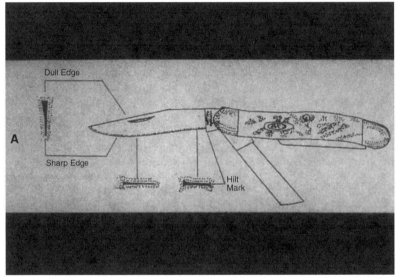

B

FIG. 4.35   **A:** A stab wound from a single-edged knife blade. In this picture, the dull portion of the blade is associated with the right wound margin of the wound and the sharp edge of the blade with the left wound margin. **B:** Diagram of a stab wound and the associated single-edged knife blade.

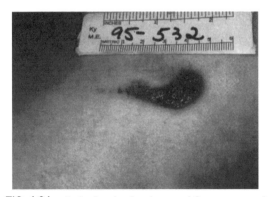

FIG. 4.36   A single-edged stab wound from a serrated knife blade. Abrasions from the blade's serrated edge are visible at the left margin of the wound. These abrasions can result from either the insertion or withdrawal of the knife blade.

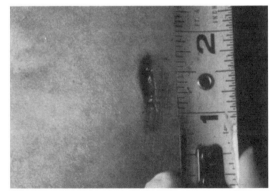

FIG. 4.37   A single-edged stab wound with a small "hilt mark" at the superior wound margin. The hilt mark occurs when the hilt of the blade (Figure 4.35B) forcefully contacts the skin.

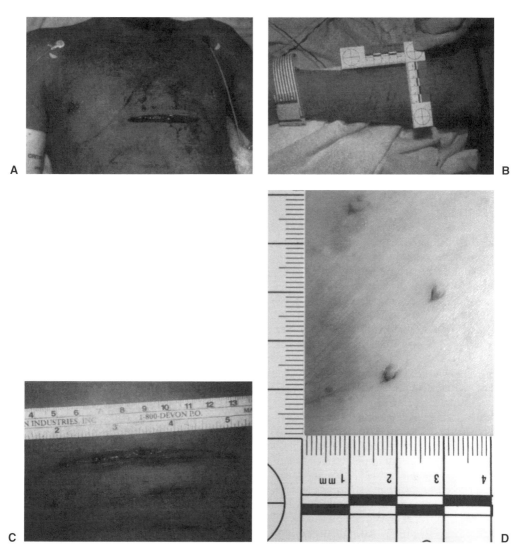

FIG. 4.38 **A:** This patient sustained 39 superficial incised wounds to his anterior thorax, reportedly inflicted by his wife. Upon pointed questioning, the patient admitted that the wounds were self-inflicted. Self-infliction behavior must be ruled out in any patient with more than one incised wound. **B:** Self-inflicted incised wounds to the wrist in a suicidal patient. The physician must reserve the use of the term "laceration" for wounds associated with blunt force trauma. **C:** A patient with four superficial incised abdominal wounds reported to police that he was assaulted with a box cutter during a robbery. Review of his medical record indicated a similar incident, with the same weapon, 3 years earlier. After pointed questioning, the patient admitted that the wounds from both "robberies" were self-inflicted. The patient was referred for psychiatric evaluation. Any patient with more than one incised wound must be evaluated for self-destructive behavior. **D:** Self-inflicted "V-shaped" puncture wounds from a scissor point.

in the gun's barrel (Figs. 4.31 and 4.32A, B). The emergency physician must try not to compromise these markings when removing a bullet from a patient (31). Bullets should be handled with gloves. Surgical instruments, such as hemostats or pickups, should be covered with gauze to ensure the preservation of these microscopic "fingerprint" marks (Figs. 4.33 and 4.34).

Radiographs may be used to locate retained projectiles and may be of evidentiary value when determining the number of projectiles and the direction of fire (11,26,27,29,31). However, they should not be exposed less than 72 in. from a bullet. Closer exposure will distort the image of the projectile and cause it to appear larger than it is. Emergency physicians should not render opinions on a projectile's caliber based solely on the radiographic image.

FORENSIC ASSESSMENT OF SHARP FORCE TRAUMA

There are two types of sharp force injuries: incised and stabbed. An incised wound is generated by a drawing motion and is therefore longer than it is deep. The stab wound is a puncture-type wound and therefore is deeper rather than wide. The wound margins of sharp force injuries are clean and lack the abraded edges of injuries generated by blunt force trauma (11,31).

Information of a forensic nature can be gleaned from the examination of a stab wound. Certain characteristics of a knife's blade, whether single- or double-edged, can be determined from visual inspection (Fig. 4.35A, B). Additional characteristics, such as whether the knife was serrated or sharp, can be determined if the blade was drawn across the skin during its insertion or withdrawal (Fig. 4.36). Serrated blades do not always leave these characteristic marks. In cases where the knife has been inserted to the proximal portion of the blade, a contusion may result from contact with the hilt (Fig. 4.37) (11,31).

Recognition of self-inflicted injuries by emergency nurses and physicians is critical to patient disposition and criminal justice. Self-inflicted injuries and associated fictitious accounts of physical and sexual assault are well documented (41). Wounds from sharp-edged implements, such as knives, scissors, razor blades, and pins, are the most common form of self-inflicted injuries. The injuries are usually superficial linear abrasions or incised wounds, uniform in nature and often parallel (Fig. 4.38A–D). When the emergency department physician encounters a patient with more than one incised wound, self-inflicted injuries must always be suspected.

SUMMARY AND CONCLUSION

It is a brave new world. The practice of medicine must evolve to meet the needs and accommodate the reality of our society. Perhaps more so in emergency medicine than in any other specialty, physicians and nurses are confronted by the fallout from a society stressed by rapid change, easy access to inexpensive weapons, and the soul-numbing bombardment of images of violence.

As before, and always, our highest calling is saving lives. It is the nature of the wounds from which we are saving patients that is changing. The medical management is not so different, yet new skills are required of us. Emergency nurses and physicians today must have a working knowledge of wound mechanics and forensic terminology. We must know how weapons wound and watch with an ever-vigilant eye for injuries indicative of self-abuse and assault. Forensics belongs in the emergency department now out of necessity, and out of an ethical obligation to fulfill a critical role in safeguarding patients.

ACKNOWLEDGMENT

I wish to thank Mr. Scott Doyle of the Kentucky State Police Crime Laboratory for his assistance and photographs.

REFERENCES

1. Smialek JE. Forensic medicine in the emergency department. *Emerg Med Clin North Am* 1983;1(3):693–704.
2. Carmona R, Prince K. Trauma and forensic medicine. *J Trauma* 1989;29(9):1222–1225.
3. Smock WS, Nichols GR, Fuller PM. Development and implementation of the first clinical forensic medicine training program. *J Forensic Sci* 1993;38(4):835–839.
4. Smock WS. Development of a clinical forensic medicine curriculum for emergency physicians in the USA. *J Clin Forensic Med* 1994;1(1):27–30.
5. Smock WS, Ross CS, Hamilton FN. Clinical forensic medicine: how ED physicians can help with the sleuthing. *Emerg Legal Briefings* 1994;5(1):1.
6. Eckert WG, Bell JS, Stein RJ, et al. Clinical forensic medicine. *Am J Forensic Med Pathol* 1986;7(3):182–185.
7. Mittleman RE, Goldberg HS, Waksman DM. Preserving evidence in the emergency department. *Am J Nurs* 1983;83(12):1652–1656.
8. Godley DR, Smith TK. Some medicolegal aspects of gunshot wounds. *J Trauma* 1977;17(11):866–871.
9. Ryan MT, Houry DE. Clinical forensic medicine. *Ann Emerg Med* 2000;36(3):271–273.
10. Goldsmith MF. US forensic pathologists on a new case: examination of living patients. *JAMA* 1986;256(13):1685–1686, 1691.
11. Smock WS. Forensic emergency medicine. In: Marx JA, Hockberger RS, Walls RM et al., eds. *Rosen's emergency medicine: concepts and clinical practice*, 6th ed. St Louis: Mosby, 2006:952–968.
12. Sharma BR. Clinical forensic medicine-management of crime victims from trauma to trial. *J Clin Forensic Med* 2003;10(4):267–273.
13. Fackler ML, Riddick L. Clinicians' inadequate descriptions of gunshot wounds obstruct justice: clinical journals refuse to expose the problem. In: Warren EA, Papke BK, eds. *Proceedings of the American Academy of Forensic Sciences*, Vol. 2. Colorado Springs, 1996:150.
14. Trunkey D, Farjah F. Medical and surgical care of our four assassinated presidents. *J Am Coll Surg* 2005;201(6):976–989.
15. Eckert W. Forensic sciences: the clinical or living aspects. *Inform* 1983;16:3.
16. Busuttil A, Smock WS. Training in clinical forensic medicine in Kentucky. *Police Surgeon* 1990;14:26.
17. Young S, Wells D, Summers I. Specific training in clinical forensic medicine is useful to ACEM trainees. *Emerg Med Australas* 2004;16:441–445.
18. Collins KA, Lantz PE. Interpretation of fatal, multiple, and exiting gunshot wounds by trauma specialists. *J Forensic Sci* 1994;39(1):94–99.

19. McLeer SV, Anwar RA, Herman S, et al. Education is not enough: a systems failure in protecting battered women. *Ann Emerg Med* 1989;18(6):651–653.

20. Breo DL. JFK's death: the plain truth from the MDs who did the autopsy. *JAMA* 1992;267(20):2794–2803.

21. Randall T. Clinicians' forensic interpretations of fatal gunshot wounds often miss the mark. *JAMA* 1993;269(16):2058, 2061.

22. DiMaio VJM, Spitz WU. Variations in wounding due to unusual firearms and recently available ammunition. *J Forensic Sci* 1972;17(3):377–386.

23. Fackler ML. Wound ballistics: a review of common misconceptions. *JAMA* 1988;259(18):2730–2736.

24. Zeichner A, Levin N. Casework experience of GSR detection in Israel, on samples from hands, hair, and clothing using an autosearch SEM/EDX system. *J Forensic Sci* 1995;40(6):1082–1085.

25. Gialamas DM, Rhodes EF, Crim D, et al. Officers, their weapons and their hands: an empirical study of GSR on the hands of non-shooting police officers. *J Forensic Sci* 1995;40(6):1086–1089.

26. Fatteh A. *Medicolegal Investigation of Gunshot Wounds.* Philadelphia, PA: JB Lippincott, 1976:88–89.

27. DiMaio VJM. *Gunshot wounds*, 2nd ed. Boca Raton: CRC Press, 1999:74–75, 86, 92.

28. Adelson L. A microscopic study of dermal gunshot wounds. *Am J Clin Pathol* 1961;35(5):393–402.

29. Dixon DS. Gunshot wounds: forensic implications in a surgical practice. In: Ordog GH, ed. *Management of gunshot wounds.* New York: Elsevier, 1988:168.

30. Andrasko K, Maehly AC. Detection of gunshot residues on hands by scanning electron microscopy. *J Forensic Sci* 1977;22(2):279–287.

31. Spitz WU. *Medicolegal Investigation of Death*, 3rd ed. Springfield, IL: Charles C Thomas Publisher, 1993: 311–412.

32. Dixon DS. Characteristics of shored exit wounds. *J Forensic Sci* 1981;26(4):691–698.

33. Matricardi VR, Kilty JW. Detection of gunshot particles from the hands of a shooter. *J Forensic Sci* 1977;22(4):725–738.

34. Wolten GM, Nesbitt RS, Calloway AR, et al. Particle analysis for the detection of gunshot residue. I: scanning electron microscopy/energy dispersive x-ray characterization of hand deposits from firing. *J Forensic Sci* 1979;24(2):409–422.

35. Wolten GM, Nesbitt RS, Calloway AR, et al. Particle analysis for the detection of gunshot residue. II: occupational and environmental particles. *J Forensic Sci* 1979;24(2): 423–430.

36. Wolten GM, Nesbitt RS, Calloway AR. Particle analysis for the detection of gunshot residue. III: the case record. *J Forensic Sci* 1979;24(4):864–869.

37. Tillman WL. Automated gunshot residue particle search and characterization. *J Forensic Sci* 1987;32(1):62–71.

38. Kee TG, Beck C. Casework assessment of an automated scanning electron microscope/microanalysis system for the detection of firearms discharge particles. *J Forensic Sci Soc* 1987;27(5):321.

39. Zeichner A, Ehrlich S, Shoshani E, et al. Application of lead isotope analysis in shooting incident investigations. *Forensic Sci Int* 2006;158(1):52–64.

40. Tugcu H, Yorulmaz C, Bayraktaroglu G, et al. Determination of gunshot residues with image analysis: an experimental study. *Mil Med* 2005;170(9):802–805.

41. Pollak S, Saukko PJ. Self-inflicted injury. In: *Encyclopedia of forensic sciences.* New York: Academic Press, 2000:391–397.

5

■ WILLIAM S. SMOCK

Motor-vehicle–related trauma claimed 42,636 lives and injured more than 2.7 million people in the United States in 2004 (1). The majority of these victims sought care and treatment in emergency departments and trauma centers. In many cases, law enforcement officials investigating these incidents had forensic questions such as those listed below for the emergency physicians and nurses caring for the injured:

> "Doc, any idea which one was the driver? They were both ejected."
> "Nurse, was any evidence from the hit-and-run vehicle transferred to the victim's clothes?"
> "What do you think took the lady's hand off? There wasn't much damage to the car."
> "Doc, any chance the pedestrian was already lying in the roadway when he was hit?"

The forensically trained emergency care provider should be able to answer these mysteries.

There are potential legal (criminal and civil) implications and consequences for these victims if an emergency physician or nurse fails to adequately document their injuries and preserve forensic evidence. Even injuries that seem superficial and not life threatening may hold the key to answering some of the investigating officer's forensic questions. Emergency care providers must be trained to provide the victim of motor vehicle trauma the same level of forensic care given to the victim of a gunshot wound, child abuse, or sexual assault (2). If, through omission or commission, we, as care givers, deny our patients access to their own short-lived "evidence," we have committed a disservice and may be culpable.

DRIVER OR PASSENGER?

The determination of a vehicle occupant's role in a serious automobile collision is an important medicolegal task. If the vehicle's occupant is pinned with his seat belt on or behind the steering wheel, the determination is easy. If the vehicle's occupants are ejected from the vehicle, the determination is much more difficult. Many impaired drivers will lie about their role, claiming to be a "passenger" to avoid liability. Evidence, some of which is short-lived, that could aid in making the determination of driver or passenger can be very fragile. There is a risk of altering or destroying evidence during the delivery of emergency treatment. The collection of material evidence should be a routine part of emergency medical care (2–4). Pattern injuries, that is, injuries that can be matched to an object, are themselves one type of "evidence." Although not life threatening, seat-belt and air-bag abrasions, steering wheel contusions, and dicing lacerations may be critical factors in determining an occupant's position in the vehicle at the time of the incident. As such, they must be recognized and documented.

In the isolation of the emergency department, the emergency physician or nurse should never render an opinion as to an occupant's position (2–4). Investigating professionals can offer such an opinion when the incident scene, the vehicle itself, and the occupants have been thoroughly assessed and analyzed. Similarly, allegations of criminal and/or civil liability must be based solely on the tangible physical evidence collected from the vehicle, its occupants, and the crash scene. Emergency personnel must refrain from rendering an opinion, as their insight is only one-third of the puzzle. Heath care providers must not set themselves up for the legal sequelae or embarrassment of rendering an opinion based on such a limited foundation. However, the medical component is fully a third of the investigative puzzle. Without this information, the incident reconstructionists will be challenged to arrive at an accurate opinion. Other potential roadblocks to determining the role of an occupant are listed below (4):

1. Occupants are removed from vehicles by well-meaning bystanders, whose statements and observations are not recorded by the investigating agencies.
2. Physical evidence of occupant movement within the vehicle and trace evidence of occupant and vehicle interaction are not recognized, collected, and documented.
3. Other occupants' injuries, including pattern injuries, are not described in the medical record or photographically documented in the emergency department.
4. Evidence standards (clothing, shoes) and biological standards (hair and blood) are not collected from all occupants.
5. An autopsy is not conducted on the deceased occupant(s).
6. Substandard analysis of the crash scene prohibits accurate reconstruction of the vehicle dynamics.

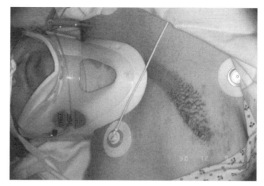

FIG. 5.2 Driver or passenger? A seat-belt abrasion over the left neck and chest indicated the patient was restrained. The abrasions could have resulted from loading the center, the left rear, or the driver's restraint but they do not prove she was the driver.

7. Vehicle components found at the crash scene are haphazardly thrown back into the vehicles, resulting in the possibility or supposition of cross-contamination.
8. Inadequate resources are committed to the evaluation of the incident.
9. An assumption is made that the owner of the vehicle is always the driver.
10. The vehicle is not preserved or is left exposed to the environment, which may lead to degradation, destruction, or loss of trace evidence.

Pattern Injuries

Matching pattern injuries with interior vehicle components will reveal an occupant's position during a portion of the vehicle's collision sequence (2–5). Common pattern injuries include contusions, abrasions, and lacerations from seat belts, steering

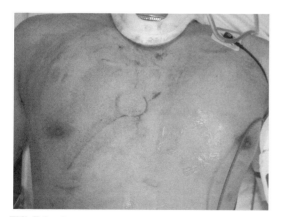

FIG. 5.1 Impact with the steering and seat belt resulted in a pattern imprint on the driver's anterior chest. This pattern injury assists in the determination of occupant role.

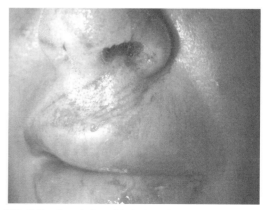

FIG. 5.3 An air-bag fabric imprint and abrasions to the upper lip.

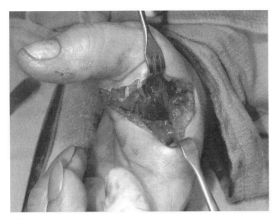

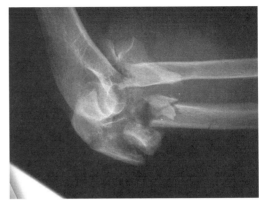

FIG. 5.4 Partial thumb amputation from impact with a deploying driver's air bag. Blood on the driver's air bag was matched to the reported "passenger."

FIG. 5.5 An open comminuted elbow fracture from impact with a deploying passenger air bag. Blood and DNA on the air bag confirmed the "passenger" was in the right front passenger seat.

wheels, air bags, air-bag module covers, window cranks, radio knobs, door latches, dashboard components, and front and side window glass (Figs. 5.1, 5.2, and 5.3) (2–4,6). An occupant's movement and subsequent contact with a vehicle's components are dictated by the forces applied to the vehicle through its interaction with the environment. Vehicle occupants, restrained or unrestrained, will initially move toward the primary area of impact (3,4). This movement within the vehicle, called *occupant kinematics*, is described as a motion parallel to and opposite from the direction of the force developed by the impacting object (3,4). Applying the principles of occupant kinematics will predict in what direction a particular occupant will move and therefore what interior component will be struck.

A deploying air bag may induce unique pattern abrasions on the face, cornea, forearms, or other exposed tissue. Pattern lacerations, specific fracture patterns, and amputations are seen when the deploying air-bag module cover impacts the hand, forearm, or feet (Figs. 5.3, 5.4, and 5.5) (6,7). The correlation of these injuries with the driver or passenger air-bag system is very helpful in assessing an occupant's role (6–8).

Both laminated (windshields) and tempered (side and rear windows) glass produce unique pattern injuries. The windshield is composed of two layers of glass laminated together with a thin layer of clear plastic sandwiched between. Laminated glass breaks into shards on impact (Fig. 5.6A,B). Tempered, or "safety," glass is a single layer of glass that breaks into small cubes when fractured. Shattered

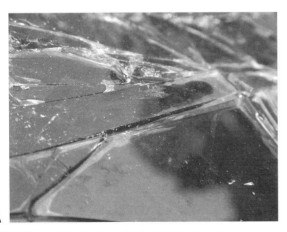

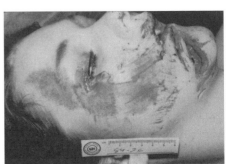

FIG. 5.6 A: The laminated windshield glass fractures into shards. Blood and hair are easily deposited during contact. B: Contact with windshield glass results in linear incised wounds.

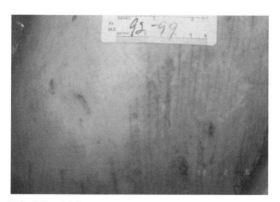

FIG. 5.7 Sliding contact with tempered glass, which is found in side and rear windows, results in "dicing" lacerations and "cube-like" wounds.

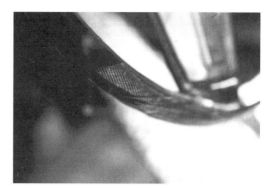

FIG. 5.9 Forceful impact of clothing against vehicle components can impart a fabric transfer. The comparison of the fabric weave from the imprint on the steering wheel assisted in determining which occupant was the driver.

tempered glass from side and rear windows imparts a "dicing" pattern to the skin (Fig. 5.7), whereas shattered laminated windshield glass causes linear incised wounds (Fig. 5.6B).

Trace Evidence

In the emergency department, an examination of clothing, shoes, and biologic standards (hair and blood) will assist in determining an occupant's role (2–5,8). Examination of the soles of leather shoes may reveal the imprint of the gas or brake pedal (Fig. 5.8). Preservation of clothing from all occupants permits comparison of clothing fibers with those fibers transferred to vehicle components during the collision (2–5,8). Imprints of fabric may also be transferred to components within the vehicle, including the steering wheel (Fig. 5.9). Contact with the windshield often transfers hair and tissue to the glass. Glass collected from within a patient's wound can be matched with a particular window within the vehicle. Clothes, shoes, and other evidence should be

collected and maintained if the role of the occupant in the collision is unclear.

Air bags and their module covers are also a tremendous source of trace evidence. Blood, hair, makeup, and skin are easily transferred to the air-bag's canvas surface during impact (Figs. 5.10 and 5.11) (6–8). The module cover will also yield transferred blood, tissue, and imprints from fabric or the soles of shoes (Figs. 5.12 and 5.13).

FORENSIC EVALUATION OF AIR-BAG–INDUCED INJURIES AND DEATHS

Designed and promoted as a lifesaving device, the air bag has made good its promise. The National Highway Transportation Safety Administration (NHTSA) estimates that nearly 19,000 lives have been spared as a result of air-bag deployment (9). Unfortunately, the same "lifesaving"

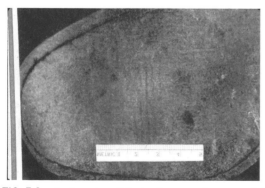

FIG. 5.8 An imprint of the brake or accelerator pedal can be transferred to leather soles. Examination of shoes can assist in the determination of an occupant's role.

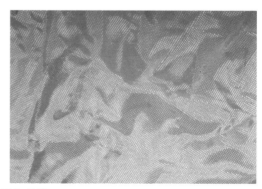

FIG. 5.10 Blood, hair, skin, and makeup are easily transferred to the air bag. An analysis of the trace evidence and their associated injuries will assist in determining an occupant's role.

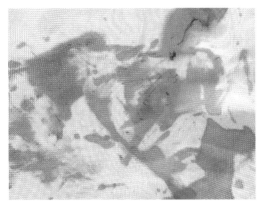

FIG. 5.11 Blood and tissue transferred to the passenger-side air bag can be correlated with the passenger's injuries.

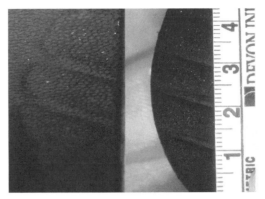

FIG. 5.13 Comparison of the imprint on the module cover and the sole of the passenger's shoe.

device has also been responsible for the deaths of at least 265 men, women, and children. Thousands of other motorists have sustained severe nonfatal injuries as a result of air-bag deployment, including cervical spine fractures, carotid artery injuries, retinal detachments, globe ruptures, cardiac rupture, closed head injuries, and comminuted fractures and amputations of the hand and upper extremity (10–21). Ironically, many of the injuries and deaths occurred in low- and moderate-speed collisions, not at high speeds.

In March 1997, NHTSA, in response to the increasing number of air-bag injuries and deaths, issued a rulemaking action that permitted automobile manufacturers to reduce the speed and force at which the bags deploy. Not surprisingly, beginning in 1998 and continuing through 2005, there has been a decline in the number of air-bag–induced serious injuries and deaths (9).

Mechanisms of Injury

Sodium azide is the toxic explosive propellant used to initiate the deployment cycle in most first-generation air bags, that is, those designed before 1998 (Fig. 5.14) (22,23). When sodium azide is ignited, the deploying air bag explodes, filling with nitrogen gas and carbon dioxide, and moves rapidly rearward toward the occupant at speeds of up to 210 mph (336 kph) (24). Second-generation air bags, generally in vehicles manufactured between 1998 and 2004, have reduced deployment speeds. Because of potential pulmonary hazards posed by the propellant sodium azide, that compound is gradually being replaced with argon gas. Third-generation air bags, found in vehicles manufactured after 2004, are equipped with special sensors that detect an occupant's position and weight and deploy at different velocities based on the severity of the collision.

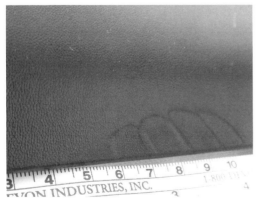

FIG. 5.12 The imprint of a shoe was transferred to the air-bag module cover. The passenger had her foot on the module cover at the moment of deployment (Fig. 5.19).

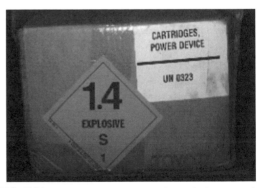

FIG. 5.14 Sodium azide is a toxic explosive material used for nitrogen generation in first-generation air bags. When not completely consumed in the inflation process, sodium azide has caused severe damage to the eyes and respiratory tract.

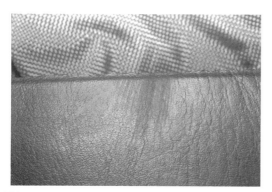

FIG. 5.15 Scuff marks on the module cover were associated with contact with the driver's right arm, which resulted in multiple fractures (Fig. 5.16).

Although the risk of injury is reduced with the second- and third-generation air bags, any body part (head, neck, chest, arms, or feet) in close proximity to the cover at the instant of deployment can still sustain severe injuries. Some of these proximity injuries have been fatal. The types of injuries that result from impact with the canvas air bag are different from those resulting from impact with its module cover (9). Reconstruction of the injuries incurred during deployment can be traced to the system component inflicting them: the canvas-covered air bag, the air-bag module cover, or both (Figs. 5.15–5.19) (14,15,25). Objects between the air bag and the occupant will be propelled rearward and inflict severe injuries (Figs. 5.20 and 5.21).

There are three basic phases to air-bag deployment: "punch out," "catapult," and "bag slap." The entire deployment process occurs in hundredths of a second. Injuries can be inflicted at any point during the air-bag deployment process (24,26).

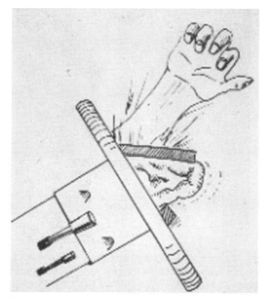

FIG. 5.17 Placement of the hand or forearm over the module cover will result in serious injuries (Figs. 5.4, 5.5, 5.16, and 5.22).

Phases of Air-Bag Deployment

1. *Punch out* is the initial stage of deployment, when the bag breaks out of its container. If the bag makes contact with an occupant at this stage, the following injuries can result: atlanto-occipital dislocation; cervical spine fracture with brainstem transection; cardiac, liver, and splenic lacerations; diffuse axonal injuries; subdural and epidural hematomas; and decapitation. Impact with the upper extremity during this phase will result in

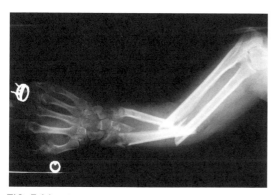

FIG. 5.16 Comminuted fractures of the wrist and mid-shaft radius and ulna from contact with the air-bag module cover of a first-generation air bag.

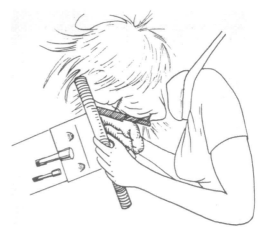

FIG. 5.18 Impact of the deploying module cover with the face can cause serious, even fatal, cranial and cervical spine injuries.

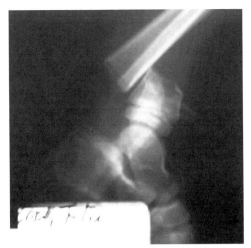

FIG. 5.19 Comminuted fractures of the distal tibia and fibula from placement of the foot on the module cover of a first-generation Ford air bag (Figs. 5.13 and 5.14).

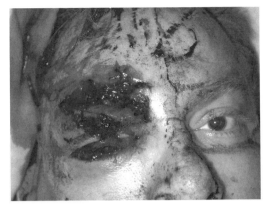

FIG. 5.21 A ruptured globe and eyelid laceration from impact with a metal cane. The cane (Fig. 5.20) was propelled rearward by the deploying passenger air bag.

massive fractures, degloving, and amputations (Fig. 5.22).

2. *Catapult* is the midstage of deployment. If the bag contacts an occupant's head during this phase, the head and neck will be driven rearward. This occurs with sufficient energy to rupture blood vessels, tear ligaments, rupture globes, and fracture cervical vertebrae. The facial and neck injuries sustained during the catapult phase occur as the result of direct trauma and cervical spine hyperextension (Figs. 5.23, 5.24, and 5.25).

3. *Bag slap* is the final stage of deployment, which occurs at the bag's peak excursion. Appropriately named, this happens when the canvas bag's fabric may "slap" the occupant's face or arms, resulting in injuries to the eye and epithelium (Fig. 5.26).

Some early first-generation air bags did not have an internal tethering system to limit the rearward excursion of the bag. Untethered air bags can extend beyond 21 in. (Fig. 5.27) compared with 12 to 14 in. of excursion in tethered models. This excessive rearward movement has been responsible for severe injuries to the face, particularly the eyes (Fig. 5.28). Even when properly restrained, properly positioned occupants can sustain severe injuries from untethered air bags (6,7,14,25).

The air-bag module covers are located in the steering wheel on the driver's side and in the dashboard panel on the passenger side. As mentioned above, in vehicles with first-generation air bags, the module cover is propelled outward at speeds of up to 210 mph (336 kph) (24). Second- and third-generation bags, although less forceful, will deploy at speeds between 100 and

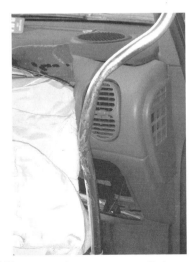

FIG. 5.20 A metal cane was propelled rearward by the deploying passenger air bag into the passenger's right eye (Fig. 5.21).

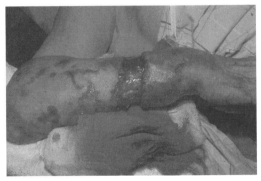

FIG. 5.22 Degloving of the forearm with comminuted fractures from impact with the module cover of a first-generation Ford air bag.

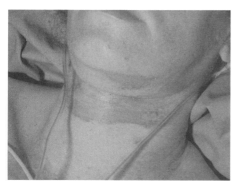

FIG. 5.23 Anterior neck abrasions from air-bag impact. Hyperextension injuries to the cervical spine are induced by the forceful rearward displacement of the head from the air bag.

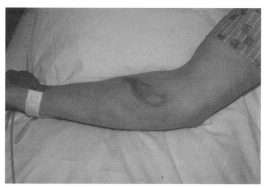

FIG. 5.26 Superficial abrasions from sliding contact with the canvas air bag.

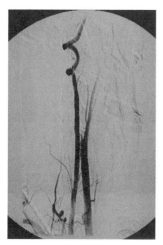

FIG. 5.24 The carotid artery was transected when the cervical spine was hyperextended during air-bag deployment (Fig. 5.23).

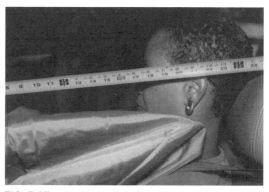

FIG. 5.27 Untethered air bags can extend rearward more than 20 in. and inflict facial injuries in properly restrained drivers and passengers. The untethered air bag in this 1989 Acura struck the driver's left eye, resulting in a lid laceration and ruptured globe.

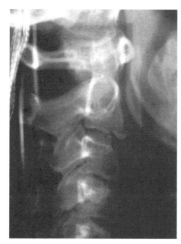

FIG. 5.25 Fracture of C-2 from air-bag–induced cervical hyperextension.

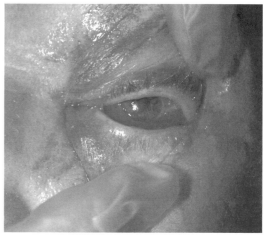

FIG. 5.28 Air bags are a common cause of ocular trauma. This patient sustained a detached retina from the blunt trauma of air-bag impact.

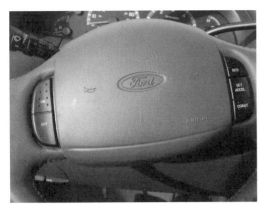

FIG. 5.29 Horn buttons located within the module cover are an invitation for hand and arm injuries if the driver attempts to blow the horn during a frontal impact.

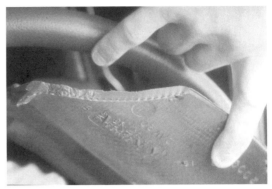

FIG. 5.31 The module cover from a 1991 Ford Taurus was torn by impact with the left side of the restrained driver's face. This force associated with air-bag deployment and module cover impact resulted in a fatal head injury.

150 mph and can induce injury. Unfortunately, most steering wheel designs incorporate and house the horn activation button within the air-bag module compartment (Fig. 5.29). This design is responsible for devastating upper extremity injuries (Figs. 5.4, 5.5, 5.16, 5.22, and 5.30). Hand and arm injuries sustained by individuals whose extremities were in contact with the horn button and module at the moment of its rupture include degloving, fracture, dislocation, fracture dislocation, and amputation (partial and complete of digits and forearms) (Figs. 5.4 and 5.30). Early module covers had considerable mass, including some with metal plate covers. Fortunately, automobile manufacturers have reduced the thickness and weight of the covers on both sides of the passenger compartment.

Beginning in 1995, automobile manufacturers began installing several types of "side air bags," including seat mounted, door mounted, window curtain, and inflatable tubular. The first reported injury from a side air bag occurred in December 1996 and involved a 3-year-old child. It was not until October 1999 that NHTSA issued a consumer advisory regarding the potential dangers of side air bags. The advisory stated "children who are seated in close proximity to a side air bag may be at risk of serious or fatal injury, especially if the child's head, neck, or chest is in close proximity to the air bag at the time of deployment" (27). As in frontal air bags, the injuries are attributed to the force of deployment of the air bag itself and/or the module cover. The risks for serious and fatal injuries to the head, neck, and the lateral thorax of both adult and pediatric occupants that lean against the side-mounted module are real (28). NHTSA has investigated 118 cases involving injuries from side air-bag deployments (28). The forensic investigator should employ the same techniques for investigating side air bag incidents as are utilized in the investigation of frontal air bag injuries.

Trace Evidence

Locards' principle regarding the transfer of physical evidence between two impacting objects is dramatically evidenced in the case of air bags. The transfer of blood, epithelial tissue, and makeup is common (Figs. 5.10 through 5.13 and 5.15). Analysis of the blood spatter pattern on the bag may assist the investigator in determining the position of the occupant and the configuration of the steering wheel at the moment of air-bag deployment.

Examination of the air-bag module cover may also reveal the presence of trace evidence. Depending on its design, the module cover may have been torn or bent, indicative of contact with an occupant's more

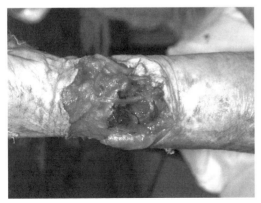

FIG. 5.30 Partial amputation of the left wrist from placement of the passenger's hand on the module cover of a 1995 Mercury Cougar.

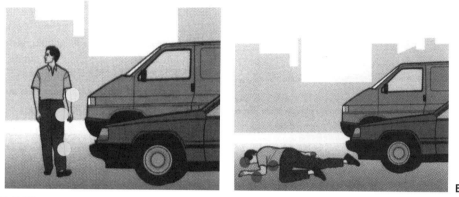

FIG. 5.32 Mechanisms of injury in an adult pedestrian struck by a car at low speed. A: Primary injuries (white bullets) are located on the victim's legs and hip, at the site of impact by the vehicle's bumper or radiator grill. B: Secondary injuries (gray bullets) occur when the victim falls on the road surface. These injuries are usually located on the head, trunk, and upper limbs. (From Payne-James J, Busittil A, Smock W, eds. *Forensic medicine: clinical and pathological aspects.* Cambridge, MA: Greenwich Medical Media, 2003, Chapter 35, Figure 35.5.)

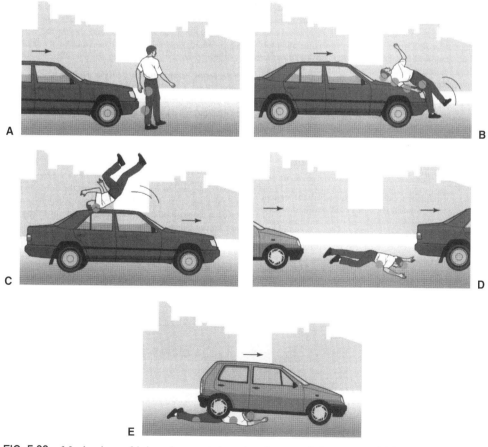

FIG. 5.33 Mechanism of injury in an adult pedestrian struck by a car at high speed (35 mph). After sustaining primary impact injuries, the victim is propelled upward (A), slides onto the hood (B), lands on the car roof (C), falls on the ground (D), and may be run over by an oncoming vehicle (E). The bullets indicate selected injury sites during the different phases of the incident. (From Payne-James J, Busittil A, Smock W, eds. *Forensic medicine: clinical and pathological aspects.* Cambridge, MA: Greenwich Medical Media, 2003, Chapter 35, Figure 35.6.)

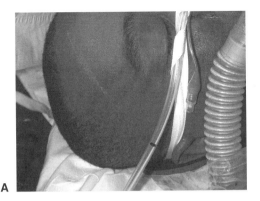
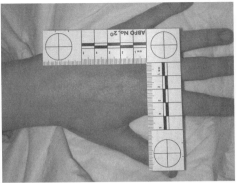
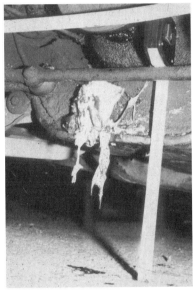

FIG. 5.34 **A:** A tire imprint located on the right temple. **B:** A tire imprint on the dorsum of the hand. **C:** The presence of skull fragments under the vehicle indicated the pedestrian was lying in the roadway when he was struck. The lack of impact injuries to the legs can indicate the pedestrian was lying in the roadway and not standing when struck.

rigid (boney) surface: face or forearm (Fig. 5.31). Scuff marks on the module cover indicate contact with an object, frequently the forearm (Fig. 5.15). Shoe imprints can occur when a passenger is resting a foot on the module cover at the moment of deployment (Figs. 5.12 and 5.13).

FORENSIC EVALUATION OF PEDESTRIAN COLLISIONS

Pattern Injuries

In 2004, approximately 4,600 pedestrians were killed and 68,000 seriously injured (1). Eighty-two percent of pedestrians are struck by a vehicle's front bumper/grill area (1). Many pedestrian incidents involve hit-and-run drivers or questions relating to

the position of the pedestrian when hit. Emergency physicians and nurses must be aware of the potential forensic issues surrounding pedestrian cases.

There are three phases of impact for a standing adult who is struck by the front of a passenger car:

1. "Primary" impact results in injuries to the pelvis and lower extremities from contact with the bumper, grill, and leading edge of the hood.
2. "Secondary" impact results in injuries to the head and torso from contact with the hood, A-pillar, and windshield.
3. "Tertiary" impact results in injuries to the head and torso from contact with the ground or other fixed objects (Figs. 5.32A,B).

Body-wide injuries, usually crushing in nature, can result from being run over (Figs. 5.33A–E). This

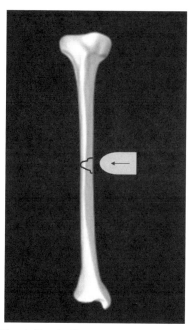

FIG. 5.35   A "wedge" type bumper fracture of the tibia. The tip of the wedge points in the direction of impact and is opposite the side of impact.

can occur if the pedestrian is already supine in the roadway or from final rest after sustaining tertiary impact. The lack of "bumper injuries" and the presence of tire marks could indicate the pedestrian was already prone or supine in the roadway when run over (Fig. 5.34A,B,C).

Bumper impacts usually cause comminuted, wedge-type fractures of the tibia and fibula and soft-tissue damage (Fig. 5.35). Pattern injuries, usually imprints of the bumper or grill, will assist in determining the orientation of the pedestrian at the moment of impact (Fig. 5.36A,B). The height of bumper injuries, measured from the heel and including the height of the patient's shoe, can be correlated with the height of the vehicle's bumper to determine whether the vehicle was braking at the moment of impact. Application of the brakes causes a vehicle's front end to dip; the presence or absence of braking may help determine the driver's intent. Emergency personnel can take such measurements before injuries are surgically repaired (destroying valuable evidence in the process). The presence of bumper injuries at one height on one leg and at another height on the other may indicate that the pedestrian was walking or running at the moment of impact, with one leg elevated. Shoe scuff marks at the scene or lateral striations on the soles may indicate the point of impact and whether the patient was dragged.

Trace Evidence

Headlight glass, windshield glass, grease, oil, and paint chips are valuable evidence in hit-and-run cases. Emergency care providers, from emergency medical technicians at the scene to physicians in the emergency department, must be aware of the potential significance of trace evidence. It is imperative the victim's clothes be preserved and inspected by an evidence technician at a crime laboratory. Glass fragments imbedded in the patient's scalp from the windshield or in the legs from the headlights must also be preserved for analysis by the crime laboratory.

CONCLUSION

The forensic aspects of motor-vehicle–related trauma are important to the care and treatment of our patients. To provide appropriate care, emergency

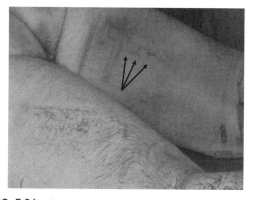

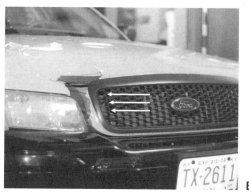

A   B

FIG. 5.36   A: A pattern imprint from the vehicle's grill is present on the posterior medial aspect of the pedestrian's right thigh. The location of the pattern contusion indicates that the victim was struck from the rear. B: The oval contusions (arrows) resulted from contact with the vehicle's grill.

care providers must receive forensic training as a component of their education. Accurate determination of an occupant's role will guarantee the guilty driver will be charged and the innocent passenger will not. Knowledge of air-bag systems and their potential to induce serious and fatal injuries will assist the emergency physician in understanding the mechanism of injury. Proper collection of evidence, in concert with precise interpretation of a pedestrian's injuries, will assist law enforcement in the investigation of pedestrian collisions.

REFERENCES

1. National Highway Traffic Safety Administration. *Traffic safety facts 2004, a compilation of motor vehicle crash data from the fatality analysis reporting system and the general estimates system* (DOT HS 809 919). Washington, DC, U.S. Department of Transportation, National Center for Statistics and Analysis, 2005.
2. Smock WS. Forensic emergency medicine. In: Marx JA, Hockberger RS, Walls RM, eds. *Rosen's emergency medicine: concepts and clinical practice*, 6th ed. Philadelphia, PA: Mosby, 2006.
3. Smock WS, Nichols GR II, Fuller PM, et al. The forensic pathologist and the determination of driver versus passenger in motor vehicle collisions: the need to examine injury mechanisms, occupant kinematics, vehicle dynamics, and trace evidence. *Am J Forensic Med Pathol* 1989;10:105–114.
4. Smock WS. Driver versus passenger in motor vehicle collisions. In: Siegel JA, Saukko PJ, Knupfer GC, eds. *Encyclopedia of forensic sciences*. San Diego, CA: Academic Press, 2000:24–32.
5. Blackbourne BD. Injury-vehicle correlations in the investigation of motor vehicle accidents. In: Wecht CH, ed. *Legal medicine annual 1980*. New York: Appleton-Century-Crofts, 1980.
6. Smock WS. Road traffic accidents, airbag-related injuries and death. In: Payne-James J, Byard R, Corey ST, et al., eds. *Encyclopedia of forensic and legal medicine*, Vol. 4. New York: Elsevier Academic Press, 2005:1–11.
7. Smock WS. Airbag-related injuries and death. In: Siegel JA, Saukko PJ, Knupfer GC, eds. *Encyclopedia of forensic science*. London: Academic Press, 2000.
8. Smock WS. Determination of driver versus passenger in motor vehicle collisions. In: Siegel JA, Saukko PJ, Knupfer GC, eds. *Encyclopedia of forensic science*. London: Academic Press, 2000.
9. National Highway Traffic Safety Administration. *Counts for frontal air bag related fatalities and seriously injured persons - counts for confirmed air bag related fatalities through 1/1/2006*. Washington, DC, U.S. Department of Transportation, National Center for Statistics and Analysis, 2006. Available at http://www-nrd.nhtsa.dot.gov/pdf/nrd30/NCSA/SCI/4Q_2005/QtrRpt/ABFSISR.htm. Accessed on February 21, 2006.
10. Huelke DF, Moore JL, Compton TW, et al. *Upper extremity injuries related to air bag deployments*, SAE Publication No. 940716. Detroit, MI: Society of Automotive Engineers, 1994.
11. Lancaster GI, DeFrance JH, Borrusso J. Air-bag-associated rupture of the right atrium [letter]. *N Engl J Med* 1993;328:358.
12. Lau IV, Horsch JD, Viano DC, et al. Mechanism of injury from air bag deployment loads. *Accid Anal Prev* 1993;25:29–45.
13. Prasad P, Daniel RP. *A biomechanical analysis of head, neck and torso injuries to child surrogates due to sudden torso acceleration*, SAE Paper No. 841656. Detroit, MI: Society of Automotive Engineers, 1984.
14. Smock WS, Nichols GN. Air bag module cover injures. *J Trauma* 1995;38(4):489–493.
15. Smock WS. Traumatic avulsion of the first digit, secondary to air bag deployment. *Proceedings of the 36th annual meeting of the association for the advancement of automotive medicine*. Des Plains, Illinois: AAAM, 1992:444.
16. Duma SM, Kress TA, Porta DF, et al. Airbag-induced eye injuries: a report of 25 cases. *J Trauma* 1996;41(1):114–119.
17. Manche EE, Goldberg RA, Mondino BJ. Air bag-related ocular injuries. *Ophthalmic Surg Lasers* 1997;28(3):246–250.
18. Ghafouri A, Burgess SK, Hrdlicka ZK, et al. Air bag-related ocular trauma. *Am J Emerg Med* 1997;15(4):389–392.
19. Walz FH, Mackay M, Gloor B. Air-bag deployment and eye perforation by a tobacco pipe. *J Trauma* 1995;38(4):498–501.
20. Perdikis G, Schmitt T, Chait D, et al. Blunt laryngeal fracture: another air-bag injury. *J Trauma* 2000;48(3):544–546.
21. Tenofsky P, Porter SW, Shaw JW. Fatal airway compromise due to retropharyngeal hematoma after air-bag deployment. *Am Surg* 2000;66(7):692–694.
22. Gross KB, Koets MH, D'Arcy JB, et al. Mechanism of induction of asthmatic attacks by the inhalation of particles generated by air-bag system deployment. *J Trauma* 1995;38(4):521–527.
23. Weiss JS. Reactive airway dysfunction syndrome due to sodium azide inhalation. *Int Arch Occup Environ Health* 1996;68(6):469–471.
24. National Highway Traffic Safety Administration. *Air-bag deployment characteristics*, DOT HS 807 869, Final Report. Washington, DC, U.S. Department of Transportation, September 1992.
25. Schubert GD. Forensic value of pattern and particle transfers from deployed automobile air-bag contact. *J Forensic Sci* 2005;50(6):1411–1416.
26. The Air-Bag Crisis: Causes and Solutions. Parents for Safer Air Bags, October 1997.
27. National Highway Traffic Safety Administration. *Consumer advisory - side impact airbags*. Washington, DC, U.S. Department of Transportation, October 14, 1999. Available at www.nhtsa.dot.gov/nhtsa/announce/press/1999/ca101499.html.
28. National Highway Traffic Safety Administration. *Special crash investigations, side air-bag cases through 1/1/2006*. Washington, DC, U.S. Department of Transportation, National Center for Statistics and Analysis, 2006. Available at www-nrd.nhtsa.dot.gov/pdf/nrd30/NCSA/SCI/4Q_2005/SummSheet/SABCSR.htm. Accessed on February 21, 2006.

FORENSIC EXAMINATION
OF ADULT VICTIMS AND PERPETRATORS OF SEXUAL ASSAULT

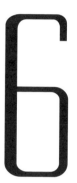

JUDITH A. LINDEN ■
ANNIE LEWIS-O'CONNOR ■
M. CHRISTINE JACKSON ■

Sexual assault is a crime of violence, which often goes unreported yet frequently has prolonged physical and emotional effects on victims. Statistics from the National Violence Against Women Survey (NVAWS), a telephone survey of 8,000 men and 8,000 women, reported a 17.6% lifetime prevalence of rape among women (1 of every 6) and a 3% prevalence rate among men (1 of every 33) (1). The National Crime Victimization Survey (NCVS) reported a sexual assault victimization rate of 0.8 per 1,000 persons aged 12 or older (2). Stated another way, a person is sexually assaulted every 2.5 minutes in the United States (3). In 1992, 16% of reported rape victims were younger than 12 (and therefore not captured in the NCVS) (4). According to the NVAWS, 3.6% of women were raped as a child, 6.3% as an adolescent, and 9.6% as an adult. Among men, 1.3% were raped as a child, 0.7% as an adolescent, and 0.8% as an adult (1). Many rapes go unreported: according to the NVAWS, only 19% of women and 13% of men who were raped after their 18th birthday reported the crime to the police (1).

Women are not convinced that reporting a sexual assault will lead to the conviction of the perpetrator. In fact, many women believe that their trauma after a sexual assault will be exacerbated if they take legal action. The 1993 Senate Judiciary Committee Report titled "The Responses to Rape" stated that 84% of reported rapes do not result in conviction (5). Of the 16% of perpetrators convicted, half are sentenced to less than 1 year in prison and 4% are not incarcerated at all (5). The NVAWS confirms this, with 46% of prosecuted rapists convicted but only 76% sentenced to jail or prison; therefore, only 13% of rapes reported to police result in incarceration (1). The sense of not being able to obtain justice from the legal system is one of the many consequences for all victims of rape. Other rape-related sequelae include posttraumatic stress syndrome, depression, eating disorders, substance abuse, and suicide (1,6–9). The tangible, out-of-pocket cost of sexual assault (excluding child sexual abuse) is estimated at $3.3 billion per year (10). For each rapist who is not convicted, there are usually subsequent victims because rapists tend to be repeat offenders. A rapist who has been caught has, on average, 14 previous victims (11). Appropriate conviction and incarceration of a rapist constitute justice served for the current victim and all prior victims; in addition, the rapist's future victims are spared.

When evaluating a victim of sexual abuse/assault, the emergency physician must not only meet strict legal standards but also provide complete medical care and emotional support. A preestablished systematic approach enables the busy emergency physician to complete an adult sexual assault examination adequately. Proper collection of evidence provides medical care for the victim as well as hope for legal recourse against the perpetrator.

Physicians who perform sexual assault evidentiary examinations must be familiar with the related legal aspects for their particular region. They must know the definition of rape and sexual assault as well as the legal time limits for evidence collection. The rights of the victim must be understood, and ensured, prior to obtaining consent for and proceeding with an evidentiary examination. To ensure the legal validity of evidence, sound procedures must be employed when collecting evidence and the chain of custody must be maintained. Failure to maintain this chain means that the collected forensic evidence can be thrown out of court, resulting in profound devastation for a victim. Because many cases depend on the forensic evidence, maintaining the chain of custody can make or break a case.

DEFINITION OF RAPE

Earlier definitions of rape typically included an act of forced vulvar penetration by a penis, object, or body part without the consent of a woman, during which ejaculation may or may not occur. This definition limits rape to women. During the past decade, many states have changed the definition to include both genders, now defining rape as an act of forced penetration of an orifice by a penis or object without a person's consent. Some states have addressed the problem of male rape by using the term *sexual assault* to broaden the coverage of unwanted sexual acts to include rape, sexual abuse, and sexual misconduct involving either gender. Sexual assault includes sexual contact of one or more persons with another without appropriate legal consent. The definition of rape and sexual assault varies slightly from state to state; although many states define rape in gender-neutral language, some states retain gender-specific language. The examiner needs to be familiar with the local jurisdiction's definitions of rape and nonconsensual sexual acts.

TIME LIMITS

In the past, the usual legal time limit for the collection of evidence was 72 hours from the time of the assault. However, recent updates in DNA analysis and sperm survival data have led some programs to extend the time limit up to 120 hours or 5 days. Victims of sexual assault presenting to a medical institution within the local jurisdiction's established specified time frame should be assigned priority in triage along with other serious emergencies, as the evidentiary examination must be conducted without delay to minimize loss or deterioration of evidence as well as immediate psychological trauma. If more than 120 hours have passed since the assault, a complete physical examination

should still be conducted to examine for injuries to the body and the genitalia, to offer treatment to prevent pregnancy and sexually transmitted infections (STIs), and to provide information for support resources. Depending on the local sexual assault protocol, a modified evidentiary examination may be indicated. On the basis of the spermatozoa survival data, there may be value in collecting cervical samples even when the patient presents more than 72 hours after the assault (12).

CONSENT/MAINTAINING CHAIN OF EVIDENCE

To protect the rights and interests of both the patient and the hospital, an appropriate signed written consent must be obtained before beginning the examination, treatment, and evidence collection. The consent form for the evidentiary examination is in the standard sexual assault evidence-collection kit. Evidence collection is never medically necessary, and it is important to know that items removed from the patient must be transferred to the police in the rare event of a warrant. In addition, body cavity searches for evidence are not medically necessary. When there is unexplained vaginal bleeding, it is medically necessary to find a cause but it is not necessary to collect evidence. When a patient signs a consent form, it means that she or he understands that evidence will be collected, preserved, and released to law enforcement authorities. Consent for the evidentiary examination includes consent for obtaining photographs of physical trauma to be used as evidence in a court of law (some jurisdictions have a separate consent form for photographs). A signed written consent for the sexual assault evidentiary examination does not replace the general consent for routine diagnostic and medical procedures that are standard with emergency treatment and done in accordance with hospital policy.

The patient may consent to an examination and/or treatment and/or evidence collection. In some states, the collection of evidence mandates a report to law enforcement officials. In other states, evidence may be collected without being reported, for a designated period of time, after which the evidence kit is destroyed if the sexual assault is not reported. When the local law enforcement agency is notified, the agency will render a complaint number and send an investigative officer to the hospital to interview the victim and generate a report. Even if the patient does not want to make a police report or have an evidentiary examination, the local enforcement agency may need to be notified to implement local procedures. In all states, the rape of minors, adults who are mentally challenged or disabled, and the elderly is subject to mandatory reporting; however, laws regarding mandatory reporting of adult victims vary from state to state (13).

When obtaining signed written consent for a sexual assault examination and evidence collection, the physician must inform the patient of his or her rights. The patient has the right to decline any or all parts of an examination that entails evidence collection. The patient needs to be made aware that evidence deteriorates over time and may be unobtainable if it is not collected and preserved promptly. In some states, evidence can be collected and the victim is given a specified period within which to report. The physician must explain that the collected body fluids and swabs may lead to the identification of the offender, especially in the light of DNA "fingerprinting" techniques and the Combined DNA Index System (CODIS) (see Chapter 13). The patient must also be informed that consent for the evidence-collection examination, once given, can be withdrawn at any time for all or part of the procedure. The patient has the right to decline the collection of reference/baseline specimens, such as pulled hair strands, blood for DNA profiling, and oral swabs.

If the patient declines to have reference samples collected at the time of the examination, it may be done at a later date. The reference specimens allow the crime laboratory to conduct a comparative analysis of the evidence in question. Patients should be informed that head hairs change over time if they are braided or dyed or if certain medicines are taken (e.g., chemotherapy).

Patients have the right to know if they are responsible for the cost of the examination. If an evidentiary examination is performed, the local government is responsible for its cost. The cost of the medical examination and treatment is the patient's responsibility (in some states [e.g., Iowa], the costs may be covered, even if a legal report is not made). Testing and treating for STIs and prophylaxis against pregnancy may also be provided without charge. Programs that do not do baseline testing for the human immunodeficiency virus (HIV) should give the patient appropriate referral information.

To maintain the chain of custody, careful and proper handling and transfer of the collected evidence are crucial. Documentation should clearly state who collected the evidence, who picked up and transported the evidence, and that it was stored appropriately and securely. A retrospective study of sexual assault evaluations performed by emergency physicians and ob-gyn residents in an urban emergency department (ED) revealed that the chain of custody was documented properly in only 6% of cases (14).

Preservation of the chain of custody is crucial to ensure that the evidence is not altered, destroyed, or lost before trial. All documentation of evidence transfers must include the following information: the name of the person transferring custody, the name of the person receiving custody, and the date and time of transfer. Transfers should be kept to a minimum, ideally limited to two persons. The evidence-collection kit is turned over to law enforcement officers by the examiner after the examination has been completed and the reference samples, swabs, and slides have been dried completely. If this is not possible, the evidence must be stored in a locked area accessible only to designated individuals. Materials that need to be refrigerated (i.e., blood and urine samples) must be locked in a refrigerated area. If some materials are still drying when the officers need to leave, a note to the crime laboratory should indicate that drying is in progress. When blood and urine collections are refrigerated, it is helpful to store the logbook in a plastic bag along with the blood. The plastic bag protects the book from spills and makes it easy to find.

THE ADULT SEXUAL ASSAULT PATIENT (FEMALES AND MALES)

Patient Intake

When a person who has been sexually assaulted comes to an ED within 120 hours after the assault, she or he should be triaged quickly, assessed for stability, and escorted promptly to a private area for the initial assessment. The triage, consent, and examination process for females is diagrammed in Figure 6.1 and the evidence-collection process is delineated in Table 6-1. The examination should be conducted without delay to minimize the loss or deterioration of evidence. A trained support person should be assigned to each victim. A patient who is taken directly to an examining room should, preferably, not change into a hospital gown until her/his clothing has been collected properly. If the patient desires evidence collection, then the protocols designated in the evidence-collection kit should be implemented. If the victim wants to report the assault, the police should be notified. In some states, the sexual assault response team (SART) is activated from triage. Law enforcement will then generate a complaint number specific to the victim. In some states, notification of police is mandatory (13).

The examiner should carefully explain the process of the examination to the patient. After the patient has been informed of her/his rights and agrees to the examination, a written consent for the examination is obtained before proceeding. The examiner should obtain the history in a nonjudgmental, warm, and professional manner,

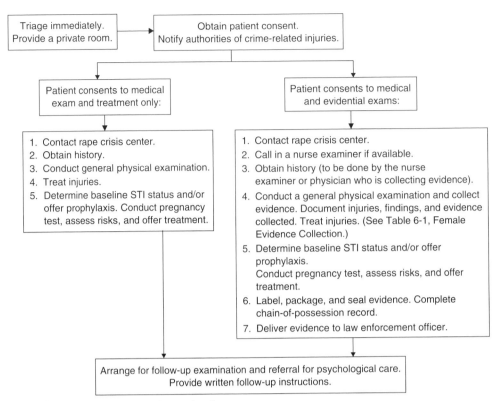

FIG. 6.1 Female sexual assault examination.

Medical Screening Examination

On arrival, the sexual assault victim needs to be assessed for unstable vital signs and must be medically and psychologically cleared before the initiation of the evidentiary examination. The clinician should determine whether there has been a change in mental status or whether there is a history of loss of consciousness. The patient should be examined to rule out serious medical/surgical injuries (including tears of the rectouterine pouch). Complaints of moderate to severe pain should alert the examiner to possible serious injuries. A review of fatal sexual assaults revealed that the most common causes of death are mechanical asphyxiation, beating, lacerations, drowning, and gunshot wounds (15). Fatal injuries are sustained by 0.1% of women who are sexually assaulted (16). Five percent to 10% of survivors of sexual assault sustain major nongenital injuries (16).

In addition to the standard trauma survey, the physician also needs to search carefully for evidence of physical injuries inflicted by the perpetrator during the assault. Findings can be documented and described on a head and/or body diagram (Figs. 6.2

realizing the emotional challenge the victim faces when recounting the details of the assault.

and 6.3.) Studies conducted during the past two decades have found that 31% to 82% of sexual assault victims sustain physical injuries (17–26), most often involving the head, face, neck, and extremities (17,19,24). Although the incidence of injuries is significant for all ages and types of victims, women younger than 50 and nonpregnant women are more likely to be physically injured during sexual assault (17,24). The risk of sustaining physical injuries also increases if the assailant was a stranger (26–28). The lack of evident physical or genital trauma does not imply consent by the victim or the absence of rape (21) (Appendix 6-1).

Slapping, kicking, beating, and biting are methods the perpetrator employs to overcome the resistance of the victim. The victim's entire body must be thoroughly examined for areas of tenderness, soft-tissue swelling, abrasions, contusions, bruises, petechiae, bite marks, lacerations, fractures, and other evidence of violence. Areas of tenderness without bruising should be documented carefully using body map or photographs. Bruises may develop 1 to 2 days later and can be photographed on follow-up examinations.

The back of the head may be banged against the ground during a sexual assault; therefore, soft-tissue swelling and lacerations may occur. The history regarding the events related to the sexual assault

TABLE 6-1

COLLECTION OF EVIDENCE FROM FEMALE VICTIMS OF SEXUAL ASSAULT
(Expansion of step 4 in evidential examination [Fig. 6.1])

Physical Examination[a,b] Female	Clinical Specimens for the Laboratory	Evidence for the Crime Laboratory (Kit comes from the police department)
4a. *Document condition of clothing worn.* Collect outer and underclothing worn during or immediately after the assault. Collect fingernail scrapings.	—	4a2. Place each piece of clothing in a separate bag. Place fingernail scrapings and foreign material found on clothing and body in separate envelopes.
4b. *General physical examination.* Scan entire body with Wood's lamp. Collect dried and moist secretions from body, head, and hair. Photograph bite marks (Figs. 6.5 and 6.6, see color plate), wounds, and any other findings. Examine the entire body. Record findings on a head and/or body diagram (Figs. 6.2 and 6.3).	—	—
4c. *Examine oral cavity.* Document findings. Swab area around the mouth. Collect oral swabs. Floss teeth. Collect GC specimen.	4c1. GC, use agar plate	4c2. Place in separate envelopes: oral swabs from external and internal surfaces, floss, foreign material
4d. *Examine external genitalia.* Scan with Wood's light. Collect dried and wet secretions and foreign materials. Cut matted pubic hair. Comb hair for foreign materials. Swab the vulvar region. Document findings.	—	4d2. Individually package dried secretions, foreign material, matted pubic hair cuttings, pubic hair combings, the comb, and swabs.
4e. *Apply toluidine dye.* Examine and document findings.	—	—
4f. *Examine vaginal and cervical area* for injury and foreign material. Collect swabs from vaginal pool. Prepare one wet mount and two dry mount slides. Collect swabs from the cervical region and vaginal walls.	4f1. GC, *Chlamydia,* and wet mount	4f2. Foreign material, vaginal swabs, and wet and dry mount slides
4g. *Examine buttock and anal region.* Collect any moist or dry secretions or foreign material. Swab anal region.	—	4g2. Dried secretions, foreign materials, and swabs
4h. *Apply toluidine dye.* Examine and document findings.	—	—
4i. *Anoscopic or proctoscopic examination* if indicated by history or examination of region. Collect anal and rectal swabs and GC swab.	4i1. GC culture	—
4j. *Clinical labs:* Pregnancy test (blood or UHCG, red-topped tube), syphilis serology (blood, gray-topped tube), HBsAG, HCsAG (blood, gold-topped 7-mL tubes), HIV[c] (blood, lavender-topped tubes)	4j1. Pregnancy and syphilis, HBsAG, HCsAG, HIV	—
4k. *Other evidence is collected at the discretion of the physician and/or law enforcement.* Alcohol (blood, red-topped tube), toxicology (blood, gray-topped tube), toxicology (50-mL urine)	4k1. Blood alcohol and toxicology and urine toxicology	—

(continued)

TABLE 6-1
(Continued)

Physical Examination[a,b] Female	Clinical Specimens for the Laboratory	Evidence for the Crime Laboratory (Kit comes from the police department.)
41. *Collect reference samples.* 25 pulled head hairs, 25 pulled pubic hairs, blood typing (yellow-topped tube)/DNA (purple-topped tube). If bloodstain cards are used, place blood on card. If bloodstain cards are not used, place the blood in a refrigerator until it is given to the police.	—	412. Reference samples
The reference samples can be collected at a later date.	—	—
Complete chain of possession record.	Send clinical specimens to laboratory.	Give evidence kit to law enforcement.
Label each envelope with the complaint number, date, time, and examiner's name. Package and seal the evidence and sign the outside envelope.	—	—

[a] All swabs and slides must be air-dried before packaging.
[b] Code corresponding swabs and slides, For example, Oral Swab No. 1/Oral Slide No. 1.
[c] In most states, counseling is mandatory before screening for HIV.
GC, neisseria gonorrhoeae culture; HBsAg, hepatitis B surface antigen; HCsAg, hepatitis C surface antigen; HIV, human immunodeficiency virus.

is crucial in guiding the examination and evidence collection. Another cause of scalp hematoma or soft-tissue swelling is violent pulling of the hair (29). Head trauma, specifically basilar skull fracture, may present as raccoon eyes or Battle's sign. If the victim experienced loss of consciousness, the Glasgow Coma Scale score should be determined at triage. A complete ophthalmic examination and evaluation of the tympanic membranes are indicated in cases of head trauma. Further evaluation for intracerebral

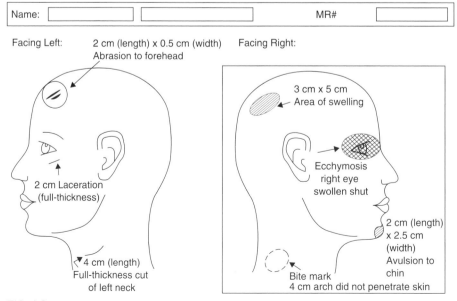

FIG. 6.2 A head diagram used to document the location and appearance of injuries.

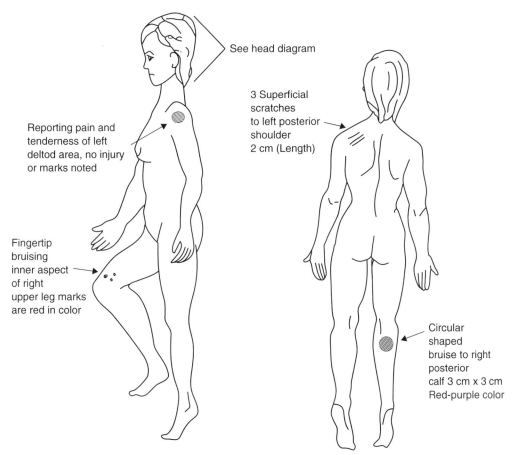

See head diagram

3 Superficial
scratches
to left posterior
shoulder
2 cm (Length)

Reporting pain and
tenderness of left
deltod area, no injury
or marks noted

Fingertip
bruising
inner aspect
of right
upper leg marks
are red in color

Circular
shaped
bruise to right
posterior
calf 3 cm x 3 cm
Red-purple color

FIG. 6.3 A body diagram used to document the location and appearance of injuries.

trauma by computed tomography scan must be considered. With blunt trauma to the head and face, associated injury to the cervical spine should be considered. Victims of sexual assault often sustain facial injuries, including mandibular fractures, nasal fractures, other facial fractures, broken or loose teeth, facial lacerations, and ocular trauma. The breasts should be examined for evidence of trauma, including contusions, lacerations, swelling, and bite marks. If the assailant pulls and twists the victim's clothing, then petechial hemorrhages or a line of punctate bruising may occur on the skin, commonly in the area of the bra strap or near the axilla (29).

The extremities should be inspected for evidence of the perpetrator's attempts to overcome the resistance of the victim. Fingernail abrasions; fingertip injuries; and bruises on the wrists, ankles, and inner/outer aspects of the arms and thighs (defense injuries) are sustained during the assailant's attempts to restrain the victim. If the perpetrator forcibly twisted the victim's wrists, erythema and point tenderness in that area may be noted (29). A careful search for patterns of injury during inspection

may reveal injuries that are not readily apparent from the initial history. If the assailant overwhelmed the victim and held her/him in restraint, then bruises and abrasions may be seen over bony prominences.

Once the trauma survey has been completed and the patient medically cleared, then a careful search for patterns of injury and evidence collection is initiated. Physical examination of the sexual assault victim focuses on the detection of physical (nongenital) injuries and genital injuries. The incidence of genital injuries varies from 6% to 65%, with most investigators reporting a range between 10% and 30% (17–21,23–26,30,31). Elderly female victims of sexual assault (age 60 to 90 years) have a 43% to 52% increased incidence of genital trauma, double that of sexual assault victims younger than 60, and their injuries are often more serious (owing to decreased or lack of estrogenation) (24,25). The most common sites of injury do not differ among victims younger or older than 50 (23). Genital injury may be more prevalent in nonpregnant victims (21% vs. 5%) (17). One must always be cognizant that lack of abnormal findings does not indicate that a sexual assault did not occur (32).

Victim Interview

It is best to begin the history taking with less invasive, general questions, such as medical and surgical history, use of medications, and drug allergies. These should have been documented in the medical chart. There is controversy over whether drug or alcohol use within the previous 120 hours should be documented, but this may be important, as it may help establish lack of consent. Positive toxicologic test results for alcohol or drugs are not uncommon and the examiner should not allow the results to place the victim's history in question (17,33). Information about anal-genital injuries sustained during the past 60 days as well as surgeries, diagnostic procedures, or medical treatment performed within that period should be documented to prevent confusion with injuries related to the sexual assault. The interview should focus on items that fulfill the legal criteria of rape, including penetration of an orifice, lack of consent, and threat or actual use of force, as well as identification of the assailant and witnesses, if possible. All recorded information is admissible in court.

The physician should document the following information (Fig. 6.4):

- The name, age, sex, and race of the victim
- The patient's vital signs
- The date, time, location, and/or physical surroundings of the assault, including odors; any witnesses
- The patient's personal hygiene (e.g., showered, bathed, brushed) since the assault
- The name(s), number, race(s), and any other identifier(s) of the perpetrator(s), if known
- The use of weapons, physical force, restraints, injuries, forced drug or alcohol use, and verbal and/or nonverbal threats
- The threats, types of force, or other methods used by the perpetrators(s) (including drug-facilitated assault) and the area(s) of the body affected
- The sexual acts committed by the perpetrator(s); the sexual acts the victim was forced to perform on the perpetrator(s)
- Details regarding the attempt to penetrate or actual penetration of the oral cavity, vagina, or rectum by penis, finger, or object and the resultant injuries
- Whether the victim recently inserted tampons or any other foreign objects into her own orifices
- The frequency and sequence of the sexual acts
- Positions used during the assault
- Whether the assailant ejaculated and the location

- The use of a condom or lubricant
- If there was more than one assailant, which perpetrator committed which act
- Whether kissing, biting, or licking occurred and the site(s) involved

A careful history must be taken, as some victims may be reluctant to describe all the acts committed, particularly anal penetration. The patient should be asked if she/he remembers injuring the assailant during the assault (e.g., by scratching or biting). Questions related to the sexual assault should be open ended (e.g., "And what happened next?"). The examiner should not ask leading questions.

Any physical injuries, sites of bleeding, and/or areas of pain described by the victim must be recorded. Injuries occurring before and independent of the assault should be identified (e.g., fractured arm, lacerations, or bruising), with clarification of all findings. If the assault occurred within 120 hours of the examination, the victim's personal hygiene activities since the assault should be noted because this information affects the laboratory analysis of evidence. The physician should ask patients if they have bathed, douched, urinated, defecated, brushed their teeth, or vomited since the assault. The date of a female victim's last menstrual period should be documented to determine whether she is menstruating at the time of the examination, to evaluate the possibility of pregnancy and to consider emergency contraception. If the patient had consenting intercourse within the past 120 hours, the approximate date and time should be recorded. This information is required by the crime laboratory because it can affect the analysis of the evidence.

Physical Examination

The patterns of injury associated with sexual assault result from restraining methods used by the perpetrator, the violent acts of the perpetrator, as well as the victim's attempt to defend her/himself. Despite evidence that sexual assault does not result in visibly detectable physical or genital injury in all cases, the criminal justice system still relies on physical evidence of trauma to convict a perpetrator. The examiner needs to be knowledgeable of forensic medicine pertaining to sexual assault to detect physical injury, document trauma, and collect evidence appropriately, all of which may increase the chances of a successful legal outcome (18,34,35). (Sexual anatomy terminology is presented in Appendix 6-2.)

Some sexual assailants use threatening behavior with guns, knives, or other weapons to overcome the resistance of the victim (36). Some use only verbal threats. Regardless of resistance efforts, the assailant's use of a weapon and/or force usually overcomes the victim (37). Cartwright retrospectively reviewed the medical records of 440 female sexual assault survivors to identify factors that correlated with injury. The risk of physical injury was greatest if the assailant's weapon was a knife or club (79%) rather than a gun (34%). If no weapon was employed, the incidence of physical injury fell between that associated with use of a knife/club and a gun (27). The patient may or may not sustain an injury from the weapon itself. The weapon may be used as a threat and the physical trauma inflicted in a different manner. The patient's history will usually guide the physician toward the detection of such injuries.

In certain circumstances, the victim may attempt to resist the assailant's attack and sustain "fight," or defense, injuries related to that effort. The victim may have contusions of the forearms or the legs, caused by self-defense movements. Injuries on the hands, especially the knuckles, can also reflect self-defense actions. If the victim was dragged over

---

Victim Information
General appearance_____
Demeanor_____
Last menstrual period_____
Recent surgeries, trauma, diagnostic procedures, or medical treatments (in the past 60 days)_____
Last consensual intercourse_____

Assault Information
Date of assault_____
Time of assault_____
Location of assault_____

Victim's Personal Hygiene
Bathed since assault   yes   no
Douched since assault   yes   no
Urinated since assault   yes   no
Defecated since assault   yes   no
Changed clothing since assault   yes   no

Perpetrator(s)
Name of perpetrator(s)_____
Number of perpetrators_____
Race of perpetrator(s)_____

Use of Force
Use of weapon   yes   no
   If yes, what?_____
Physical force   yes   no
   If yes, what?_____
Restraints   yes   no
   If yes, what?_____
   If yes, where?_____
Verbal threats   yes   no
   If yes, explain_____
Non-verbal threats   yes   no
   If yes, explain_____
Other types of force used? yes   no
   If yes, explain_____

Wounds inflicted on assailant?   yes   no
   If yes, where?_____

FIG. 6.4 History checklist.

Alcohol/Drug Use

Alcohol use	yes		no		

If yes, amount?_____

If yes:	forced use		consensual use	both

Drug use	yes		no		

If yes, what?_____Route?_____

If yes:	forced use		consensual use	both

Sexual Acts

		yes	no	attempted	unknown
Oral penetration		yes	no	attempted	unknown
Vaginal penetration					
Penis		yes	no	attempted	unknown
Finger		yes	no	attempted	unknown
Foreign object		yes	no	attempted	unknown
Rectal penetration					
Penis		yes	no	attempted	unknown
Finger		yes	no	attempted	unknown
Foreign object		yes	no	attempted	unknown

Frequency and sequence of the above acts/positions_____
_____

Ejaculated	yes	no	unknown

If yes, where?_____

Difficulty maintaining an erection?	yes	no	
Kissing/licking	yes	no	unknown

If yes, where?_____

Biting	yes	no	unknown

If yes, where?_____

Use diagrams to document foreign material, excretions, trauma, physical injuries, and Wood's lamp findings.

Evidence/Injuries

Clothes torn	yes	no

If yes, where?_____

Clothes stained	yes	no

If yes, where?_____

Physical injuries	yes	no

If yes, where?_____

Fractures	yes	no

If yes, where?_____

Lacerations	yes	no

If yes, where?_____

Cuts	yes	no

If yes, where?_____

Abrasions/ecchymosis	yes	no

If yes, where?_____

Bite mark(s)	yes	no

If yes, where?_____

Size_____Shape_____

Foreign bodies found?	yes	no

If yes, where?_____

If yes, type?_____

FIG. 6.4 (Continued)

a rough surface, she/he may have longitudinal abrasions on the limbs or trunk. Dirt particles may be embedded in the skin. The victim's fingernails may be broken if she/he scratched the assailant or defended herself/himself during the attack. The victim's clothing may have been torn during attempts to resist the assault (28).

The amount of resistance by the victim is affected by many variables, one of which is fear instilled by the assailant's verbal threats and/or threats with weapons. A victim held at gunpoint is less likely to have injuries associated with resistance. Although there is some consensus that resistance increases the chance of aborting rape, it is inconclusive whether the victim's physical resistance alters the risk of being physically injured (16,37). The risk of physical injury correlates with the assailant's aggression, not with more forceful resistance by the victim (38).

Evidentiary Examination

A full evidentiary examination includes collecting clothing; debris; samples from under the patient's nails; pubic and scalp hair samples; reference blood; swabs from the skin, sites of injury (bite marks), and bodily orifices; and control swabs. Before collecting evidence, the examiner should moisten a set of control swabs with the same vial of sterile water used to moisten the evidence-collection swabs. Saline should *not* be used to moisten the swabs because it can destroy DNA evidence. The sterile water vial becomes the control. After the swabs dry, they should be returned to the sleeve and placed in an envelope labeled as such. Some kits come with "control swabs." In this case, controls need not be prepared.

Collection of Clothing

After arrival at the ED, the patient should remain clothed until it is time to conduct the examination, if possible. Once a patient consents to evidence collection, the steps delineated in the evidence-collection kit should be followed. A thorough history of the sexual assault should be obtained (see the bulleted list under Victim Interview on page 92). The patient's general appearance and demeanor should be documented objectively. Along with the vital signs, the patient's height, weight, and color of eyes and hair should be noted. Once evidence collection begins, the examiner should wear gloves to prevent DNA contamination. The patient's clothing should be observed for rips, tears, odors, stains, and other foreign materials, including fibers, hair, twigs, grass, soil, splinters, glass, blood, and seminal fluid. Before the patient's clothing is collected, it should be scanned for fluorescent exudates (using a Wood's lamp), and positive areas should be noted in the examination report. All clothing worn during and immediately after the assault should be collected and labeled and its collection should be documented (Table 6-1). If the victim is not wearing the clothing worn at the time of the assault, then only the items that are in direct contact with the victim's genital area need to be collected. The police officer in charge should be informed to arrange for collection of the clothing worn at the time of the assault.

The proper method of collecting the clothing is to have the patient stand on two sheets of clean paper on the floor, one sheet on top of the other. The disposable paper placed routinely on examination tables can be used for this process. The purpose of the bottom sheet of paper is to protect evidence on the clothing from being contaminated by debris or dirt on the floor. The top sheet is submitted to the crime laboratory. The patient should remove her/his shoes prior to stepping on the paper for disrobing to avoid contamination of loose trace evidence with nonevidential debris from the shoe soles. The shoes should be collected and packaged separately. The victim's clothing should not be shaken, because microscopic evidence could be lost. Holes, rips, or stains in the victim's clothing must not be disturbed by cutting. In the case of a ligature, the knot should not be untied (see the explanation in the next section).

Skin Survey

A thorough head-to-toe skin surface survey must be conducted. The skin should be searched grossly for evidence of bleeding, lacerations, abrasions, bruises, erythema, edema, scratches, bite marks, burns, stains, moist and dried secretions, and foreign materials. Different patterns of trauma are associated with an assailant's efforts to stop the victim from screaming: clamping the hand over the mouth, use of adhesive materials over the mouth, gagging, and strangulation. The mouth and lips must be inspected for evidence of trauma or residual adhesive material. Marks of brute force or strangulation should be sought. The presence of ligature marks, bruises, abrasions, or scratches on the neck should be noted. Swabbing these areas for DNA using a wet and then a dry swab has led to an increase in DNA findings. Gagging and strangulation both lead to asphyxia and may result in physical evidence, such as scattered petechial hemorrhages over the face and the eyelids. Subconjunctival hemorrhages and retinal hemorrhages may also result from attempted strangulation (29,39).

The perpetrator may have used ligatures or tape (e.g., duct tape) to restrain the victim. If ligatures are still in place, the entire ligature and its placement (including the knot) should be photographed before its removal. Then the ligature can be cut away from the knot, taking care not to destroy the knot, which may be a signature of the assailant. The physical signs of restraint, usually on the ankles and/or wrists, vary and depend on the tightness, resistance, and the length of time the victim was restrained. The patterned abrasion or bruise at the site of the restraint may range from tenderness to slight erythema of the skin to a deeper skin lesion with distal edema (29).

With the lights darkened in the room, the entire body should be scanned with a long-wave ultraviolet light (Wood's lamp/Bluemaxx light), searching for fluorescent exudates. The ultraviolet light reveals evidence of dried or moist secretions, stains, fluorescent fibers, and subtle injuries (such as rope marks and contusions) not readily visible in white light. If findings are noted, their location, size, and appearance should be documented in the text and on the schematic figures of the body. Photographs of the skin trauma should be taken. If photographs are to be taken of injuries that are visible only in ultraviolet light, the examiner may want to rely on local crime laboratory experts. Photographic documentation of these subtle injuries requires a longer exposure time and the use of a stationary tripod in a darkened room. Photographs of bruises may be helpful in defining the object that inflicted the injury (patterned injury).

With the proper technique, photographs of bite marks assist in identifying the perpetrator. If the bite mark has broken or perforated the skin, the creation of a cast by a forensic odontologist, if available, may be indicated. This evidence can be compared with court-ordered impressions and wax bites from the suspect. A typical human bite mark is a round or oval ring-shaped lesion with two opposing, often symmetric, U shapes with open spaces at the bottom. The intensity of force behind the bite affects the pattern depth and characteristics (i.e., the pattern may have abrasions, contusions, or lacerations in the area of the teeth) (40) (Figs. 6.5 and 6.6, see color plate). The classic bite mark shape is not always present, so if a bite mark is suspected, then forensic evaluation of the lesion is indicated. In documenting the bite mark, the site, size, shape, color, and type of injury are noted (e.g., contusion with ecchymosis, abrasion, laceration, incision, avulsion, petechial lesion). Findings such as smooth skin or indentation of the skin by teeth should be noted. If the patient gives a history of being bitten in a certain area but tenderness is the only physical sign noted, the clinician must remember that bruises and bite marks may not be apparent immediately following an assault but can develop later. A recommendation should be made to the police to arrange for a follow-up examination and additional photographs by the crime laboratory after the bruising

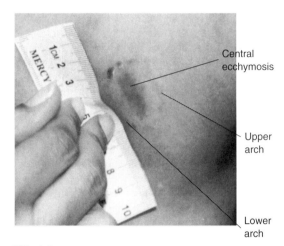

FIG. 6.5   Bite mark on the breast (see color plate).

has developed more fully. Serial photographs have been recommended by law enforcement and should be taken for 6 days at 24-hour intervals, because bruises and bite marks become more evident with time.

The perpetrator's saliva and residual epithelial cells on bite mark wounds should be collected using the two-swab technique for the collection of dried secretions. The outside border of the bite mark should be swabbed toward the center of the bite mark, first with the wet swab, then the dry one. Some local protocols specify the use of two moist swabs together. The greatest amount of saliva is usually deposited in the area of the bite mark caused by the lower teeth. Both swabs must be allowed to dry thoroughly, the wet swab for at least 1 hour. Then both swabs are submitted for the forensic analysis of DNA.

Collection of Foreign Material

Along with textual, diagrammatic, and photographic documentation, evidence on the patient's body (e.g., foreign materials, dried and moist secretions, and stains) should be collected properly. Foreign materials include fibers; hair; grass; dirt; and thicker stains of semen, saliva, or blood. A separate "miscellaneous" envelope should be used for each location on the body from which foreign material is collected. The envelope should be labeled with the term "debris" and the materials and the site of collection should be noted. The separate foreign material envelopes are sealed and placed in the main miscellaneous evidence-collection envelope. Location of the foreign material should be recorded in the text and marked on the diagram. For the collection of foreign materials, a tweezer, a glass slide, or the dull side of a scalpel blade can be used to gently loosen or scrape the foreign substance onto the opened and flat miscellaneous paper collection

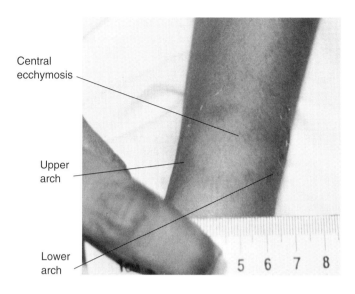

Central ecchymosis

Upper arch

Lower arch

FIG. 6.6 Bite mark on the wrist (see color plate).

envelope. Sometimes the use of a cotton-tipped swab moistened with sterile water can be helpful. The paper envelope should be refolded in a manner to retain the scraping and debris. If heavily crusted semen or blood is found on the pubic hair, the matted hairs bearing the specimen should be cut out and placed in a collection envelope, which is then labeled and sealed.

If the victim gives a history of scratching the assailant or if foreign material is observed under the nails, fingernail scrapings should be collected, as they may contain blood and/or tissue of the perpetrator or other evidence from the crime scene. The right- and left-hand collections are performed as separate procedures. Most sexual assault examination kits provide the two fingernail scrapers and the collection envelopes required for the procedure. Each of the victim's hands should be held over an unfolded, flat collection paper. Then scrapings are taken from under all five fingernails and the debris is allowed to fall onto the paper. The used scraper is placed in the center of the paper, which is then refolded to retain the debris and the scraper and placed in a labeled envelope. The two envelopes are identified as containing "right-hand fingernail scrapings" or "left-hand fingernail scrapings." The nails may also be swabbed using a cotton swab moistened with sterile water.

Evidence specimens of thin secretions and stains from blood, semen, and saliva need to be collected properly to improve the forensic yield when they are subjected to genetic typing tests, most importantly DNA testing. The method of collecting evidence from moist secretions or stains differs from that involving dried secretions or stains. Both methods use swabs supplied in the sexual assault evidence kit. If the number of swabs is not sufficient, a sterile cotton-tipped swab can be used. Each suspicious

moist or dried secretion, stain, or fluorescent area needs to be approached as a separate procedure with separate swabs and labeled in detail. When bloodstains are present, the stain pattern should be photographed before the evidence is collected. The area is swabbed, and injuries that might be associated with the blood should be noted.

The two-swab technique is used for dried secretions or stain areas noted on the gross visualization examination and with the light-scanning procedure (41). The first swab is moistened with sterile distilled water and then used to swab the evidence area. When wetting the swab with sterile water, one drop should be used, if possible, rather than saturating the swab. The amount of moisture applied to the swab can be controlled by using a 10-mL syringe into which distilled water has been drawn. This technique is generally adequate for obtaining the specimen and facilitates drying in a timely manner. Both swabs must be dried thoroughly—the wet swab for at least 1 hour with either a stream of cool air or on a drying rack. The second swab is left to dry and is used to swab the same site as the wet swab. Once the wet swab has dried, both swabs from one evidence site are packaged together in the original wrapper. The wrapper is labeled with the evidence-collection site and placed in the main miscellaneous evidence-collection envelope. If evidence is collected from a moist area of secretion or stain, a dry swab is used to avoid dilution of the evidence. The swab is allowed to air-dry for at least 1 hour and is then placed in a labeled envelope or tube, which is then sealed. If the swabbed area (moist or dried) was found with the use of a Wood's lamp, "W.L." should be marked on the envelope. The findings are recorded, and the locations of the secretions or stains are noted in the text and on the diagram of the body.

Sometimes a hand or arm print will show up on the Wood's lamp examination. It is important to swab and document these areas because they may contain epithelial cells from the assailant.

Dried semen stains have a characteristic shiny, mucoid appearance and tend to flake off the skin. Under an ultraviolet light, semen usually exhibits a blue-white or orange fluorescence and appears as smears, streaks, or splash marks. Because freshly dried semen may not fluoresce, each suspicious area should be swabbed, whether it fluoresces or not, with a separate swab. Not all fluorescent areas observed under ultraviolet light are indicative of seminal fluid; therefore, forensic confirmation of the findings is necessary.

Reference Samples

Reference samples, including blood and head and pubic hair, are collected to determine whether the specimens are foreign to the patient. They are also used for comparison with specimens from potential suspects. Plucking of hairs from the patient's head permits the evaluation of hair length as well as the variation of natural pigment or hair dyes from the root to the tip of the strand. Patients should be given the option of pulling out their own hair reference samples, as this gives them the feeling of having more control over the situation. A minimum of five full-length hairs should be pulled from each of the following scalp locations (total of 25 hairs): center, front, back, left side, and right side. The hairs should represent variations in length and color. They are placed in an envelope, which is labeled and sealed. (If a patient has attached synthetic hair, samples of both the synthetic hair and the real hair should be collected, and a notation made on the outside of the collection envelope that both have been included.)

Reference samples of pubic hair can be collected simultaneously with the pubic hair evidence collection. A sheet of paper should be placed beneath the patient's buttocks. The pubic hair is combed forward from the mons pubis toward the vaginal area first, to remove any loose hairs or foreign materials that may have transferred from the assailant to the patient during the assault. The loose hairs, foreign materials, pubic hair, and comb are placed in the sheet of paper, which is then folded with the contents inside. The folded paper and its contents are placed in a large labeled envelope, which is then sealed. Then, samples of the patient's pubic hairs are needed for comparison with the suspect's hairs. The patient or the examiner needs to pluck at least 10 to 15 hairs of various lengths and color from the pubic area (42). The hairs can be compared microscopically, and if hairs foreign to the victim are identified, they can be tested utilizing polymerase chain reaction (PCR) DNA. (Some crime labs request that the hairs be plucked later, when requested by laboratory personnel.)

Forced Oral Penetration

If the patient reveals that oral penetration occurred as part of the assault, the mouth and perioral area should be examined for evidence of trauma. The lips should be inspected for contusions, lacerations, and moist or dried collections of seminal fluid. Any evidence of ecchymosis and/or petechiae in the oral cavity, most commonly seen in the posterior pharynx or on the soft palate, should be noted. Erythema or hemorrhagic findings on the palate may be a result of the negative pressure associated with oral penetration, direct trauma, or, occasionally, infectious diseases (e.g., candidiasis, gonorrhea). Oral penetration may also tear the frenulum under the tongue, cause other lacerations, and loosen teeth. All three frenula should be inspected for injury. If denture devices are present, they should be removed and swabbed. However, in most cases, few, if any, physical findings are detected after forced oral penetration, because this act usually does not produce clinical lesions or trauma (43).

If the assault involved oral penetration and/or if the assailant placed his hand over the victim's mouth, and if the assault occurred less than 24 hours before the examination, the area around the mouth and the oral cavity must be swabbed for evidence of seminal fluid or epithelial cells. Two swabs should be used to collect evidence from the oral cavity. Using each swab individually, the inside of the left and right cheek area, and the upper gum lines, are swabbed with enough pressure applied to the buccal cavity to retrieve a good sample of epithelial cells and saliva for crime laboratory analysis. Two dry mount slides are then prepared—one from each swab—and labeled "Swab/Slide No. 1" and "Swab/Slide No. 2"; a fixative is not recommended. The swabs are allowed to air-dry for at least 1 hour; the slides are then packaged in the miscellaneous collection envelopes, which are labeled and sealed.

Forced Vaginal Penetration

A woman presenting after forced vaginal penetration needs a careful physical examination of the introitus and the vagina. This examination should be conducted even if the patient denies vaginal complaints. The external genitalia should be inspected for evidence of foreign materials and collections of dried and/or moist secretions. Dried secretions may appear as areas of matted pubic hair. The external genitalia, fossa navicularis, posterior fourchette (Fig. 6.7, see color plate), and vestibule should be examined for evidence of trauma. If

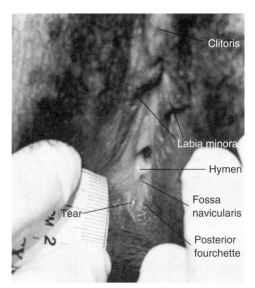

FIG. 6.7 Tear to posterior fourchette. Female Tanner 4 sexual assault patient (see color plate).

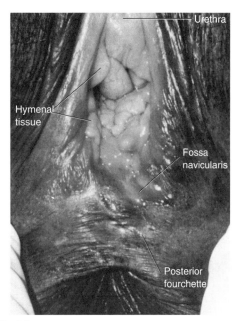

FIG. 6.8 Female sexual assault victim Tanner 5 before toluidine blue dye testing (see color plate).

the hymen is particularly redundant, and its edges are not clearly visible on labial retraction, a Foley balloon technique or a wet cotton-tipped swab is utilized to thoroughly assess the hymen prior to the insertion of a speculum. Toluidine blue should then be applied, if indicated, before the speculum examination (see the following section for details) (44).

Then a speculum examination of the vagina is performed to inspect for signs of internal trauma. The cervical os is the site for collecting the first swab (endocervical); because if sperm are present beyond 72 hours, this is where they are most likely to be collected (45).

Vaginal pool secretions, exocervical swabs, vaginal wall swabs, and swabs of the perivaginal area should be collected for the detection of spermatozoa, acid phosphatases, p30 (an antigen derived from the prostate epithelial cells and found in seminal plasma and urine from men, including those who have had a vasectomy) (12), and DNA testing. Any bleeding, abrasions, fissures, lacerations, petechiae, ecchymosis, edema, contusions, or hematomas observed on the external genitalia or internally should be photographed as well as documented in the narrative note and on the appropriate body diagram. The most common areas of injury are the posterior fourchette, fossa navicularis, labia, and vagina (20,22,24,30,31).

Enhanced Technology

In many states, enhanced technology such as special stains, colposcopy, and video documentation is used to supplement the visual inspection done during the

speculum examination of the sexual assault victim. Documentation of the trauma sustained during sexual assault has improved with the introduction of toluidine blue dye and colposcopic examination with photography (Figs. 6.8 through 6.10, see color plate).

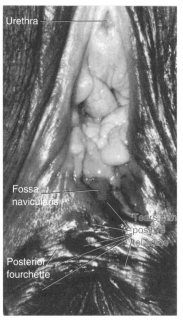

FIG. 6.9 Female sexual assault victim Tanner 5 after toluidine blue dye testing (see color plate).

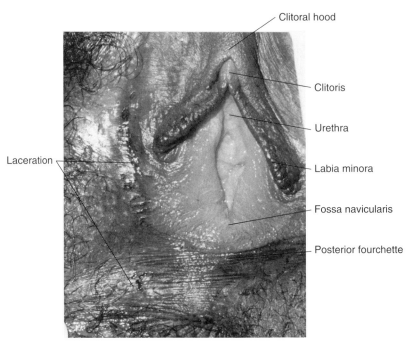

Clitoral hood

Clitoris

Urethra

Laceration

Labia minora

Fossa navicularis

Posterior fourchette

FIG. 6.10   Female sexual assault victim Tanner 5 after toluidine blue dye testing (see color plate).

Lauber and Souma (46) introduced the use of a 1% aqueous solution of toluidine blue dye, a nuclear stain, to improve the identification of genital microlacerations during the examination of rape victims. They found that microlacerations occurred in 40% of the victims of sexual assault and in only 5% of patients with a history of recent consensual sexual intercourse. Normal vulvar skin does not contain nuclei and therefore does not bind the dye. Disruption of the normal vulvar skin by the trauma of sexual assault allows the dye to bind to nuclei in the deeper layers of the skin. During the pelvic examination of a rape victim, a 1% aqueous solution of toluidine blue dye is applied to the posterior fourchette area with gauze or by using cotton-tipped applicators (Table 6-2). After a few

seconds, the dye is wiped away with lubricating jelly and 4 × 4-in. gauze squares or cotton balls, and the microlacerations are noted as linear areas of blue dye uptake. Diffuse uptake or no uptake of the toluidine blue dye is considered a negative examination. However, deeper lacerations that are still oozing will not take up the toluidine dye and should not be interpreted as a negative finding. Because the dye is not absorbed systemically, it has a low-risk profile and can therefore be used in pregnant women.

The timing of the toluidine blue dye examination depends on the local sexual assault evidentiary examination protocol. In some areas, the protocol calls for the toluidine blue dye examination only after the anogenital examination has been performed and forensic samples have been collected. Other areas call for the dye examination to be performed before the speculum examination to exclude the possibility of trauma during insertion of the speculum. From a legal standpoint, the latter is the preferred method (44).

McCauley et al. (47) compared the incidence of genital microlacerations detected in sexual assault victims with gross visualization alone against that with the addition of toluidine blue dye in the same patients. The detection of injuries increased substantially—from 4% to 58%—with toluidine blue dye testing. Their control group of patients had only 10% positive uptake with the toluidine blue dye

TABLE 6-2

STEPS FOR THE APPLICATION OF TOLUIDINE DYE, 1% AQUEOUS SOLUTION

1. Apply to posterior fourchette or rectal area with a cotton-tipped applicator.
2. Let dry.
3. Remove with lubricating gel and 4 × 4 gauze.
4. Do not apply to mucosal surfaces (Figs. 6.8 and 6.9, see color plate).

testing, and most of those patients complained of dry and painful intercourse. The increased positive uptake of toluidine blue dye on testing in the sexual assault group suggests a lack of consent.

The ability to diagnose vaginal trauma after sexual assault is also significantly enhanced by colposcopy (48) and video documentation (such as with a MedScope). A colposcope is an instrument that allows up to 30 times binocular magnification with excellent lighting and has the capacity to take still photographs or video films without additional lighting or flash. It looks like a large microscope mounted on wheels. The main purpose of the colposcope in sexual assault evaluations is to improve the detection and documentation of injuries of the vaginal introitus, vagina, and cervix. The injuries can then be documented in the text of the chart, on diagrams of the female body, and by photographs of the injuries. The photographs can be reviewed later by medical experts for legal purposes.

Slaughter and Brown (49) added colposcopy to the standard sexual assault protocol to improve the detection of injuries sustained during sexual assault. Again, the most common sites of injury were the posterior fourchette, fossa navicularis, hymen, and labia minora. Tears were noted most often on the posterior fourchette and the fossa navicularis, abrasions on the labia, and ecchymosis on the hymen. Lenahan et al. (23) compared differences in the detection of genital injuries when using the standard gross visual genital examination versus the addition of colposcopy. The detection of injuries increased more than eightfold when colposcopy was added to the gross visual examination in the same patients.

Enhanced technology methods such as colposcopy and the use of special stains are becoming the preferred method for evaluating sexual assault victims and are currently used by centers established strictly to perform medical and forensic evaluations of victims of sexual assault or the suspects of the crime. In these centers, the main examiner is usually a nurse (a sexual assault nurse examiner [SANE], sexual assault forensic examiner [SAFE], or forensic nurse examiner [FNE]) with specific training in the medical and forensic evaluation of the sexual assault victim. With increased recognition that the physician's role is to examine the sexual assault victim not only medically but also forensically, efforts have been made to incorporate forensic aspects of the sexual assault examinations into continuing medical educational programs and resident training curriculums.

Anogenital Examination

A thorough and carefully documented anogenital examination follows. If the victim has bathed, showered, or douched since the assault, the examiner would collect samples from the appropriate body orifices to attempt to preserve trace evidence. To prevent the loss of evidence from the genital area through wiping or washing, the patient should not void before the examination. If the patient must urinate, a specimen container should be provided and the urine sent to the hospital laboratory to be examined for motile or nonmotile sperm. The patient should be instructed either not to use toilet tissue to wipe herself or to place the used tissue in an envelope. The tissue is then dried, labeled, and submitted with the other evidence.

The external genitalia should be examined for foreign material, bleeding, or evidence of trauma. Injuries may include abrasions, lacerations, ecchymoses, hematomas, edema, contusions, or petechiae. A common finding after recent coitus is erythema and superficial abrasion of the posterior fourchette. Most genital injuries from sexual assault involve the fossa navicularis and the posterior fourchette. Any extensive tears or bleeding should be evaluated and repaired surgically, if necessary, by a gynecologist. Findings on gross visual examination should be documented on the body diagram and in the text. The location of the anogenital findings should be documented by using the face of a clock and the patient in anatomic position as a reference (e.g., midline injuries at the entrance to the vagina over the posterior fourchette at the 6 o'clock position).

Foreign materials and dried or moist secretions on the external genitalia are collected as evidence. Foreign bodies found in the vagina should be removed, photographed, and dried. For evidence collection, the two-swab technique is used for dry secretions and the one-swab technique for moist secretions. The area is scanned with a long-wave ultraviolet light (Wood's lamp/Bluemaxx light), and any findings are recorded in the text and on the body diagram. On the diagram, "W.L." should be written next to the findings noted with a Wood's lamp or ultraviolet light.

Before the speculum examination, the area should be swabbed for DNA from epithelium that may be present in the perineum, using a two-swab (moist then dry) technique. Then, toluidine blue dye should be applied to the external perineal area and the findings recorded (see the previous section for the technique). Areas that retain the royal blue dye are interpreted as having tested positive. The findings should be recorded and abnormalities photographed. The area must be wiped completely dry to avoid the entry of toluidine blue or lubricating jelly into the vagina and thereby prevent the contamination of subsequent forensic tests. As stated in the preceding text, in some states and jurisdictions, the protocol calls for the collection of forensic specimens from the vaginal pool, cervical os, and anus before the use of toluidine blue dye to prevent the contamination

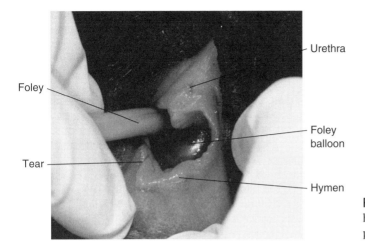

Foley

Tear

Urethra

Foley
balloon

Hymen

FIG. 6.11 Use of a Foley balloon to show hymen tear on a 14–year–old sexual assault patient (see color plate).

of specimens. The method chosen depends on local forensic protocols. The preferred order is to proceed from external examination, application of toluidine blue, to the internal examination, and Foley balloon if needed, and then the speculum examination of the cervix and swabs.

The Foley balloon technique (used only in postpubescent females) may be used when the hymen is very redundant or thickened secondary to estrogen changes. For this technique, the examiner inserts a Foley catheter into the vagina and then inflates the balloon with 20 to 30 mL of air (water is too heavy) (Fig. 6.11, see color plate). The catheter is pulled out slowly until the hymenal edges rest on the surface of the balloon, where the injury can be evaluated. The balloon is then deflated and the catheter removed (50). The balloon catheter is included in the evidence-collection kit in a separate labeled envelope.

The speculum examination is done to observe trauma and collect evidence from the vaginal/cervical area. A nonlubricated speculum moistened with warm water is used for this examination. Care should be taken in selecting the speculum size: special consideration should be given if the woman is elderly, is an adolescent, or does not ordinarily have sexual relations with male partners. A speculum should not be used to examine a girl or woman who is less than Tanner 3. For Tanner 1 and 2, gentle traction on the labia majora along with good positioning is usually sufficient for the visualization of the vagina and cervix and for obtaining evidence. If more visualization is needed because of bleeding, a tear, or other forensic findings, the examination should be performed under anaesthesia.

In Maryland, the sexual assault kit has four swabs. The first swab is used to swab the cervical os, the cervix, and the vaginal walls and pool. This swab is used to prepare a slide that the crime laboratory

will examine for the presence of sperm. It is then dried and labeled as the first swab. After the slide has air dried (without a cover slip), it is immersed in 70% ethanol for a minimum of 30 seconds. (Some crime labs do not want the hospital to prepare slides from the evidence swabs.) Specimens are then collected from the cervix (exocervical), cervical os (endocervical) (in some areas these swabs are collected and labeled separately), and the vaginal walls and pool. The number of swabs collected depends on the local protocol and the contents of the state's sexual assault kit. For evidence collection of the vaginal pool, two swabs are held together as a unit and then inserted into the pool. The swabs are rotated to ensure uniform distribution of the sample on them. If extra swabs are needed, sterile cotton swabs on wooden sticks can be used. The swabs and the slide are labeled and placed in the envelope labeled "Vaginal Swabs and Smears" (e.g., "Vaginal Swab No. 1," "Vaginal Slide No. 1").

After the collection of the vaginal swabs, separate specimens of the perianum may be collected for the detection of spermatozoa as well. If the clinician chooses to prepare a separate slide to look for spermatozoa at the hospital, one swab is used on the entire vaginal area and then a wet mount slide is prepared using normal saline, which is examined immediately for motile and nonmotile sperm. This slide should not be discarded! It should be heat preserved and placed in a separate miscellaneous evidence envelope labeled as such (51). Although nonmotile sperm can be detected for up to 3 days in samples from the vaginal pool and up to 5 to 7 days in the cervix after coitus, they are infrequently identified by hospital clinicians. Some jurisdictions request that the examiner not look for sperm because crime laboratory personnel will examine the slide. Any conflict between the crime laboratory's finding and the examiner's observation can pose a problem in court.

Sperm or ejaculate may be absent if the assailant used a condom, did not ejaculate, or had a vasectomy (52).

Colposcopy, if available, should be performed to visualize signs of minor injury to the genital area. The magnification setting on the colposcope should be recorded. Many colposcopes have photographic capability; if injuries are found, they should be photographed. In addition, the findings should be documented in the text and on the diagram of the female body. Although some experts recommend collecting specimens for gonorrhea culture and other STIs as indicated, from the cervical os as a baseline, this practice remains highly controversial. Most protocols recommend prophylactic treatment for STIs (discussed in the next section) (53).

The anorectal area should be examined for signs of injury and foreign materials. If the victim's history indicates that anal penetration occurred, then the physical examination proceeds beyond the standard inspection of the anus and the perianal area to include a careful examination of the distal anus using an anoscope (Figs. 6.12 and 6.13, see color plate). Some programs use an anoscope only if the victim has active bleeding from the anus and/or is experiencing severe pain. Moist or dried collections of secretions, fecal mater, bleeding, lubricants, or other foreign material in the perianal area may be seen with gross visualization and with the assistance of a Wood's lamp or Bluemaxx light. Foreign material should be deposited in a separate, labeled envelope. Any suspicious substance or fluorescent area should be swabbed. Semen tends to collect at the anal mucocutaneous juncture. Injuries may include edema, abrasions, ecchymoses, contusions, petechiae, lacerations, and fissures. The application

of toluidine blue dye around the rectal area before the anoscopic examination aids in the visualization of injuries. Injuries should be photographed at the time of their detection (e.g., before the use of swabs in the anorectal area). The anorectal findings are documented in the text and on the body diagram. Anoscopy, and in some cases proctoscopy, is indicated when rectal trauma is suspected. Ecchymoses, petechiae, focal edema, internal fissures, lacerations, and excoriations may be seen with anoscopy. Proctoscopy, with an appropriately sized instrument, is indicated when significant rectal trauma is suspected. If a colposcope is available, trauma should be identified and described in the text. If the history indicates, anal swabs are collected using two swabs together. The swabs should be moistened with sterile water, because dry swabs entering the anus can be extremely uncomfortable. A slide is prepared without a cover slip and allowed to air-dry. The swabs and slide are labeled as the "anal swabs" and "anal swab slide" and placed in the evidence-collection envelope.

In most programs, rectal swab evidence is collected only if the assault occurred 24 hours or less before the examination. The first step in the collection of rectal swabs requires swabbing the area around the anus for DNA using a two-swab technique and then cleaning the area to prevent the transfer of semen that may be present on the perianal area. The sphincter is dilated using a small, nonlubricated speculum moistened with warm water or by offering the patient the choice to move to a lateral decumbent or prone knee-to-chest position. Sometimes, gently placing a finger next to the sphincter and applying gentle pressure for about

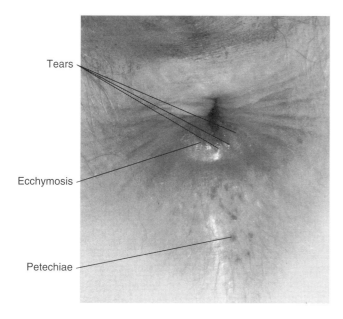

Tears

Ecchymosis

Petechiae

FIG. 6.12 Anal trauma in a female with a history of anal penetration (see color plate).

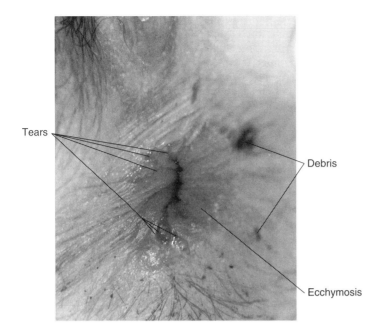

Tears

Debris

Ecchymosis

FIG. 6.13 Anal trauma in a female with history of anal penetration (see color plate).

a minute will cause the sphincter to relax. During the collection of seminal fluid from the anal columns and the distal rectum, the swab should be introduced slowly and rotated 360 degrees. The swab should be moistened with sterile water; saline solution should not be used. Two slides are prepared from the rectal swabs. They are then air-dried and labeled "anal swab" and "anal slide" and placed in the original wrapper and then in the evidence-collection envelope along with the anal swab and slide.

Documenting the Examination

Violent sexual acts (e.g., forced vaginal intercourse, oral penetration, or anal penetration) may or may not cause physical or anogenital injuries. A negative examination does not imply that sexual assault did not occur (21,54). However, because positive findings on examination are legally important in the prosecution of the perpetrator, the emergency medicine physician needs to do a careful examination and document all findings.

Conclusions about the examination should be limited to statements of the findings. Inferences about the findings should not be a part of a report. Inference statements can be made during a trial, when the examiner, identified as an expert witness, is asked what the findings indicate.

Blood Testing

Before the completion of the evidence examination, a sample of venous blood is obtained, most commonly in a lavender-topped tube, as a reference specimen

for the patient's DNA. In some states, buccal swabs are used for this purpose. The advantages of a buccal swab are that anyone can be trained to do it and it is easy to obtain. The disadvantages are the small sample size and, if a person has poor oral hygiene, contamination of the sample with bacteria, requiring multiple samples to be collected. The advantages of the blood sample are the larger sample size and avoidance of contamination. The disadvantages of a blood sample are that a nurse or trained phlebotomist must collect it and that, because of some disease states, it may be very difficult to acquire blood from some people. It can be especially difficult to draw blood from babies and small children.

In Baltimore City, blood samples are collected as part of the SAFE procedure. The blood is placed on an UltraStain card (Whatman, Inc., Clifton, New Jersey), a circular piece of filter paper, approximately 2 in. in diameter, with four circles on it. Using a pipette from the evidence kit, the examiner places two drops of blood in the center of each circle. The rest of the blood is discarded, and the card is dried, labeled, and placed into the kit. The UltraStain card does not need to be refrigerated; therefore, if the kit is not refrigerated in a timely manner, the blood DNA is still preserved. Other jurisdictions use the fluorescent treponemal antibody (FTA) cards (Tri-Tech, Inc., Southport, North Carolina), which fix the DNA to a matrix in the paper. In the opinion of the Baltimore City Crime Lab, the UltraStain cards are as effective as the more expensive FTA cards in the preservation of blood samples.

A blood (preferably) or urine sample should be sent to the hospital laboratory for pregnancy testing.

Testing for syphilis serology may be done at the time of blood collection. The need for STI testing has become a controversial subject (see the next section). Testing for baseline hepatitis B antibodies and HIV may also be done, depending on the local hospital protocol (HIV testing requires written consent).

Urine toxicologic testing is also controversial. Advocates are concerned that a positive drug test will hurt the patient's case when it goes to court. Most EDs test for only alcohol and common drugs (which may have been ingested voluntarily by the victim). Labs usually do not test for drugs such flunitrazepam (Rohypnol) or γ-hydroxybutyrate (GHB), known for their use as "date-rape drugs." For cases of suspected drug-facilitated assault, some states (e.g., Massachusetts) have protocols that include confidential comprehensive toxicology testing by the state crime laboratory, with results made available to the victim, regardless of whether she/he reports to the police or not, through the local rape crisis center. The patient needs to be made aware that the results of any test done on the patient are admissible in court.

An individual who is intoxicated or is under the influence of any mind-altering substance is at a heightened risk of assault. Forensic examiners must help courts and juries appreciate that a person's use of a mind-altering substance does not give anyone the right to assault or rape that individual.

PATIENT SUPPORT

Sexual assault may cause severe psychological as well as physical trauma. Victims have a wide range of possible demeanors. They may be calm and show little emotion or anxious and hysterical. All behaviors should be accepted by the staff as the victim's means of coping with a violent experience. The sexual assault evaluation and examination is a potentially degrading and humiliating experience for any patient. It is essential that it be carried out in a manner that is both competent and compassionate. Before the start of the examination, the patient should be asked whether she or he would like an advocate to be present during the evidentiary examination. Offering the choice of an advocate helps the patient regain a feeling of having control over what is happening. An advocate may be a nurse, a social worker, a trained person from a crisis-intervention team (preferable), or a physician. The advocate gives emotional support to the victim and acts as a liaison with family and friends. Someone should stay with the victim at all times during the evaluation to ensure a sense of safety. The facility and staff should provide privacy for the victim during the entire examination. Only the primary examiner and the advocate (if requested) should be present for the examination. If an advocate is not available, then a staff nurse should be assigned to that role for the entire evidentiary examination.

The primary examiner should introduce herself/himself and ask the patient how she/he prefers to be addressed. Throughout the evidentiary examination, the examiner should explain the reasons for the questions that must be asked and the evidence-collection process. Only questions pertinent to the evidentiary examination should be asked. Questions regarding the patient's reasons or motivations must be avoided. Before posing emotionally sensitive questions, the examiner should establish rapport with the patient. As the physical examination proceeds, the clinician should inform the patient of the findings. The patient can be involved in decisions regarding treatment, follow-up care, and notification of family or friends. The patient should be told about the benefit of counseling after sexual assault and given appropriate referral information. The staff must show confidence in the victim's ability to recover from such a violent crime.

The concept of trauma-informed care has been used to describe complete, compassionate care of patients in substance abuse and mental health treatment, taking into account recent and past traumatic events (including physical and sexual abuse) and the strong association with the development of mental health and substance abuse disorders (55,56). This concept can also be applied to the emergency treatment of the rape victim because many sexual assault victims have been previous victims as well. These previous experiences will affect the victim's current reaction/coping skills and the services needed. Victims should be encouraged to express their emotions, and the staff should acknowledge the traumatic nature of the experience. The primary examiner and staff must demonstrate behavior that is both empathetic and nonjudgmental to help reduce the victim's acute psychological trauma. A sexual assault evaluation must not only address the medical and legal aspects of the assault but also include treatment for the psychological trauma sustained by the victim.

The psychological aspects of the assault should be addressed as soon as the victim arrives. Victims should be treated promptly and with regard to helping them regain self-esteem. Trauma-informed care includes an assessment of past or current exposure to abuse or violence and an assessment of symptoms of post-traumatic stress disorder (PTSD) and related behavioral symptoms. Many victims of actual or attempted sexual assault will experience symptoms of PTSD: the persistent, involuntary reexperiencing of distress, emotional numbing, detachment from other people, and hyperarousal (e.g., irritability, insomnia, fearfulness, and nervous agitation) (57). The provider interacting with victims and survivors of violence needs to be respectful of safety issues and should emphasize personal strengths and identify social supports. Information related to intervention and referral should be presented in an authentic manner that does not stigmatize the victim and does not suggest that her/his reaction is a pathologic condition.

MEDICAL TREATMENT

The sexual assault victim's injuries must be evaluated and treated. Patient stability is the priority. The collection of forensic evidence should proceed only after significant injuries have been addressed. The treatment of wounds includes tetanus prophylaxis. The surgery or gynecology service should be consulted if the victim has moderate or severe physical or genital injuries.

During evaluation of the female sexual assault patient, a pregnancy test must be performed to rule out preexisting pregnancy. If the patient is not pregnant, she should be counseled regarding options for preventing pregnancy (53).

The risk of becoming pregnant from a rape is approximately 5% but varies depending on time of assault during the menstrual cycle. The risks and benefits of postcoital contraceptive medication should be explained. The patient must be informed that the prophylactic regimens are approximately 98% effective if started within 24 hours and are recommended only if the victim is seen and treated within 120 hours after the assault. The prophylactic regimen has a 1% to 2% failure rate and may have teratogenic effects. Some hospitals require a separate consent form for emergency contraceptive pills. Contraceptive pill regimens include the following:

- *Norgestrel (Plan B)*: two pills together immediately or one pill immediately and one in 12 hours (When taken within 72 hours, norgestrel reduces the risk of pregnancy by 89% (58–60).)
- *Norgestrel/ethinyl estradiol (Ovral) (50 mg)*: two pills taken immediately and two pills in 12 hours
- *Norgestrel (Lo-Ovral) (or other low-dose hormone)*: four pills immediately and four pills in 12 hours

The sexual assault victim should be counseled about exposure to and prophylaxis for STIs. The risk of acquiring an STI because of sexual assault is unknown, as it is difficult to determine whether the infection was present before the assault. Jenny et al. (61) studied STIs in victims of rape to focus on the incidence of newly acquired disease after the assault against the incidence of preexisting disease. They concluded that, for victims of rape, the prevalence of preexisting STIs is higher than the incidence of acquiring an STI

because of the assault. The most common preexisting STIs detected with screening (in descending order) were bacterial vaginosis and infection with *Trichomonas vaginalis, Chlamydia trachomatis*, cytomegalovirus, *Neisseria gonorrhoeae*, herpes simplex virus, *Treponema pallidum*, and HIV. The newly acquired diseases detected on return visit (in decreasing order) were bacterial vaginosis, trichomoniasis, *N. gonorrhoeae* infection, and chlamydial infection (61). Other studies revealed a similar transmission rate for gonorrhea and syphilis after sexual assault: 2.5% to 13.3% and 0% to 2%, respectively (19,62). Although HIV-antibody seroconversion has been reported among persons with sexual assault as the only known risk factor, the risk of acquiring HIV infection through sexual assault is low. This risk is influenced by the risk factors of the assailant(s), type of sexual acts during the assault (e.g., oral, vaginal, or anal), and whether ejaculation occurred (63). Other risks include multiple assailants, known or potential HIV risk of the assailant(s), and a bloody assault.

Screening cultures are controversial, because the patient is often treated prophylactically for common STIs. Proponents of screening argue that they are treating the patient like any other patient on whom they perform a pelvic examination, who states that he or she may have an STI, and that negative cultures can help relieve their anxiety because STI is one of the main fears of rape victims. Positive cultures offer the opportunity to check for a resistant strain and to encourage the patient to inform her/his current sexual partner(s) about the infection.

It is very difficult to correlate a victim's STI with an assailant. Finding an STI in a presumed suspect does not mean that he had the infection at the time of the assault; similarly, a negative test for STI does not mean that the assailant did not have an infection when the assault occurred. An assailant with an STI may have it treated before he is apprehended, thereby giving him a negative STI result. Those in favor of not culturing argue that, because the patient is being treated anyway, the culture serves little purpose, and there is concern that a positive test could be used against a victim in court by suggesting promiscuity and thereby helping the defense. The American College of Emergency Physicians (ACEP) (64) states that because the cultures are not forensically indicated, one management strategy is that no culture be taken acutely unless obvious signs of STIs are present. However, in cases of chronic sexual abuse, cultures should be obtained because chronic infection may be asymptomatic. The ACEP notes that a positive result of the initial STI testing of adult sexual assault victims may or may not indicate new infection.

During the establishment of standards and guidelines for a SAFE program, the pros and cons of any testing need to be evaluated, e.g., performing STI cultures, hepatitis evaluation, HIV testing and prophylaxis, and pulling hair samples. After these decisions are made, the protocol needs to be written down and understood by the staff.

Other infections and conditions associated with sexual activity, such as hepatitis B and C, head lice infestation, venereal warts, and nonspecific urethritis in males, should also be considered when establishing protocols. Follow-up visits are very important because some diseases that can be transmitted to the victim will not show up for weeks or months after the assault.

If cultures are obtained from any site of penetration by the assailant(s), they should be tested for *N. gonorrhoeae* and *C. trachomatis*. A wet mount and culture can be obtained to test for *T. vaginalis*, bacterial vaginosis, *Trichomonas*, and yeast infection. The victim's serum is used to establish a baseline for syphilis, hepatitis B, hepatitis C, and HIV infection. A separate consent form needs to be signed for HIV testing, and counseling should be provided before and after testing in accordance with local protocols and laws.

Routine preventive therapy for the most common STIs should be administered at the time of the initial evaluation. Only 30% to 53% of sexual assault victims return for follow-up appointments, so the initial examination may be the only opportunity for STI prophylaxis (19,62). The Centers for Disease Control (CDC) recommend prophylactic treatment against hepatitis B, *Chlamydia*, *N. gonorrhoeae*, *Trichomonas*, and bacterial vaginosis (65). A postexposure hepatitis B vaccination (without hepatitis B immunoglobulin) at the time of the initial evaluation should provide adequate protection against this virus. The recommended antimicrobial regimen is ceftriaxone (125 mg IM, single dose) plus metronidazole (2 g orally, single dose) plus azithromycin (1 g orally, single dose) or doxycycline (100 mg orally twice a day for 7 days). If there is a contraindication to this treatment regimen, CDC guidelines should be consulted (65). If the sexual assault victim is pregnant, erythromycin (500 mg orally 4 times a day for 7 days) or azithromycin may be used instead of doxycycline to prophylactically treat for *Chlamydia* infection. If the patient is pregnant and allergic to cephalosporins, then spectinomycin (2 g IM, single dose) may be an alternative prophylactic against *N. gonorrhoeae*.

Although the risk of acquiring HIV infection through sexual assault is low, concern about transmission remains because the consequences are grave. The risk of transmission of HIV following sexual assault and the efficacy of prophylaxis are unknown. Prophylaxis may be considered in certain high-risk situations, such as an assailant known or highly suspected to be HIV positive, multiple assailants who induced physical trauma, and rectal penetration (63). A starter pack of antiretroviral medications should be given, with concrete plans for follow-up and blood testing. The rate of follow-up among sexual assault victims treated with HIV prophylaxis is very low (66).

The examiner should follow local protocols regarding prophylaxis against HIV infection. If prophylaxis is considered, the risks and benefits of treatment with antiretroviral agents must be explained to the patient. If the patient decides to take postexposure prevention for HIV, the guidelines for nonoccupational exposure, or, in the absence of such a local protocol, occupational mucous membrane exposure should be followed (63). Treatment currently consists of two-drug therapy with Combivir (zidovudine and lamivudine). The addition of a protease inhibitor such as nelfinivir (Viracept) or lopinavir/rionavir (Kaletra) may be considered in certain very high risk scenarios (56). Because drug treatment recommendations change frequently, providers should follow their local protocol, consult their local expert, call the CDC "warm line" (800-933-3413), or consult the CDC website (www.ucsf.edu/hivctr). Sexual assault victims should be scheduled for follow-up in 14 days to ensure successful prophylaxis. Repeat tests for syphilis and HIV should be obtained 6, 12, and 24 weeks after the assault, because their incubation period is longer than that of the more common STIs. Follow-up doses of the hepatitis B vaccine should be given 1 or 2 months and 4 to 6 months after the initial dose (65).

The influence of drugs must be considered in each sexual assault case. The victim may have altered mental status on presentation or poor recollection of the assault because of the effects of illicit drugs, medications, or alcohol. The assailant may have given the victim a drug such as flunitrazepam (Rohypnol) or GHB to diminish resistance. Neither drug is legal in the United States. During the forensic examination, if a drug-facilitated assault is suspected, urine (and serum if less than 24 hours have elapsed since the assault) should be collected, with the victim's consent, to screen for drugs. The urine must be collected within 72 hours of drug ingestion and tested immediately or the specimen needs to be frozen until the test is performed.

PHOTOGRAPHY

Photographs are a valuable form of evidence, especially for situations that cannot be documented adequately in diagrams (e.g., bite marks or massive injuries) (see Chapter 17). When the patient signs the consent for collection of evidence, the examiner needs to explain that photographs will be taken for the purpose of documenting injuries. Some hospitals require a separate consent for photographs. Other hospitals consider photographic documentation to be a part of medical treatment or a forensic examination, such as that done with plastic surgery, and do not require a separate consent form. Ideally, photographs should be taken before medical treatment of the wounds. Any camera may be used, as long as it can be focused for nondistorted close-up shots and provide an accurate color rendition. A 35-mm camera is recommended, although digital photography is gaining acceptance in the judicial system (67). Adequate lighting is essential, whether the source is natural, flood, or flash. Rules of three include medium, close, and close-up photographs of wounds and bite marks. The camera should be held perpendicular to the body surface being photographed. This is essential to avoid photographic distortion of wounds or bite marks, especially those on curved surfaces of the body. The photograph should be arranged to include a ruler or scale near the injury for size reference and a label with the patient's name for identification purposes. The lesion must not be obscured by the ruler or label. At least one or two photographs should be taken without the scale to orient the lesion and to demonstrate that the scale has not obscured important evidence. The scale should be retained for later reference to enable the photographic laboratory to produce an accurate, life-size (1:1) photograph. The photograph(s) can then be compared with evidence (e.g., suspect dental casts for bite marks or object[s] that may have inflicted the injury). The name of the photographer should be recorded on the film evidence envelope.

The photographs may be taken in the hospital by the sexual assault examiner or by the crime laboratory, in accordance with local law enforcement policies. The patient's rights need to be remembered when the photographs are taken. The patient must understand that the photographs will be used in court as evidence. The patient's sensitivity about being undressed for photography must be addressed. Patients should always be draped appropriately. Also, the person taking the photographs should be the most likely to minimize the victim's discomfort (e.g., for a female victim, a female law enforcement officer, a crime laboratory staff member, or a female nurse trained in forensic photography).

Review of Camera Systems

Many photographic systems are available to forensic professionals (Table 6-3). This review focuses on systems available for documenting interpersonal violence examinations.

TABLE 6-3

CONTACT INFORMATION FOR MANUFACTURERS OF PHOTOGRAPHIC EQUIPMENT AND DOCUMENTATION SOFTWARE

XamStation
Lightyear Multimedia Studios
Leesburg, Virginia
http://unilnk.net/lightyearstudios_com/xamstation.htm

TACT System
Infosys Business Solutions
http://infosysbiz.com/TACT.htm

Wallach Surgical Devices, Inc.
Orange, Connecticut
www.wallachsurgical.com

MedScope/Second Opinion
ALLPRO Imaging
Hicksville, New York
www.allproimaging.com

Canon Cameras
usa.canon.com

Sony Cameras
sonystyle.com

The trend toward digital recording of images has created a flood of new products and the digitization of existing systems. There is also a trend toward computer documentation and storage in an effort to reduce paper-based storage needs and associated costs. The retrieval and transmission of medical records has increased the need for encryption software to allow the electronic movement of sensitive information.

A purchase decision should not be based solely on the current practice environment but with a view to program needs in 5 to 10 years. The cost of many systems is considerable, and careful thought should go into the capability for its growth. Representatives of law enforcement agencies and the state's attorney's office should be involved in this decision to determine their plans for document sharing and computer upgrades. It may be unwise for a smaller program to invest large sums in advanced equipment that may not be fully utilized by other members of the justice community. Personnel in risk management should be consulted for their advice on compliance with regulations set forth in the Health Insurance Portability and Accountability Act (HIPAA) and in responding to requests for the production of documents during litigation.

In a hospital setting, it may be necessary to have in-house Internet technology staff review the intended purchase for compatibility and maintenance of components. Even if the system will not be connected to the hospital server, it is likely that the technicians will be called on to service the components after warranty periods. It is a professional courtesy to solicit their input on the purchase of systems they might be required to maintain. Many hospitals mandate that all equipment be inspected and registered as part of the fire safety plan to ensure compliance with grounding capability and safe wiring.

Many programs need a handheld film or digital camera for taking whole-body and macro images. This type of camera can be used during examinations at remote sites. There is a definite advantage in using a digital camera for forensic evaluations, because most of them allow the images to be viewed immediately and thereby indicate whether the shot was adequate. Film cameras generally require bracketing exposures to ensure that a properly exposed image is obtained—a technique seldom mastered by the average user. A malfunction with a film camera will not be discovered until processing and can cause a "moment in time" to be lost forever.

The method used to store images in the digital camera should be given careful consideration. Cameras that burn the images to a minidisk have been in use for some years now. However, problems related to the number of moving parts and the sensitivity of the disc tray have been identified. Handling and storage of the disc can affect the retrieval of images. Programs that choose this method of documentation should be aware of limitations inherent in this medium. Consumer-quality discs have great variation in the length of time the disc can be archived without loss of image quality. Some camera systems recommend discs made by the manufacturer. Use of other brands can have mixed results in retrieving images. Programs would do well to purchase medical-grade archival discs. Storage must address both archival and chain of custody concerns, with careful surveillance for possible exposure to magnetic fields. If images that appear to have been recorded cannot be viewed later, assistance can be obtained from companies that retrieve forensic documentation from disks and hard drives (for a fee).

For cameras using a flash card, consideration should be given to capacity. The goal is to maximize image quality while balancing the number of images stored on each disk. Some programs issue a card to each examiner, thereby limiting unintentional overlap without proper identifiers separating the cases. A locked storage area should be provided to house the discs between examinations. As each case is completed, staff should be designated to download or print the images as required and clear the memory for reuse. A policy should be written to clearly state the handling and storage procedures.

Most digital systems provide a way to merge the images with a documentation format or computer storage. Some programs need to have the images sent to other sites for review or casework. Hospital-based programs may have access to encryption services. Programs without that level of support can purchase adequate encryption mechanisms to protect the data. A web search will yield many products that meet this need. A program should purchase the best system it can afford that will interface with other equipment. Most sites have technical support links that can be used to ask the manufacturer about suitability.

Even if the images will not be exported over the Internet, a tracking system should be installed. There are many photo management systems on the market. At a minimum, the system should be able to record any manipulation of the image, a capability that enhances its admissibility at the trial, because the system tracks every keystroke associated with the image. This permits re-creation of how the image has been stored and displayed, dispelling concerns about manipulation to hide or enhance the subject.

Several systems link a camera with a computer, laptop, or printer. Most of them are configured on a cart or rack to provide mobility in the examination room. A purchase decision should consider features such as durability, ease of use, cleaning, troubleshooting, and service package. The vendor's record of service response and technical support should weigh heavily in product selection.

Systems that use a camera lens on an umbilical-type flexible shaft are very popular. Modified from systems commonly used for dental imagery, they have the advantages of small size and mobility. In comparing systems, a feature that controls the light intensity at the lens is desirable. The number of lights surrounding the lens greatly affects the ability to secure excellent images. Overuse of strong secondary light sources such as goosenecks or examination lights can cause some on-lens lights to automatically dim, defeating the desired effect. A footswitch as well as a stand are essential to hold the lens for hands-free capture. A bonus offered by some systems is the ability to "film" continuously and then pull only the best images later for incorporation into the case. This is a vast improvement over old print systems that required almost a minute per capture to print.

Some manufacturers provide documentation software that allows a digital camera to be linked to a computer. At the time of this writing (late 2005), the industry standard for digital cameras is 7 to 8 megapixels, which delivers adequate quality for the enlargements needed for trial purposes.

When considering cameras to be used predominantly in macro situations, SANE/SAFE program representatives should do extensive trials before committing to the purchase, if possible. The macro setting on some cameras will not allow the lens to focus on the cervix; instead, it focuses on the outer edge of the speculum. Some cameras require a change in the focus brackets to allow a narrow target area on the cervix. On-camera flashes at close focusing distances have a very narrow beam. If the camera flash is off-center from the lens, unacceptable shadows can be thrown onto the target area. To properly light a subject at close distances, some manufacturers recommend a ring flash that encircles the lens. In most cases, a separate battery pack is required to supply power to the flash, which adds bulk and weight to the system, a factor that many consider a serious drawback.

The use of a pelvic training mannequin is invaluable in assessing the suitability of a camera/lens combination, as multiple settings can be tried without causing discomfort to a live model. Thought must be given to the photographic skills of the examiners, so that settings are simple and easily reproducible each and every time. It is best to test the camera in the same lighting as it will be mainly used in practice. It is advantageous to install color-balanced lighting in the examination room's fixtures whenever possible to render more accurate skin tones.

Another feature of some new systems is the ability to use diagrams or body maps. Somewhat of a holdover from the days of film, when it was not known if images were captured correctly, many examiners still consider the drawings to be a vital part of the documentation process. There is some wisdom in maintaining drawings because there is always a risk of lost or unrecoverable data or images that are too graphic to be admitted for trial. It is unlikely that a drawing would be excluded for being too graphic. Some software manufacturers provide a means of making a notation or reference to an injury on the body map, whereas others allow the examiner to use simple drawing tools to represent findings or injuries.

A final consideration in system selection is the ultimate storage of the data. Sensitive information should not be stored on a personal computer or laptop. Even with the best firewalls and prevention software, any system can be hacked and laptops can be stolen. A possible solution is to purchase an external hard drive of good quality and capacity. This device plugs into a port on the computer or laptop and data can be downloaded at regular intervals. This device is compact and can be locked away in a secure cabinet. Again, a data-storage policy should be in place if the program's practices must be questioned at trial. Only a limited number of staff should have administrative access to the data so that accountability is ensured.

FOLLOW-UP

After the evidentiary examination is completed, the patient's environment should be assessed for safety. The patient should be asked if she/he knows someone to call and has a safe place to stay. The patient should be given options for follow-up counseling and should be encouraged to obtain it. The addresses and telephone numbers for rape crisis centers and victims' programs should be provided as well as information about crime victim compensation. The medical and counseling follow-up plans should be established clearly before the patient leaves the facility. Counseling improves the patient's long-term prognosis. The hope is to help the victim regain a sense of well-being and to limit the effects of PTSD (see Chapter 2).

ADULT MALE SEXUAL ASSAULT VICTIM

During the past 30 years, concerns about the violent crime of rape have focused on female victims—the "forced vaginal penetration of the woman by a male assailant." This definition ignores the possibility of a male being a rape victim. The term *rape* is now accepted in most states to mean the forced penetration of either female or male victims. In efforts to be gender neutral and encompass a broader range of violent sexual acts (e.g., penetration and sodomy), the term *sexual assault* is now used in many states.

Although female victims of sexual assault outnumber males 3:1 each year in the United States, the number of sexual assaults against males is alarming. In 1998, the National Institute of Justice reported that approximately 93,000 males were forcibly raped in the United States (1). Adult men represent <5% of reported adult sexual assault cases (68,69), but they seem to sustain more severe physical injury, as observed in the SAFE Program in Baltimore City and documented in a study done in Toronto (70). Making this type of assault gender neutral has allowed more treatment options for male victims (e.g., treatment in a sexual assault center). However, most male victims in prisons cannot obtain the benefit of sexual assault centers and follow-up care.

The protocols for evaluation of male sexual assault victims are similar to those of female victims. The victim should be triaged as a priority to protect the quality of the evidence (Fig. 6.14). He should remain clothed until the time of the evidence examination.

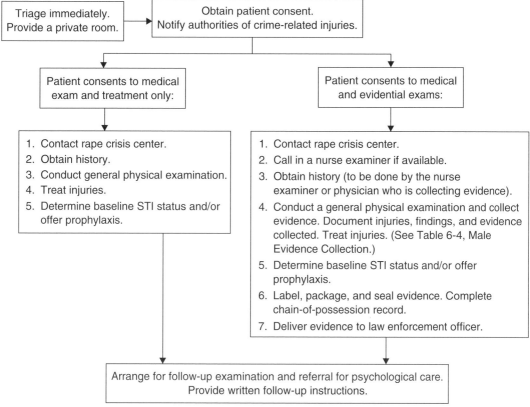

FIG. 6.14   Schematic of male sexual assault examination.

An advocate for the victim should be involved early in the process. The victim needs to sign a consent form after being informed of his rights. Much of the history and evidence collection is similar to that used for female victims (see the section on the adult sexual assault patient in the preceding text). Many males are reluctant to discuss specific sexual acts, so an extra measure of compassion and sensitivity will be needed if the examiner has to elicit this information regarding the assault. In some cases, assuring a heterosexual male who has been sexually assaulted that this attack will not make him homosexual can be helpful. Male sexual assault is a violent crime that affects heterosexual men as much as homosexual men. The crime has no relation to the sexual orientation of the attacker or the victim, and the assault does not make the victim survivor gay, bisexual, or heterosexual (71).

During the physical examination (Table 6-4), any congenital abnormalities of the penis should be documented and a note should be made as to whether the patient is circumcised. The number of testicles palpated, or the absence of testicles, should be recorded. The presence of dried and moist secretions, lubricants, feces, foreign materials, and

venereal lesions must be noted. In uncircumcised males, foreign materials may be retained on the penis, particularly on the glans or in the sulcus. Any foreign material, including matted pubic hair, should be collected and placed in the appropriate envelope, which is then labeled and sealed. Dried secretions are collected with the two–swab technique and moist secretions with the one–swab technique. The area is scanned with a Wood's lamp and the fluorescent areas swabbed. The sites of secretions should be documented on the male traumagram; secretions detected with a Wood's lamp should be marked with "W.L."

The patient's pubic hair should be combed, and the comb should then be placed on the paper sheets under the patient's buttocks for collection later. Reference samples of the pubic hairs (20–30 hairs) should be collected at this time (however, some programs do not collect any hair reference samples until a later date, when requested by the crime laboratory). Penile swabs must also be collected. The number of swabs varies with different protocols; most of the protocols require one swab from the urethral meatus and one from the glans. A swab taken from the penile shaft may be indicated. The

TABLE 6-4

COLLECTION OF EVIDENCE FROM MALE VICTIMS OF SEXUAL ASSAULT
(Expansion of step 4 in evidential examination [Fig. 6.14])

Physical Examination[a,b] Male Victim	Clinical Specimens for the Laboratory	Evidence for the Crime Laboratory (Kit comes from the police department)
4a. *Document condition of clothing worn.* Collect outer and underclothing worn during or immediately after the assault. Collect fingernail scrapings.	—	4a2. Place each piece of clothing in a separate bag. Place fingernail scrapings and foreign material found on clothing and body in separate envelopes.
4b. *General physical examination.* Scan entire body with Wood's lamp. Collect dried and moist secretions from body, head, and hair. Photograph bite marks (Figs. 6.5 and 6.6, see color plate), wounds, and any other findings. Examine the entire body. Record findings on a head and/or body diagram (Figs. 6.2 and 6.3).	—	—
4c. *Examine oral cavity.* Document findings. Swab area around the mouth. Collect oral swabs. Floss teeth. Collect GC specimen.	4c1. GC, use agar plate	4c2. Place in separate envelopes: oral swabs from external and internal surfaces, floss, and foreign material
4d. *Examine external genitalia.* Scan with Wood's light. Collect dried and wet secretions and foreign materials. Cut matted pubic hair. Comb hair for foreign materials. Swab the base, shaft, and glans of the penis. Collect cultures. Document findings.	4d1. GC and *Chlamydia* cultures	4d2. Individually package dried secretions, foreign material, matted pubic hair cuttings, pubic hair combings, the comb, and swabs.
4e. *Examine buttock and anal region.* Collect any moist or dry secretions or foreign material. Swab anal region.	—	4e2. Dried secretions, foreign material, and swabs
4f. *Apply toluidine dye.* Examine and document findings.	—	—
4g. *Anoscopic or proctoscopic examination* if indicated by history or examination of region. Collect anal and rectal swabs and GC swab.	4g1. GC culture	4g2. Swabs
4h. *Clinical labs:* Syphilis serology (blood, gray-topped tube), HBsAG and HCsAG (blood, gold-topped 7-mL tubes), HIV[c] (blood, lavender-topped tubes)	4h1. Syphilis, HBsAG, HCsAG, HIV	—
4i. *Other evidence is collected at the discretion of the physician and/or law enforcement.* Alcohol (blood, red-topped tube), toxicology (blood, gray-topped tube), toxicology (50 mL urine)	4i1. Blood alcohol and toxicology and urine toxicology	—
4j. *Collect reference samples.* 25 pulled head hairs, 25 pulled pubic hairs, blood typing (yellow-topped tube)/DNA (purple-topped tube). If bloodstain cards are used, place the blood on card. If bloodstain cards are not used, place the blood in a refrigerator until it is given to the police.	—	4j2. Reference samples

(continued)

TABLE 6-4

(Continued)

Physical Examination[a,b] Male Victim	Clinical Specimens for the Laboratory	Evidence for the Crime Laboratory (Kit comes from the police department)
The reference samples can be collected at a later date.	—	—
Complete chain of possession record.	Send clinical specimens to laboratory.	Give evidence kit to law enforcement.
Label each envelope with the complaint number, date, time, and examiner's name. Package and seal the evidence and sign the outside envelope.	—	—

[a] All swabs and slides must be air dried before packaging.
[b] Code corresponding to swabs and slides, For example, Oral Swab No. 1/Oral Slide No. 1.
[c] In most states, counseling is mandatory before screening for HIV.
GC, neisseria gonorrhoeae culture; HBsAg, hepatitis B surface antigen; HCsAg, hepatitis C surface antigen; HIV, human immunodeficiency virus.

swabs are moistened before evidence is collected. (If a condom was worn during the assault, the examiner will also want to collect swabs from the base of the penis.) The presence of fecal matter is noted. The swabs are air-dried for at least 1 hour and then labeled as to location. If indicated, a specimen is obtained for *N. gonorrhoeae* and *Chlamydia* culture from the urethra as a baseline and prophylactic medication is offered to the patient. Other STI cultures are obtained as indicated.

If the patient reports anal penetration, then a thorough anorectal examination is indicated to expose evidence of trauma, such as bleeding, abrasions, ecchymoses, edema, contusions, petechiae, lacerations, and fissures. Microscopic or magnified examinations can be performed with a magnifying lens or colposcope to confirm signs of minor injury. Any trauma should be photographed. Any dried or moist secretions noted in the perianal area with either gross visualization or a Wood's lamp should be collected using the two-swab technique if dry and the one-swab technique if moist. The swabs are air-dried for at least 1 hour. The collections are documented in the text and the sites of the collections marked on the male traumagram. If the secretion was noted only with the Wood's lamp, "W.L." is marked next to it on the traumagram. Any foreign material is collected in a "debris" envelope, which is then labeled and sealed. Two anorectal swabs are collected, and two dry mount slides are prepared from them, labeled "Swab No. 1/Slide No. 1" and "Swab No. 2/Slide No. 2."

An anoscopic examination is performed, using an anoscope lubricated with water to inspect the rectum for trauma. If a colposcope is available, injuries can be photographed and the findings noted in the

text. When the examination is completed, the paper beneath the patient's buttocks is folded with the comb inside and placed in a miscellaneous evidence-collection envelope, which is then labeled and sealed.

The patient should be referred for follow-up for both physical and psychological sequelae of the assault. The aftermath on a male victim can be devastating, so all patients should be referred for counseling by professionals trained to address the psychological trauma related to sexual assault.

SUSPECT EXAMINATION PROTOCOL

Most sexual assault suspects are male. The forensic examination of the suspect is similar to that of the male victim of sexual assault, with a few modifications (Table 6-5). The suspect is usually brought to a sexual assault evaluation center by the police. For the safety of the staff, and for the purpose of having a second person verify collection of the evidence, the police should be present during the entire evaluation and collection of evidence. Either consent is obtained from the suspect or the court-ordered search warrant is reviewed before beginning the examination. It is best to have a court order because, without the order, the evidence collected can be considered inadmissible if the suspect changes his mind about his consent. Ideally, a court-ordered search warrant specifically orders the medical examination, collection of specimens, screens for STIs and HIV, and collection of clothing. The examiner may collect only what is specified on the search warrant. SAFE programs should nurture a good working relationship with the police department so that the clinician can advise the officers regarding the information that should

TABLE 6-5

EVIDENTIAL EXAMINATION OF THE MALE SEXUAL ASSAULT SUSPECT

Physical Examination[a,b] Male Suspect	Evidence for the Crime Laboratory (to be given to law enforcement)	Clinical Specimens for the Hospital Laboratory
Obtain history and authorization for examination from law enforcement officer.	—	—
Establish security.	—	—
Prevent contact between the victim and the suspect.	—	—
1. Note condition of clothing worn on arrival. Collect outer and underclothing worn during or immediately after the assault. Collect fingernail scrapings if indicated.	1a. Place each piece of clothing in a separate bag. Place fingernail scrapings and foreign material found on clothing and body in separate envelopes.	—
2. Conduct a general physical examination. If <24 h have passed since the alleged assault, scan the entire body with Wood's lamp. Collect dried and moist secretions from body, head, hair, and scalp. Document findings.	—	—
3. Examine the oral cavity for injury. Document findings. If <24 h have passed since the alleged attack and if indicated by the history, swab the area around the mouth. Collect two oral swabs and prepare a dry slide mount. Collect specimen for GC analysis.	3a. Two swabs from oral cavity, two dry mount slides, one swab from around the mouth	3b. GC
4. Examine external genitalia for injury. If <24 h have passed since the alleged assault, scan with Wood's lamp. Collect dried and moist secretions and foreign materials. Document findings. Cut matted pubic hair. Comb pubic hair to collect foreign materials. Swab the shaft of the penis and the glans penis.	4a. Any dried secretions, foreign material, matted pubic hair cuttings, pubic hair combings, the comb; one swab from the shaft of the penis and one from the glans penis	4b. GC and *Chlamydia*
—	—	—
5. If <24 h have passed since the alleged attack, examine the buttocks, perianal skin, and anal folds for injury. Collect dried and moist secretions and foreign material. Document findings. If indicated by the history or findings, collect two rectal swabs of the external area with two dry mount slides.	5a. Dried secretions, foreign material, and rectal swabs	—
—	—	—
6. Collect three blood samples (syphilis serology [red-topped tube], alcohol/toxicology [gray-topped tube], blood typing [yellow-topped tube]). Collect 50 mL of urine. Collect reference samples: saliva specimen, 25 head hairs, 25 pubic hairs, 25 body hairs.	6a. Blood alcohol/toxicology, blood typing, urine specimen; reference samples	6b. Syphilis tests

(continued)

TABLE 6-5

(Continued)

Physical Examination[a],[b] Male Suspect	Evidence for the Crime Laboratory (to be given to law enforcement)	Clinical Specimens for the Hospital Laboratory
7. Document injuries, findings, and evidence collected. Label, package, and seal the evidence. Complete the chain of possession record.	—	—
—	Give evidence kit to law enforcement.	Send clinical specimens to laboratory.

[a] All swabs and slides must be air dried before packaging.
[b] Code corresponding swabs and slides, For example, Oral Swab No. 1/Oral Slide No. 1.
GC, neisseria gonorrhoeae culture.

appear on a search warrant with respect to different situations that arise with suspects. For example, a search warrant should not request a semen sample. For DNA analysis, the court order should request a blood sample.

The examiner is allowed to record any utterances from the suspect during the examination. If a search warrant is not provided, the suspect can later state that he did not agree to give the evidence. Then any evidence collected is not admissible in court. If a court order has been received and the suspect is in the ED or clinic but refuses to allow evidence collection, the suspect must not be forced into compliance by physical restraints or other means. The police officers should take the suspect to a controlled environment (prison), where there is sufficient help for collecting the evidence.

Examination of the suspect requires the use of a sexual assault examination kit when the perpetrator is brought in within a reasonable time after the assault. An exact time frame needs to be established by the local judicial system. The examiner obtains the history from the police and the suspect. Information from the suspect should include medications, allergies, major medical history, congenital abnormalities, surgeries, implantation devices, STI history, HIV-screening history, vasectomy history, and recent history of urinary tract infections and anogenital problems.

The search warrant should state that all of the suspect's clothing is to be collected for forensic evaluation. The suspect's clothing is collected in the same manner as a victim's clothing.

When a suspect is brought in within 24 hours of the assault, the physical examination and the evidence examination are conducted in the same manner as a sexual assault forensic examination of a male victim. For suspects brought in after 24 hours, appropriate modifications of the examination should

be implemented. When a suspect is brought in after 72 hours, it may be necessary to collect only reference samples (pubic, head, and body hair and blood).

The examiner must look for physical identifiers (e.g., tattoos or scars) and for physical signs of high-risk behavior that would place the victim at greater risk of contracting a disease from the suspect (e.g., needle marks from intravenous drug abuse). Evidence of physical trauma inflicted by the victim's attempts to resist should be sought (e.g., scratches). The rest of the nongenital and genital evidence examination is identical to the sexual assault examination protocol. If the suspect is a male, the examiner should document if he is circumcised or not, if he has implantation devices or congenital abnormalities, and if he has one, two, or no testicles. Photographs should be taken of evidence of trauma. Specimens are obtained for laboratory analysis: blood alcohol, urine toxicology, syphilis serology, HIV testing, hepatitis panel. Cultures for *N. gonorrhoeae* are taken from the throat, the urethra, and, if indicated, the rectum. *Chlamydia* cultures from the urethra and the rectum may be obtained if this procedure is part of the local protocol.

Collection of Reference Samples from the Suspect

Most perpetrators are apprehended several months after an assault. During that time, any number of conditions may develop in the victim: venereal warts, condylomata lata (secondary syphilitic lesions in the perineum, anal cleft, or axilla), positive HIV titer, syphilis, chlamydial infection, gonorrhea, *Trichomonas*, herpes simplex, hepatitis B, bacterial vaginosis, or pregnancy. Males cannot be tested for bacterial vaginosis, and trichomoniasis testing on males is almost always negative, so a court order should not request tests for them.

The examiner should note the length of time between the reported assault and the collection of reference samples. If hair samples are being collected, the clinical record should note if the subject has undergone chemotherapy, had any major illnesses, dyed his hair, or had his hair altered in any way (e.g., had fibers braided into the hair) since the time of the assault. When samples are collected for *Chlamydia*, gonorrhea, or herpes simplex cultures, the examiner must realize that the suspect may have received treatment for STIs during the time since the assault and will now have negative results. In people with herpes simplex, lesions may not be present and blood tests may or may not be positive in this case. In addition, blood tests cannot differentiate sexual from nonsexual causes of herpes simplex.

The most accurate method of testing for syphilis is dark-field microscopy, but this technique is of value only if lesions are present (i.e., in primary, some secondary, and early congenital syphilis that has not been treated). Serologic tests for syphilis are of two general types. The oldest are the nontreponemal antigen tests such as the Venereal Disease Research Laboratory (VDRL) test, the Kolmer test, and the rapid plasma regain (RPR) test (72). These are good screening tests for most stages of syphilis, and their titer is a good measure of disease activity; however, they can have false-negative results in individuals with early primary syphilis, in those with late syphilis, and in some people with HIV (73). False-positive results are associated with Lyme disease; autoimmune diseases; viral, chronic bacterial, and parasitic infections; multiple blood transfusions; tuberculosis; and advancing age (73). Most patients with seropositive primary and secondary syphilis become seronegative 6 to 12 months after treatment. Patients who remain seropositive 2 years after appropriate treatment will have low VDRL titers (73). Therefore, it is important for the examiner to know that if the assault occurred more than 6 months before the examination and if the person being tested has been treated for syphilis, the test results could be negative now but the suspect could have had syphilis at the time of the assault.

A positive VDRL or RPR test result always needs to be confirmed with a treponemal antigen test—the second type of serologic test used to diagnose syphilis. Primary in this group is the fluorescent treponemal antibody, absorbed (FTA-ABS) test, which uses lyophilized *T. pallidum* as an antigen in an indirect florescent antibody technique (72). The treponemal antigen tests rarely yield false-positive results. If the FTA-ABS test is reactive, it is diagnostic of syphilis or other treponemal diseases (yaws, pinta, bejel). Treponemal tests remain positive after adequate therapy. Therefore, if an examiner strongly suspects that the individual being tested had syphilis but the RPR test is negative, then the FTA-ABS test should be requested but a lower titer should be expected if the suspect has received treatment. Beaded, nonreactive, and borderline outcomes are not diagnostic of syphilis (74).

The results of blood tests for HIV and for hepatitis A, B, C, and D need to be evaluated with respect to time. SANE/SAFE program representatives who are asked to testify in court will need to be able to explain the test results and would be wise to take an infectious disease textbook along to the courtroom for reference.

Venereal warts may emerge on the victim several weeks after a sexual assault. To demonstrate that the causative papillomavirus came from the suspected perpetrator, both the victim and the perpetrator must be tested through biopsy. Understandably, it is difficult to obtain an agreement to the collection of specimens. A simpler method of obtaining specimens from a male is to scrape lesions on the urethral and anorectal areas. Males with papillomavirus infections frequently have lesions in the perianal region, but lesions can also be found on the shaft of the penis, on the scrotum, and in the urethral meatus. When obtaining the scrapings, a sufficient number of cells must be collected without causing bleeding (the presence of blood makes it difficult to detect the human papillomavirus [HPV] genome). Scrapings can be obtained with a cervical brush; the specimens should be labeled according to the site from which they were obtained. Biopsy specimens must be frozen but scrapings can remain at room temperature for a couple of hours and then need to be refrigerated or frozen so that they are easier to handle. The turnaround time for results is 2 to 4 weeks. Only a limited number of laboratories test for the HPV, so if this evaluation is necessary, the examiner must tell the state's attorney's office where to send the scrapings. The chain of custody must be maintained.

DNA test results must be read carefully, because genome typing is used primarily for the evaluation of cervical cancer and what is read as negative for cervical cancer may be positive for HPV. HPV has more than 100 known genotypes (75). If the HPV genome is the same on the victim and the suspect, the examiner can confidently infer, during courtroom proceedings, physical contact between the two people.

When samples are to be collected from a suspect several weeks after an assault, the SAFE/SANE has time to consult with the state's attorney to ensure that the warrant is worded correctly. The examination can be scheduled during the day, when

TABLE 6-6

EXAMPLE OF DOCUMENTATION OF SUSPECT EVIDENCE COLLECTION

Date:	December 10, 2005
Time:	10:05 a.m.
Location:	Mercy Medical Center
	Baltimore, Maryland
Police complaint	No. 05-4L1234
10:05 a.m.	Mr. John Q. Public, 40 y/o W/M (DOB 03/23/65), brought to Mercy Medical Center by Detectives Stone and Jones of the Sex Offense Unit for collection of evidence per search and seizure warrant. Placed in Exam Room 8 for evidentiary examination.
10:10 a.m.	Identity positively verified by photograph provided by Detective Stone. State Identification Number on photo/ID bracelet worn by Mr. Public: 234–567.
10:14 a.m.	Buccal swabs collected from right and left buccal cavity. Swabs labeled and placed in swab dryer to air-dry per policy.
10:18 a.m.	One tube of blood obtained from right antecubital area, after site was prepped per policy, and placed in purple-topped tube. Blood transferred to blood card by a pipette; blood card labeled and placed in swab dryer to air-dry. Small dressing placed on venipuncture site.
10:25 a.m.	Four swabs obtained from the base, shaft, and glans of penis. Swabs labeled and placed in swab dryer.
10:37 a.m.	Five digital photographs taken of superficial scratches on right posterior shoulder. Scratches (x3) are 4 cm in length. Three swabs obtained from scratches and placed in swab dryer to air-dry (areas of scratches and swabs obtained are documented on body diagram).
10:50 a.m.	Mr. Public left in custody of Detectives Stone and Jones. Mr. Public was cooperative with the above procedure.
11:30 a.m.	All swabs air dried, removed, and placed in appropriate provided envelopes. All envelopes sealed and placed in suspect evidence kit. Suspect kit sealed with evidence tape and secured in evidence locker, to be retrieved at a later time by law enforcement. Chain of custody form completed.

Suspect evidentiary examination performed by this writer: Mary L. Smith, RN, BSN, FNE-A

---

it is convenient for everyone involved. Sample wordings for a warrant are listed below:

- External examination of the genitals and anus for warts. Scrapings to be obtained from any warts, the urethral orifice, and the anorectal region.
- Application of 3% acetic acid to the penis, scrotum, and perianal region for further screening. Any suspect areas will be reexamined in 2 days with scraping of any new lesions that are noted. (*Editors' note:* Acetic acid is a white vinegar solution that causes some wart surfaces to turn white. Its application is not painful.)
- Routine blood sampling for syphilis testing. Two tiger-topped tubes for the collection of laboratory samples. (*Editors' note:* This phrasing gives the examiner leeway to use the vials and quantities recommended by the laboratory. In

general, an RPR test will be done for initial screening and, if the result is positive, then an FTA-ABS test will be done to ascertain a titer or ratio that will indicate whether the suspect has been treated and the stage of syphilis.)

The examination of the suspect should be documented in great detail and a male traumagram should be used to note the sites of the findings (Table 6-6 and Fig. 6.15). When summarizing the findings, the examiner should not render an opinion as to whether the suspect is indeed the assailant. The evidence should be carefully collected, dried, labeled, and sealed. A copy of the court-ordered search warrant should be enclosed in the evidence envelope. The chain of custody must be maintained during the entire process and the transfer of evidence must be documented.

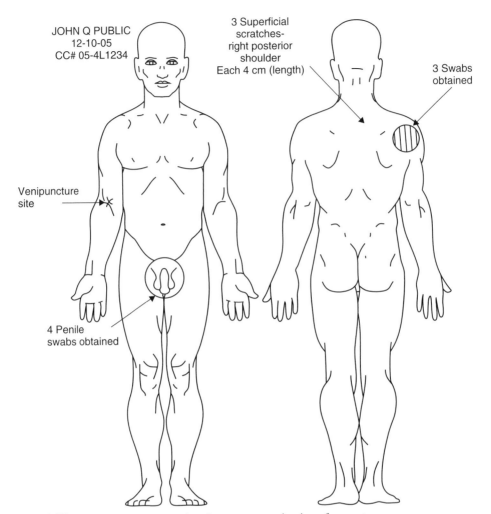

FIG. 6.15   Male traumagram used to document examination of suspect.

APPENDIX 1
FEMALE SEXUAL RESPONSE[a]

Masters and Johnson first described the human sexual response in 1966, and their work was updated in 1988 by Kolodny.[b] These authors described the physiologic response that occurs in men and women when they engage in consensual sexual intercourse. The entire process can be separated into five phases: desire, excitement, plateau, orgasm, and resolution. Lack of the normal response in the female explains some of the vaginal injuries that occur in rape victims.

The desire phase is referred to as the "springboard for sexual arousal" and is initiated by cognitive cues (such as interpersonal attraction), general mood, situational receptivity, and general health. Approximately 70% of sexual arousal is believed to be psychological. The desire phase induces no physical changes but triggers the excitement phase. During the excitement phase, vaginal lubrication begins: the labia majora flatten and move back from the vaginal orifice; the labia minora thicken; the cervix and the uterus move upward; and the heart rate, blood pressure, and respiratory rate increase. The excitement phase is followed by the plateau phase, in which there is continual lubrication. The inner two thirds of the vagina lengthens and expands, and the cervix and the uterus are further elevated. This phase is followed by orgasm, when heart rate, blood pressure, and respiratory rate reach a peak. Then follows the resolution phase, when the woman's physiology returns to normal. When these physiologic changes do not occur, a woman is more likely to sustain vaginal trauma during a sexual assault.

---

[a]The female sexual response is often referred to by lawyers during a trial and is frequently used to explain why vaginal injuries occur because of sexual assault or are absent in women alleging sexual assault. Using the findings reported by Masters and Johnson, defense lawyers may imply that the lack of trauma means that the act was consensual, which is not a conclusion that follows logically from the study data, because only consenting adults, not assaulted women, were examined and because the investigators did not look for trauma after consensual sex acts.
[b]Masters WH, Johnson VE, Kolodny RC. *Heterosexuality*. New York: HarperCollins, 1992.

APPENDIX 2
SEXUAL ANATOMY TERMINOLOGY

Anus (Male/Female)

Anus	Terminal orifice of the alimentary canal; opening to the rectum; 4 cm in length; pain sensitive; surrounded by the sphincter muscles
Anal verge	The tissue overlying the subcutaneous external anal sphincter at the most distal portion of the anal canal and extending to the margin of the anal skin
Perianal skin fold (rugae)	Wrinkles or folds of the anal verge skin, radiating from the anus, which are created by the contraction of the external sphincter
Rectal ampulla	The dilated portion of the rectum just proximal to the anal canal
Gluteal cleft	A naturally occurring groove between the buttocks
Tag	Extra skin that usually develops after trauma or laceration
Venous pooling	Dilatation and sometimes bulging of the veins around the anus (also called venous engorgement)

Female

Acts committed	Coitus, penile-labial (also called vulvar coitus or simulated vaginal intercourse); coitus, full penetration; fellatio, oral-penile; cunnilingus, oral-vaginal; sodomy, usually refers to penile-anal, but has many definitions; analingus, oral contact with the anal area.
Bartholin's glands	Two oval racemose glands lying one to each side of the lower part of the vagina at 4 and 8 o'clock positions, which secrete a lubricating mucus
Cervix	Narrow lower or outer end of the uterus; neck of uterus
Cervical os	Opening of cervix (endocervix)
Clitoris	Small erectile organ at the anterior or ventral part of the vulva; sole purpose is sexual stimulation; homologous to the penis
Fold	Redundant skin often found at the 12 and 6 o'clock positions
Fossa navicularis	Concave area immediately below the hymen, extending outward to the posterior fourchette
Hymen	Fine membranous tissue that partially or (rarely) completely covers the vaginal orifice. Separates the external genitalia from the vagina. Located at the junction of the vestibular floor and vaginal canal. All females have this structure; however, wide anatomic variations exist. During the forensic examination, hymenal configuration, symmetry, narrowing, and injuries are documented. Terms such as "intact," "not intact," and "virginal" are NOT used today.
Hymenal findings (may represent normal variations)	
Bump	Small rounded projection, which may indicate where a septate bridge once attached, an area of attachment of vaginal rugae, or a chronic inflammatory change (also called mound)
Cleft	V-shaped indentation, not extending to base (junction of the hymen and vestibule) (also called notched)
Fimbriated	Uneven edges with small projections
Gaping	Extra large hymenal diameter without stretching
Rolled	Tissue folded over on itself either inwardly or outwardly
Scalloped	Rounded series of half-circle tissue (also called ruffled)
Smooth	No breaks, bumps, or notches (also called regular)
Thickened	Fatter and less elastic
Transected	Torn, cut, or divided (usually used to describe a healed tear with edges that have not grown back together)
Hymenal shapes	
Annular	Ring shape: smooth, unfolded, 360 degrees
Crescentric	Half moon; the anterior rim of tissue extending from 1 to 11 o'clock position may be absent
Cribriform	Multiple small openings
Elongated	Vertical diameter is longer than horizontal length
Fimbriated	Ruffled, redundant, uneven tissue
Imperforate	No opening; the vaginal orifice cannot be visualized
Microperforate	Small opening
Septated	Band of tissue crossing the vaginal orifice
Sleevelike	Ventrally displaced hymenal tissue with circular orifice; "kangaroo pouch"
Intervaginal rugae	Transverse folds of the mucous membrane of the vagina (also called longitudinal folds or ridges)
Labia majora	Outer skin folds to the vagina; covered with pubic hair after menarche
Labia minora	Inner skin folds to the vagina
Midline commissure	Midline fusion external from the posterior fourchette; used in anatomic descriptions of children
Midline sparing	White avascular linear area posterior to the hymen at the 6 o'clock position

Mons pubis	Rounded eminence of fatty tissue on the pubic symphysis
Pectinate line	Anal papilla and columns interdigitate with the anal verge tissue (where squamous cells meet columnar cells)
Perineal body	Mass of muscle and fascia that separates the lower end of the vagina from the rectum
Perineum	Region bounded by the vulva in front, by the buttocks behind, and laterally by the medial side of the thighs. A line drawn transversely across in front of the ischial tuberosities divides the space into two portions: the posterior (anal region) contains the termination of the anal canal and the anterior (urogenital region) contains the external urogenital organs. The perineum is sometimes raised, rough, and/or pigmented. Its deep boundaries are the pubic arch and the arcuate ligament of the pubis in front, the tip of the coccyx behind, the inferior rami of the pubis and ischium on either side, and the sacrotuberous ligament
Periurethral tissue	The immediate 360-degree area around the urethra, not including the urethral meatus
Periurethral vestibular bands	Bands lateral to the urethra, connected to the vestibule wall; support bands
Posterior fourchette	Area below the fossa navicularis; the point of fusion of the posterior labia minora
Skene's glands	Located on the upper wall of the vagina, around the lower end of the urethra. They drain into the urethra and near the urethral opening. These glands are also known as the lesser vestibular or paraurethral glands and as the Gräfenberg (G) spot; the general area is the urethral sponge. Homologous with the prostate gland in males.
Tissue	
Attenuated	Decrease in amount of tissue (also called thinning)
Estrogenized	Pubertal changes to hymen: light pink/white color, with increased redundancy and elasticity
Flap	Loose movable tissue protrusion
Nonestrogenized	Translucent
Redundant	Containing an excess or superfluous amount
Remnant	Residual tissue left after chronic trauma
Tag	Fingerlike projection that may occur after a break or separation of the septated bridge
Thickened	Fatter and less elastic
Velamentous	Veil-like, thin, delicate (also called membranous, translucent, wispy)
Vestibular papillae	Nipple- or fingerlike projections involving the medial aspects of the labia, introitus, and lower vagina, in the area lateral to the hymen, from the base of the hymen to the labia minora (also called micropapillomatosis labialis)
Tanner stage	Development assessment used to stage gonadal maturation in terms of acquisition of secondary sexual characteristics. For females, breast size and pubic hair distribution are assessed to categorize the stage of development. For males, scrotal, penile, and pubic hair distribution is used to stage development.
Pubic hair	

1. No hair or fine vellus (peach fuzz) hair
2. Sparse, long pigmented hair
3. Increased density; dark, coarse, curly hair
4. Abundant hair, sparing medial thighs
5. Abundant hair, spreading to medial thigh

Urethral meatus	Orifice for the urethra
Vagina	Tubular structure or canal extending from the hymen to the cervix
Vestibule	Space between the labia minora, into which the urethra and vagina open (also called vestibulum vaginae)

Vulva	Region of the external genital organs of the female (including the labia majora, labia minora, and mons pubis)
Male	
Dorsal vein	Vein that runs along the dorsal surface of the penile shaft
Epididymis	A highly coiled tubing network folded against the back surface of each testis. Sperm cells spend several weeks in the epididymis while they mature. The epididymis then passes to the vas deferens.
Glans	Head of the penis, which is an expansion of the corpus spongiosum, covered by a loose skin (foreskin or prepuce), which enables it to expand freely during erection; also called the balanus.
Median raphe	Seamlike union extending from the scrotum to the rectum
Penis	External organ consisting of three parallel cylinders of erectile tissue that run the length of the penis; consists of the glands, prepuce, corona, shaft, and frenulum. Two of the tissue masses lie alongside each other and end behind the head of the penis. The third tissue mass lies beneath them and contains the urethra. The average length of a nonerect penis is 8.5 to 10.5 cm and the length of an erect penis averages 16 to 19 cm, with a diameter of 3.5 cm.
Perineal body	Mass of muscle and fascia that separates the lower end of the urethra from the rectum
Perineum	Region bounded by the scrotum in front, by the buttocks behind, and laterally by the medial side of the thighs (See Female, Perineum, for further definition)
Prepuce or foreskin	Fold of skin that covers the glans of the penis; circumcision is the surgical removal of this skin
Prostate	Located directly below the bladder and surrounding the urethra. Normally about the size of a chestnut; consists of a muscular and a glandular section. The prostate produces approximately 30% of the seminal fluid; the remaining 70% is produced by the seminal vesicles.
Rectum	Terminal part of the intestine from the sigmoid flexure to the anus; not sensitive to pain
Scrotum	Thin loose sac of skin under the penis, which contains the testicles
Seminal fluid	The whitish sticky material, also called semen, that carries mature sperm from the body. Semen is discharged at sexual climax. A single discharge, about 3.5 mL of semen, contains 120 million to 600 million spermatozoa. (After a vasectomy, sperm is no longer present in the ejaculate, but the quantity of seminal fluid remains the same.)
Shaft	Long cylindric area of the penis below the glans
Spermatozoa	Mature male sperm cells. A sperm is only 1/1,500 in. long and is visible only by microscope. A spermatozoon resembles a tadpole and is made up of three sections: a head, a midpiece, and a tail that propels the sperm with a lashing movement.
Testes	The male reproductive organs. The testes have two functions: production of hormone and production of sperm. The entire process of sperm production takes 70 days. The male produces billions of sperm annually from puberty until death; in contrast, the female creates no new eggs after birth.
Urethral meatus	External orifice for the urethra, at the tip of the shaft in the center of the glans
Vas deferens	The 16-in. tube that connects the epididymis to the urethra; this tube is cut and sutured off during a vasectomy.

ACKNOWLEDGMENT

The authors thank Joyce Faust, RN, FNE, for her substantive contributions to the photography section of this chapter.

REFERENCES

1. Tjaden P, Thoennes N. *Extent, nature and consequences of rape victimization: findings from the national violence against women survey*. Washington, DC: US Department of Justice, Office of Justice Programs, 2006. NCJ 210346, Available at www.ncjrs.org/pdffiles1/nij/210346.pdf. Accessed on February 13, 2006.

2. Catalano S. *Criminal victimization, 2003. Bureau of Justice statistics. national crime victimization survey*. Washington, DC: U.S. Department of Justice, 2004. NCJ 205455 September 2004.

3. Rape, Abuse & Incest National Network. *The facts about rape*. Washington, DC: RAINN, 2005, Available at http://www.rainn.org/statistics.html. Accessed on August 23, 2005.

4. United States Department of Justice. *Child rape victims, 1992*. Crime Data Brief, NCJ-147001, 1994.

5. *The responses to rape: detours on the road to equal justice*. Washington, DC: U.S. Congress, Majority Staff of the Senate Judiciary Committee, 1993.

6. Dansky BS, Brewerton TD, Kilpatrick DG, et al. The National Women's Study: relationship of victimization and posttraumatic stress disorder to bulimia nervosa. *Int J Eat Disord* 1997;21(3):213–228.

7. Ullman SE, Brecklin LR. Sexual assault history and suicidal behavior in a national sample of women. *Suicide Life Threat Behav* 2002;32(2):117–130.

8. Kilpatrick DG, Edmonds CN, Seymour AK. *Rape in America: a report to the nation*. Washington, DC: National Victim Center, Charleston, South Carolina: Medical University of South Carolina, 1992.

9. Campbell J. Health consequences of intimate partner violence. *Lancet* 2002;359:1331–1336.

10. Miller T, Cohen M, Wiersema B. *Victim costs and consequences: a new look*. Washington, DC: National Institute of Justice, U.S. Department of Justice, 1996.

11. Holmes ST, Holmes RM. *Sex crimes: patterns and behaviors*, 2nd ed. New York: Sage Publications, 2001.

12. Green WM. *Rape: the evidential examination and management of the adult female victim*. Lexington, MA: DC Health, 1988.

13. Houry D, Sachs CK, Feldhaus KM, et al. Violence inflicted injuries: reporting laws in the fifty states. *Ann Emerg Med* 2004;39(1):56–60.

14. Jackson MC, Groleau G, Kimmel C. Comparison of the quality of medical documentation for findings related to sexual assault prior and post the development of a sexual assault forensic examination program [abstract]. *Acad Emerg Med* 1999;34(4 Pt 2):S40.

15. Deming JE, Mittleman RE, Wetli CV. Forensic science aspects of fatal sexual assaults on women. *J Forensic Sci* 1983;28:572–576.

16. Marchbanks PA, Lui KJ, Mercy JA. Risk of injury from resisting rape. *Am J Epidemiol* 1990;132(3):540–549.

17. Satin AJ, Hemsell DL, Stone IC, et al. Sexual assault in pregnancy. *Obstet Gynecol* 1991;77(5):710–714.

18. Rambow B, Adkinson C, Frost TH, et al. Female sexual assault: medical and legal implications. *Ann Emerg Med* 1992;21:727–731.

19. Tintinalli JE, Hoelzer M. Clinical findings and legal resolution in sexual assault. *Ann Emerg Med* 1985;14(5):447–453.

20. Cartwright PS, Moore RA, Anderson JR, et al. Genital injury and implied consent to alleged rape. *J Reprod Med* 1986;31:1043–1044.

21. Bowyer L, Dalton ME. Female victims of rape and their genital injuries. *Br J Obstet Gynecol* 1997;104(5):617–620.

22. Slaughter L, Brown CR, Crowley S, et al. Patterns of genital injury in female sexual assault victims. *Am J Obstet Gynecol* 1997;176(3):609–616.

23. Lenahan LC, Ernst A, Johnson B. Colposcopy in evaluation of the adult sexual assault victim. *Am J Emerg Med* 1998;16(2):183–184.

24. Ramin SM, Satin AJ, Stone IC Jr. Sexual assault in postmenopausal women. *Obstet Gynecol* 1992;80(5):860–864.

25. Cartwright P, Moore R. The elderly victim of rape. *South Med J* 1989;82:988–989.

26. Sugar NF, Fine DN, Eckert LO. Physical injury after sexual assault: findings of a large case series. *Am J Obstet Gynecol* 2004;190(1):71–76.

27. Cartwright PS. Factors that correlate with injury sustained by survivors of sexual assault. *Obstet Gynecol* 1987;70(1):44–46.

28. Ruback RB, Ivie DL. Prior relationship, resistance, and injury in rapes: an analysis of crisis center records. *Violence Vict* 1988;3(2):99–111.

29. Heger AH. Sexual violence In: Mason JK, Purdue BN, eds. *The pathology of trauma*, 3rd ed. Boston, MA: Little, Brown, 1998:176–190.

30. Biggs M, Stermac LE, Divinsky M. Genital injuries following sexual assault of women with and without prior sexual intercourse experience. *Can Med Assoc J* 1998;159(1):33–37.

31. Kindermann G, Carsten PM, Maassen V. Ano-genital injuries in female victims of sexual assault [article in German]. *Swiss Surg* 1996;1:10–13.

32. Kellogg ND, Menard SW, Santos A. Genital anatomy in pregnant adolescents: "normal" doesn't mean "nothing happened". *Pediatrics* 2004;113:e67–e69.

33. Fitzgerald N, Riley KJ. *Drug facilitated rape: looking for the missing pieces*. 2006. Available at http://www.ncjrs.gov/pdffiles1/jr000243c.pdf. Accessed on February 12, 2006.

34. Rogers D. Physical aspects of alleged sexual assaults. *Med Sci Law* 1996;36(2):117–122.

35. Campbell R, Patterson D, Lichty LF. The effectiveness of sexual assault nurse examiner (sane) programs: a review of psychological, medical, legal, and community outcomes. *Trauma, Violence, Abuse* 2005;6(4):313–329.

36. Perkins C. *Weapon use and violent crime. National Crime Victimization Survey 1993–2001*, NCJ 194820, 2003. Available at http://www.ojp.usdoj.gov/bjs/pub/pdf/wuvc01.pdf Accessed on February 12, 2006.

37. Bart PB. A study of women who both were raped and avoided rape. *J Social Issues* 1981;37:123.

38. Ullman SE, Knight RA. A multivariate model for predicting rape and physical injury outcomes during sexual assaults. *J Consult Clin Psychol* 1991;59(5):724–731.

39. Purdue BN. Asphyxial and related deaths In: Mason JK, Purdue BN, eds. *The pathology of trauma*, 3rd ed. Boston, MA: Little, Brown and Company, 1998:230–252.

40. Bowers CM, Bell G. *Manual of forensic odontology*, 3rd ed. Montpelier, VT: American Society of Forensic Odontology, 1995.

41. Sweet D, Lorente M, Lorente JA, et al. An improved method to recover saliva from human skin: the double swab technique. *J Forensic Sci* 1997;42(2):320–322.

42. Deedrick D. Hairs, fibers, crime, and evidence. In: *Forensic science communication*, Vol. 2, No. 3. Washington, DC: U. S. Department of Justice, Federal Bureau of Investigation, 2000.

43. Damm D, White D, Brinker M. Variations of palatal erythema secondary to fellatio. *Oral Surg* 1981;52:417.
44. Hochmeister MN, Whelan M, Borer UV, et al. Effects of toluidine blue and destaining reagents used in sexual assault examinations on the ability to obtain DNA profiles from postcoital vaginal swabs. *J Forensic Sci* 1997;42(2):316–319.
45. Office on Violence Against Women. *A national protocol for sexual assault medical forensic examinations: adults/adolescents.* Office on Violence Against Women, NCJ 206554, September 2004. Available at http://www.ncjrs.org/pdffiles1/ovw/206554.pdf. Accessed on May 2005.
46. Lauber AA, Souma ML. Use of toluidine blue for documentation of traumatic intercourse. *Obstet Gynecol* 1982;60(5):644–648.
47. McCauley J, Guzinski G, Welch R, et al. Toluidine blue in the corroboration of rape in the adult victim. *Am J Emerg Med* 1987;5(2):105–108.
48. Sommers MS, Schafer J, Zink T, et al. Injury patterns in women resulting from sexual assault. *Trauma, Violence Abuse* 2001;2(3):240–258.
49. Slaughter L, Brown CR. Colposcopy to establish physical findings in rape victims. *Am J Obstet Gynecol* 1992;166 (1 Pt 1):83–86.
50. Jones JS, Dunnuck D, Rossman L, et al. Adolescent Foley catheter technique for visualizing hymenal injuries in adolescent sexual assault. *Acad Emerg Med* 2003;10(9):1001–1004.
51. Khaldi N, Miras A, Botti K, et al. Evaluation of three rapid detection methods for the forensic identification of seminal fluid in rape cases. *J Forensic Sci* 2004;49(4):749–753.
52. Burgess AW, Groth AN. Sexual dysfunction during rape. *N Engl J Med* 1997;297(14):764–766.
53. Lewis-O'Connor A, Franz H, Zuniga L. Limitations of the national protocol for sexual assault medical forensic examinations. *J Emerg Nurs* 2005;31(3):267–270.
54. Adams JA, Harper K, Knudson S, et al. Examination findings in legally confirmed child sexual abuse: it's normal to be normal. *Pediatrics* 1994;94(3):310–317.
55. Clark HW, Power AK. Women, co-occurring disorders, and violence study: a case for trauma-informed care. *J Subst Abuse Treat* 2005;28:145–146.
56. Domino M, Morrissey JP, Nadlicki-Patterson T, et al. Service costs for women with co-occurring disorders and trauma. *J Subst Abuse Treat* 2005;28:135–143.
57. Kessler RC, Sonnega A, Bromet E, et al. Posttraumatic stress disorder in the National Comorbidity Survey. *Arch Gen Psychiatry* 1995;52:1048–1060.
58. FDA approves progestin-only emergency contraception. *The Contraception Report* 1999;10(5):8–10.
59. Rodrigues I, Grou F, Joly J. Effectiveness of emergency contraceptive pills between 72 and 120 hours after unprotected sexual intercourse. *Am J Obstet Gynecol* 2001;184(4):531–537.
60. Van Look PFA, Stewart F. Emergency contraception. In: Hatcher RA, Trussell S, Stewart E, et al., eds. *Contraceptive technology*, 18th ed. New York: Ardent Media, 2004.
61. Jenny C, Hooton TM, Bowers A, et al. Sexually transmitted diseases in victims of rape. *N Engl J Med* 1990;322(11):713–716.
62. Schwarcz SK, Whittington WL. Sexual assault and sexually transmitted diseases: detection and management in adults and children. *Rev Infect Dis* 1990;12(Suppl 6):S682–S690.
63. Smith DK, Grohskopf LA, Black RJ, et al. Antiretroviral postexposure prophylaxis after sexual, injection-drug use, or other nonoccupational exposure to HIV in the United States: recommendations from the U.S. Department of Health and Human Services. *MMWR* 2005;54(RR-2):1–20.
64. American College of Emergency Physicians. *Evaluation and management of the sexually assaulted or sexually*

abused patient. Dallas, TX, ACEP, 1999:109. Available at http://www.acep.org/NR/rdonlyres/11E6C08D-6EE7-4EE2-8E59-5E8E6E684E43/0/sxa_handbook.pdf. Accessed on December 28, 2005.
65. Centers for Disease Control. Sexually transmitted diseases treatment guidelines—2002. *MMWR* 2002;51(RR-06):1–80.
66. Linden JA, Oldeg P, Mehta SD, et al. HIV post-exposure prophylaxis in sexual assault: current practice and patient adherence to treatment recommendations in a large urban teaching hospital. *Acad Emerg Med* 2005;12:640–646.
67. Kershaw S. *Digital photos give the police a new edge in abuse cases.* New York Times, 2002.
68. Riggs N, Houry D, Long G, et al. Analysis of 1,076 cases of sexual assault. *Ann Emerg Med* 2000;35(4):358–362.
69. Read KM, Kufera JA, Jackson MC, et al. Population-based study of police-reported sexual assault in Baltimore, Maryland. *Am J Emerg Med* 2005;23(3):273–278.
70. Stermac L, Del Bove G, Addison M. Stranger and acquaintance sexual assault of adult males. *J Interpers Violence* 2004;19(8):901–915.
71. National Center for Victims of Crime. *Male rape.* Washington, DC, National Center for Victims of Crime, 1997. Available at http://www.ncvc.org/ncvc/Main.aspx. Accessed on December 28, 2005.
72. Jacobs DS, Demott WR, Oxley DK. *Jacobs & demott laboratory test handbook with key word index*, 5th ed. Hudson, OH: Lexi-Comp, Inc., 2001.
73. Perine PL, Bell TA. Syphilis and the endemic treponematoses. In: Strickland GT, ed. *Hunter's tropical medicine and emerging infectious diseases*, 8th ed. Chapter 48, Philadelphia, PA: WB Saunders, 2000:354–364.
74. Ferri FF. *Ferri's clinical advisor: instant diagnosis and treatment.* Philadelphia, PA: Mosby, 2005:1255.
75. Molijn A, Kleter B, Quint W, et al. Molecular diagnosis of human papillomavirus (HPV) infections. *J Clin Virol* 2005;32(Suppl 1):S43–S51.

SUGGESTED READINGS

Aiken MM, Speck PM. Sexual assault and multiple trauma: a sexual assault nurse examiner (SANE) challenge. *J Emerg Nurs* 1995;21(5):466–468.
Arndt S, Goldstein S. *SART/SANE orientation guide.* Santa Cruz, CA: Forensic Nursing Services, 1993.
Burgess AW. *Violence through a forensic lens.* King of Prussia, PA: Nursing Spectrum, 2000.
Burgess AW, Holstrom L. *Rape, crisis and recovery.* Bowie, MD: Robert J. Brady Co: A Prentice-Hall Company, 1979.
DiNitto DM, Martin PY, Maxwell MS, et al. Rape treatment programs: delivering innovative services to survivors. *Med Law* 1989;8(1):21–30.
Douglas JE, Burgess AW, Burgess AG, et al. *Crime classification manual: a standard system for investigating and classifying violent crimes.* San Francisco: Jossey-Bass, 1997.
Edwards L. *Genital dermatology atlas.* Philadelphia, PA: Lippincott Williams & Wilkins, 2004.
Fagan JA, Stewart DK, Hansen KV. Violent men or violent husbands? In: Finkelhor D, Gelles RJ, Hotaling GT et al., eds. *The dark side of families: current family violence research.* Beverly Hills, CA: SAGE Publications, 1983:1–25,49–67.
Giardino AP, Girardin BW, Faugno DK, et al. *Sexual assault victimization across the life span: a clinical guide and color atlas.* Philadelphia, PA: WB Saunders, 2003.
Golden G. Use of alternative light source illumination in bite mark photography. *J Forensic Sci* 1994;39(3):815–823.
Hazelwood RR, Burgess AW. *Practical rape investigation.* Boca Raton, FL: CRC Press, 1995.

Herman JL. *Trauma and recovery*. Basic Books: A Member of Perseus Books Group, 1997.

Ledray L. *Sexual assault nurse examiner, development and operation guide*. U.S. Department of Justice Office of Justice Programs, Office for Victims of Crime. 1999. Available at www.sane-sart.com/index.php?topic=Pubs. Accessed on May 20, 2005.

Ledray L, Netzel L. DNA evidence collection. *J Emerg Nurs* 1997;23(2):156–158.

Ledray LE. *Recovering from rape*. New York: Henry Holt, 1994.

Lenehan GP. Sexual assault nurse examiners: a SANE way to care for rape victims. *J Emerg Nurs* 1991;17(1):1–2.

Lynch VA. *Forensic nursing*. Virginia, VA: Mosby, Elsevier, 2005.

Ogle RR. *Crime scene investigation and reconstruction*. Prentice Hall, 2003.

U.S. Department of Justice. *A national protocol for sexual assault medical forensic examinations adults/adolescents*, NCJ 206554, September 2004. Available at http://www.ncjrs.org/pdffiles1/ovw/206554.pdf. Accessed on May 2005.

West M, Barsley RE, Friar J, et al. Ultraviolet radiation and its role in wound pattern documentation. *J Forensic Sci* 1992;37(6):1466–1479.

West MH, Barsley RE, Hall JE, et al. The detection and documentation of trace wound patterns by use of an alternate light source. *J Forensic Sci* 1992;37(6):1480–1488.

Williams RM. Few convictions in rape cases: empirical evidence concerning some alternative explanations. *J Crim Justice* 1981;9:29.

7

SEXUAL ABUSE AND SEXUAL ASSAULT OF ADOLESCENTS

■ V. JILL KEMPTHORNE

In the past several decades, it has become apparent that sexual victimization is widespread both in the United States and abroad. Until recently, efforts to address and prevent sexual abuse and sexual assault have focused primarily on the needs of children and women, and less so on those of adolescents specifically. This may reflect the difficulties in both identifying and understanding adolescent sexual victimization. Adolescents are typified as rebellious, curious, and risk-takers in all aspects of their lives, particularly in their sexual attitudes and behaviors. This will color not only the adolescent's perception of possible sexual victimization but also societal response to this victimization. Fortunately, this historical bias has been shifting, and the topic of adolescent sexual victimization has received more focused attention in recent years (1–4).

To better address key issues, this chapter is organized into five sections: (a) Epidemiologic Considerations, (b) The Unique Vulnerability of the Adolescent, (c) The Clinical Approach to the Adolescent Patient, (d) The Diagnosis and Treatment of Sexually Transmitted Infections (STIs), and (e) The Mental and Psychosocial Consequences of Sexual Assault and Sexual Abuse in the Adolescent Patient.

EPIDEMIOLOGIC CONSIDERATIONS

Adolescent sexual victimization is a significant problem. It is estimated that by 18 years of age, 10% to 30% of females and 5% to 10% of males will have been sexually victimized (5). In the 2003 Centers for Disease Control (CDC) Youth Risk Behavior Survey of high-school students, 12% of the female respondents and 6% of the male respondents gave a history of having been forced to have sex (6).

The nature of sexual victimization changes from childhood to adolescence (Fig. 7.1). Younger teens are more commonly the victims of sexual abuse; i.e., victimized by persons in a position of caring for the teen. In fact, sexual abuse most commonly starts in the preteen years. In one study, the risk of sexual abuse increased markedly between the ages of 6 and 10 (7); and in another study, sexual abuse started on average at the age of 7.5 years and continued until the age of 13 (8).

By early to mid adolescence, sexual abuse begins to taper off and sexual assault increases. Older teens are more often the victims of sexual assault and experience violence by intimate partners rather than assault by strangers (9). A 1994 crime data brief from the U.S. Department of Justice reports that almost half the sexual assaults on girls younger than 12 years were by a family member, whereas for girls 12 to 17 years of age this percentage dropped to 20% and, for women 18 and older, to 12% (10). The 1998 National Crime Victimization Survey found that the rate of sexual assault increases through the teen years and peaks at around age 20 (11), supporting the observation that the risk of sexual assault for women is highest during the college years.

These published statistics do not portray the true scope of the problem. First, the relation between sexuality and violence goes beyond the usual definitions

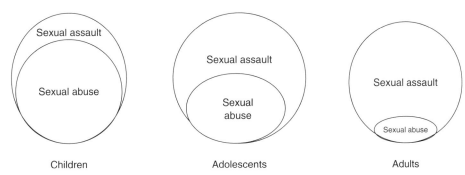

FIG. 7.1 Relative prevalence of sexual abuse in different age-groups.

of sexual victimization. In many cases, intimate-partner violence follows rather than precedes sexual intimacy. In an analysis of a national longitudinal study of adolescent health (the AdHealth study), Kaestle and Halpern found that 37% of the respondents had experienced verbal or physical aggression *following*, not *preceding*, sexual intercourse (12). Such instances may not be reported as sexual assault, yet they have similar negative effects on the adolescent's well-being and trajectory of life.

Second, nondisclosure of sexual victimization is extremely common, and most, if not all, surveys and criminal reports have significant underreporting bias. Of those teens surveyed in the 1997 Commonwealth Fund Survey on the Health of Adolescent Girls, 30% of girls and 50% of boys with a history of physical or sexual abuse had told no one (13). In a national telephone survey of children aged 10 to 16 years, Finkelhor found that the rate of sexual assault for 12- to 15-year olds was three times higher than the rate reported in the comparable National Crime Survey (14). In a study of sexual aggression on college campuses, 27% of college women surveyed indicated that they had been victims of sexual assault, yet none had contacted the police (15). In a report on sexual crime statistics, the U.S. Department of Justice cites National Crime Victimization Survey data showing that two thirds of sexual assaults are not reported to law enforcement agencies (16).

Nondisclosure is more common (a) if the victim knows the perpetrator (17), (b) among males than females (13–18), and (c) among African American youth (19). Also, for teens who do disclose, delayed disclosure is common. In one study of adolescent girls, a mean time of 2.3 years had elapsed from the initial assault to disclosure (20). In another study of 125 adult sexual assault victims (average age 36 years) receiving care at the sexual assault centers in Maryland, almost 80% had been victimized by a family member, and the average time elapsed to disclosure was 15.5 years (21).

The reasons for nondisclosure or delayed disclosure are many and include the following:

- The adolescent's failure to recognize victimization (22) or the adolescent's assumption that coercion is a normal part of the sexual experience (23, 24). In one study, nearly one third of the adolescents interpreted a scene with violent behavior as love and less than 5% interpreted it as hateful (25).
- There are occasions when the adolescent does not remember the assault. Most often this happens if the adolescent is intoxicated. It can also happen if the adolescent has been given the so-called "date-rape drug," flunitrazepam (Rohypnol), a benzodiazepine with significant sedative and amnesiac effects (26). (See Chapter 12.)
- The emotional burden of shame, guilt, and fear. These sentiments are common following a date rape, particularly if alcohol or drugs are involved, on college campuses and high schools (17,27,28).
- A sense of futility. In one study of adolescents who had not disclosed a history of sexual assault to their parents, half of them thought their parents would not believe them (20).
- Fear of the consequences of disclosure, e.g., placement in a foster home, separation from parents or the sexual partner, threats of harm or retribution.

THE UNIQUE VULNERABILITY OF THE ADOLESCENT

Many of the defining qualities and unique characteristics at the adolescent stage of life may increase the risk of sexual victimization in this age-group, as discussed in the subsequent text.

Adolescent Maturation, Decision-making, and Risk-taking Behavior

Adolescence has been described as maturation in three different domains: physical, cognitive, and psychosocial. The timing and tempo of these maturational changes are important in shaping adolescent sexuality and they vary widely from one child to the next. Puberty, or the development of secondary sexual characteristics, is an early and mid-adolescent process. It tends to start earlier in girls than in boys and may actually start in the preteen years. In fact, in a recent study involving data from private practice sites, the American Academy of Pediatrics reported that normal girls as young as 8 or 9 years may show pubertal breast development or pubic hair growth (29). Cognitive maturation, or the maturation of abstract reasoning capability, also tends to occur in early and mid adolescence. On the other hand, psychosocial maturation, or the maturation of social relationships and behaviors, extends past the mid adolescent years into late adolescence and sometimes into young adulthood.

Competent decision-making requires a certain degree of cognitive and psychosocial maturity; however, particularly in the early and mid adolescence, this maturity may be lacking. With the appearance of secondary sexual characteristics in the early and mid adolescent years comes a heightened interest in sexual experimentation. Risky sexual behavior can emerge, given a combination of limited life experience, limited self-awareness of sexual feelings, and relatively immature psychosocial skills. This trajectory is seen in studies showing that girls who enter puberty early exhibit more high-risk sexual behavior than girls who enter puberty late (30,31).

Extreme Risk-taking Behavior: Perceived Normalcy and Links to Maltreatment

Although adolescent behaviorists in the early 1900s considered adolescent turmoil and rebellion to be a necessary part of the adolescent experience, recent studies have shown that adolescence is typically not a tumultuous time (32), and that the rate of behavioral disturbance in adolescence is similar to that in the other stages of life (33). Although some risk-taking behavior is essential to adolescent development (34), extreme risk-taking behavior is not. Moreover, extreme risk-taking behavior is not that common in adolescence, contrary to popular perception. A 1993 American Medical Association report on adolescent maltreatment cites numerous studies showing that extreme risk-taking behavior is more common in adolescents who have been abused or neglected and that this behavior itself increases the risk of future maltreatment and victimization (35). This same report states: "Adolescents experience maltreatment at rates equal to or exceeding those of younger children. Recent increases in reported cases of maltreatment have occurred disproportionately among older children and adolescents. However, adolescents are less likely to be reported to child protective services and are more likely to be perceived as responsible for their maltreatment" (35). Perhaps it is too easy for the parents, the neighborhood, or the community to see extreme risk-taking as normal adolescent behavior and to see adolescent maltreatment as a "deserved" consequence of this behavior.

Clearly, there are unique challenges in identifying and addressing adolescent maltreatment. However, there are few, if any, adolescent-focused units as part of child protection. In 1996, a telephonic survey of the 24 county-based child protection offices in the State of Maryland found no evaluation and treatment programs designed specifically to serve maltreated adolescents (E. Kelly, *personal communication*, 1996). Typically, abused adolescents are served through an array of other programs, as summarized in Figure 7.2.

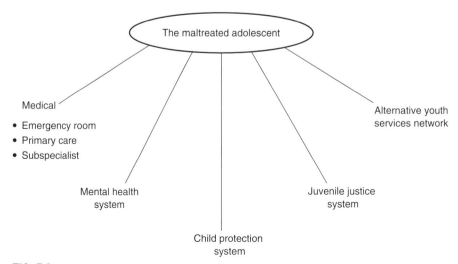

FIG. 7.2   Services for the maltreated adolescent.

The Teen–Parent Relationship

An adolescent's risk-taking behaviors and the consequences of those behaviors are strongly influenced by family dynamics. The teen–parent relationship that leads to risk-taking behaviors in the first place can lead to escalation of these behaviors (Fig. 7.3). Increased risk-taking behaviors are seen in authoritarian families in response to excessive restriction and discipline and in permissive families in response to lax parental control and "benign neglect." Also, parents may be the models for the very attitudes and behaviors their teenage children display, and their failure to acknowledge this may contribute to the problem.

Concerns with Confidentiality and Access to Health Care

Several issues limit health care access for adolescent patients and hence increase their vulnerability. Chief among these are concerns about confidentiality. Numerous studies have documented that adolescents may not seek medical care for reproductive health issues if parental consent is required (36,37). Recognizing this, the American Academy of Pediatrics, the American Academy of Family Physicians, and the American Academy of Obstetricians and Gynecologists have all endorsed the importance of confidentiality in adolescent health care (38,39). In addition, federal law mandates that adolescents have the right to access family planning services, and each state has legislative statutes that allow the provision of reproductive health care services to adolescents without parental consent (40). These "minor consent statutes" were formulated in the 1960s and 1970s after it was recognized that adolescents younger than 18 may self-limit their use of needed reproductive health care services if parental consent is required. These statutes notwithstanding, concerns about confidentiality may determine whether an adolescent decides to seek care following sexual abuse or sexual assault. These concerns are not unfounded.

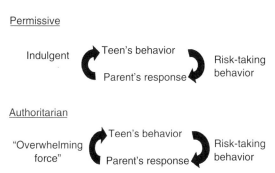

FIG. 7.3 Parenting styles.

If an adolescent seeks care following sexual abuse, the case must be reported to child protection. If an adolescent seeks care following sexual assault, the provider may feel that it is in the best interest of the adolescent to inform the parent. (See section on the clinical approach to the adolescent patient, in the subsequent text, for further discussion of confidentiality.)

Another issue is whether adolescents have access to health care providers they trust. This is problematic for the teen who sees a particular physician for the first time. How will the teen know whether the provider is comfortable providing confidential care to adolescents? How will the teen decide whether to talk about sensitive sexual health concerns? Can the teen trust the provider to keep these concerns confidential and not tell the parent? Access can also be problematic if the adolescent's family has been going to the same physician for many years. In such situations, the adolescent may be concerned that the physician will decide that the parents' need to know is more important than the teen's need for privacy.

A final issue of access to care is payment for services. This is a problem for both uninsured and insured patients. Adolescents may not understand the importance of health insurance or have the necessary funds to pay for health care out of pocket. If they seek care in an emergency department, problems with insurance and payment may not directly affect their receipt of care, although an itemized bill may be sent to their parents. Parents, in turn, are under no obligation to pay for services that are confidential and provided without their consent, unless the care provided was for an emergency (38,41). If adolescents go to a clinic without active insurance or cash to cover the visit, they are often denied care and referred to an emergency department. This scenario is not infrequent because adolescents and young adults are more likely to be uninsured than individuals from any other age-group (42–44).

Even insured adolescents have problems. For adolescents who are covered under their parents' private insurance, an itemized bill may be sent to the parent following the health care visit. To avoid this, the adolescent may need to arrange to pay for the visit out of pocket. In addition, some private insurers do not pay for family planning. Also, for the adolescent who is on medical assistance, some plans cover family planning services but not the cost of testing and treatment for sexually transmitted diseases.

These health care-access issues are all significant forces shaping the utilization of health care by the adolescent. In many instances, adolescents simply do not go to a physician even though they have significant health care needs. They also may preferentially use the emergency department for any reproductive health care needs because most emergency departments provide care regardless of insurance coverage.

Legislation has been enacted to address some of the issues of access to health care for the acute sexual assault victim. The Violence Against Women Act of 1994 mandates that states provide forensic examinations free of charge in order to receive federal funds. Despite this, women are sometimes charged for these examinations and are unaware that it should have been free (21).

Increased Vulnerability

Substance Abuse

Many teens abuse drugs and alcohol, and the prevalence increases as the teen grows older. The CDC 2003 Youth Risk Behavior Survey found that more than 75% of high-school students surveyed had consumed alcohol in the past, 37% of high-school seniors had engaged in binge drinking, and 40% of high-school seniors had used marijuana (6). Many studies have shown that substance abuse and coercive sexual experiences commonly occur at the same time (45). In one study of college-aged women, 72% of those who had been raped were intoxicated at the time of the rape (46).

Adolescents with a History of Childhood Sexual Abuse

Adolescents with a history of childhood sexual abuse are at increased risk of early-onset sexual activity, unprotected intercourse, multiple partners, and sexual assault (47,48). One study found that the severity of childhood sexual abuse (e.g., penetration, use of force, frequency of sexual encounter) was directly correlated with the degree of subsequent high-risk sexual behavior (49).

Adolescents Who Are "Cognitively Challenged"

A special group of adolescents at increased risk for sexual victimization are those with developmental disabilities or mental retardation (50,51). Like normal adolescents, these teens often experience a heightened interest in sexuality as they go through puberty. However, they are especially ill equipped to process these feelings because cognitive and psychosocial maturation are both significantly compromised. These teens are more easily coerced into sexual activity but less likely to disclose any sexual experience or seek help if they are confused or scared. Adults need to be alert to changes in their behavior or mood as possible clues to inappropriate or unwanted sexual experiences. An interview may be difficult or impossible once these teens are brought for medical attention, and a complete physical assessment may require conscious sedation (see subsequent text).

An Older Partner: Statutory Rape

Another group at increased risk for sexual victimization are younger adolescents involved with older partners. In state law, the term "statutory rape" is applied to such relationships. Specific details, including the age of the teen and the age difference between the teen and the older partner, differ from one state to the next. For example, in the State of Maryland, statutory rape occurs if the teen is under 16 and the partner is at least 4 years older.

In statutory rape, the risk of coercion or exploitation is high, simply because of the teen's relative immaturity and the difference in age between the teen and the sexual partner. Yet, these relationships are usually consensual and may provide both emotional and material comforts. Parents may implicitly or explicitly support the relationship as a welcome sign of emerging autonomy and independence.

Statutory rape is not uncommon, although providers and parents may be unaware that it is occurring, especially when the teen and the sexual partner do not appear to be much different in age. Some data suggest that statutory rape is more common with younger teens. A 1988 National Maternal and Infant Health Survey found that fathers of newborn babies were at least 5 years older than the mothers in 24% of births to 17-year olds, 27% of births to 16-year olds, and 40% of births to 14-year-olds (52).

THE CLINICAL APPROACH TO THE ADOLESCENT PATIENT

Including the Parent: When, Why, and How

The adolescent years span a period marked by significant change not only in sexual knowledge, attitudes, and behaviors but also in the teen–parent relationship. The care of the adolescent patient who has been sexually victimized will often involve the parents, and it is therefore important to understand the basic legal rights and responsibilities of both parents and teens and how these change as the teen grows older.

When care is provided to an adolescent patient, it is important to know the parents' role in the visit. Has the adolescent come to the health care provider alone or with a parent or guardian? Who initiated the visit? Is it the adolescent who wants to be seen or the parent who wants the adolescent to be seen? Does the adolescent have a specific health complaint or is the adolescent there because the parent has concerns, e.g., does the parent want an examination to see if the adolescent has been sexually active? If the adolescent comes in alone, does the parent know about the visit, or does the teen want everything to be kept confidential? Is the adolescent old enough that any reproductive health concerns, including those following sexual abuse or sexual assault, do not have to be communicated to the parent? Is the adolescent an emancipated minor? The answers to these questions are often not straightforward and will require the provider to consider the specific circumstances and applicable state law.

By law, in most states the age of majority is 18. Once the teen has reached this age, parental consent for health care services is not needed, and in most cases he or she must give permission for any sensitive health information to be shared with the parent.

As discussed earlier in this chapter, all states have minor consent statutes that allow the provision of care to adolescents below the age of majority for certain reproductive health care needs, including care for sexual abuse or sexual assault. In addition, in some states, additional statutes apply for the "emancipated minor," i.e., the adolescent who is below the age of majority and yet considered to be legally autonomous owing to circumstances of life (e.g., is married or is in the armed forces). The emancipated minor may consent for any and all health care, including that needed following sexual assault or abuse.

However, in caring for adolescents, and especially for those who have been sexually victimized, consent does not imply confidentiality. If sexual abuse has occurred, state law mandates reporting the matter to child protection or the police. If statutory rape has occurred, some would argue that the parent has a right to know and an obligation to intercede. In fact, in the State of Maryland, parental failure to intercede knowing that statutory rape has occurred is considered child neglect. If an adolescent under 18 presents to the emergency department following a self-identified coercive sexual assault and does not want the parent to know, the physician may still decide that it is in the best interest of the adolescent to contact the parent. In Maryland, specific legislative statutes give care providers the right (but not the obligation) to share sensitive reproductive health information with the parents of minors.

In all cases, if an adolescent discloses a history of sexual victimization and wants this to be kept confidential, it is important to ask why. The provider must bear in mind that some teens have valid concerns about sharing information with their parents. For example, if there is a nondisclosed history of maltreatment, the teen may justly fear further abuse if the parents are informed of sexual misadventures or victimization. If there is any concern about contacting the parents, then consultation with a social worker is critical to help address these issues and arrange appropriate follow-up care.

Sometimes it will be clear from the very start that the parent should be included in the clinical encounter. At other times, it will not be clear and the provider will have to decide how to involve the parent as the visit unfolds. In general, if the adolescent is brought to the visit by a parent or guardian, the adolescent should be interviewed alone at some point during the course of the visit. Also, if the adolescent is younger than 18, it may be appropriate to ask the guardian or parent about specific concerns they may have. The provider may decide to interview the parent alone at some point. If this happens, it will be important to talk with the teen afterward to allay fears of being talked about "behind their back." This being said, if the adolescent has been sexually abused, in most cases the parent will need to be involved, and if the adolescent has been sexually assaulted, in most cases the parent should be involved. In all situations, clinical skill, time, and private space are needed to provide the necessary clinical services in an effective manner that balances the parent's rights and need to know and the adolescent's rights and need for confidentiality and autonomy.

Obtaining the History

General Considerations

Most adolescent victimization is identified through the history. Sometimes the history is elicited without much difficulty. For instance, the patient presenting to the emergency department following acute sexual trauma may disclose assault or abuse with little prompting. More often, considerable interviewing skill is needed to elicit a history of sexual abuse or assault. The patient may present with vague somatic complaints, depression, or substance abuse and be hesitant to disclose a history of sexual victimization for reasons of guilt, shame, or even fear of retribution. Figure 7.4 details a few of the many medical and psychological consequences of sexual victimization. When a patient presents with these complaints or histories, it is imperative that the care provider ask about sexual victimization.

It is also important to ask about sexual abuse and assault during routine well-child visits. In the 1997 Commonwealth Fund Survey of the Health of American Girls, almost 50% of those who responded felt that their physician should inquire about any history of abuse, yet only 13% reported that their physician had done so (13).

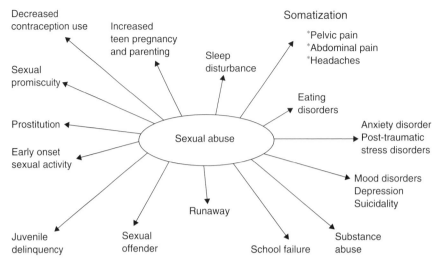

FIG. 7.4 Psychosocial consequences of sexual abuse in the adolescent patient.

Specific Guidelines

In taking a history from the adolescent patient, the clinician should follow these guidelines:

- The history should be obtained with the adolescent fully clothed and comfortable.
- Good eye contact should be maintained, and the seating for the examiner and the adolescent should place them at the same eye level.
- Note-taking should be limited to minimize distracting the adolescent.
- Limits of confidentiality should be discussed, and no promise of unconditional confidentiality should be given.
- The teen should be interviewed without the parents present for matters regarding sexuality, a possible history of abuse, and high-risk behaviors.
- In approaching the psychosocial interview, the least intimate questions, such as those pertaining to the home, education, and activities, should be asked initially. These can be followed by questions regarding mental health, sexual activity, and abuse.

The sexual history should include the following:

- Is there any history of consensual sexual activity?
  - Age at first experience
  - Number of lifetime partners
  - The patient's sexual orientation
  - Contraceptive use
  - Condom use
  - Age of partners
  - Use of drugs or alcohol by partner or patient
  - Any coercive elements in the sexual experience
- Is there any history of STIs?
  - When?
  - Was the patient treated?
  - Was the partner treated?

- Is there any history of clinical symptoms suggesting an STI?
  - Penile or vaginal discharge?
  - Pain with urination?
  - Abdominal or testicular pain?
  - Painful sores or wartlike lesions?
- For girls, a complete menstrual history should be obtained.
  - Age at first menses
  - Menstrual pattern (frequency, duration, regularity)
  - Any heavy or painful menses
  - Date of last menstrual period
- For girls, is there any obstetric history?
  - Any prior pregnancy?
  - Any living children?
  - Any prior abortions?
- Is there any history of sexual abuse or sexual assault?
  - When did it start and has it stopped?
  - What was the frequency and degree of sexual contact?
  - Was force used?
  - Does anyone know?
  - Was a report made to child protection or the police?
  - Has the patient received counseling?
  - Is the patient safe, or is there risk of further contact with the perpetrator?

Particularly for younger, sexually inexperienced adolescents, a sexual abuse history may be vague. The teen may not remember many details of the experience, or it may not have seemed coercive at the time. The sexually inexperienced female adolescent may not appreciate the difference between vaginal penetration and vulvar coitus, the latter being when the penis is forced between the labia majora and the labia minora but not past the hymen into the vaginal vault. The patient also may not be able to distinguish between sodomy, or penetration through the anus, from intercrural coitus, whereby the penis is forced between the buttocks but not into the rectum. The patient may not know when ejaculation has occurred. In one study, seminal fluid was detected in 7 of 16 patients who denied vaginal penetration or ejaculation (53).

The Physical Examination

General Guidelines

With pubertal maturation comes a heightened sense of privacy and increased embarrassment with the physical examination, especially for the younger adolescent. The following guidelines should be used when examining the adolescent patient.

- A chaperone should be present whenever possible.
- If the adolescent expresses a gender preference for the examiner, it should be accommodated if at all possible.
- If the adolescent prefers that the parent be present, this should be accommodated.
- If the parent insists on being present, the adolescent should be asked what he or she wants. The adolescent's preference should be followed if at all possible.
- The adolescent should be asked whether he or she has ever had a genital examination. If not, the physician should outline the examination before proceeding.
- Appropriate draping should be used, including a gown and a sheet over the lap.
- If the adolescent refuses any or all of the genital or perianal examination, gentle counseling may help relieve anxiety. If the adolescent still refuses, the physician may need to outline the need for forensic evidence if the adolescent wants to press charges. If he or she still refuses, the examination cannot be forced on the adolescent.
- If failure to do the examination could pose a significant health risk (e.g., failure to diagnose and treat a significant injury), then conscious sedation should be offered.
- In the developmentally delayed teen who needs a thorough genital examination, conscious sedation may be necessary so the examination can be performed without traumatizing the teen.

Pubertal Assessment

When examining the breasts and genitalia in the younger adolescent patient, it is important to ascertain whether the child is in early, mid, or late

TABLE 7-1

PUBERTAL TIMING

	Onset (Age in Years)	Completion (Age in Years)	Duration (Years)
Females	8.5–13	12–19	1.5–6.0
Males	9.5–13.5	13–17	3–5

Data from Marshall WA, Tanner JM. Variations in pubertal changes in girls. *Arch Dis Child* 1969;44:291–303 and Marshall WA, Tanner JM. Variations in the pattern of pubertal changes in boys. *Arch Dis Child* 1970;45:13–23.

puberty (Tables 7-1 and 7-2). The common approach is to assign Tanner stages. In the late 1960s, Tanner and Marshall studied several thousand school children in England and devised the Tanner classification scheme to describe pubertal changes. For boys, Tanner stages are based on pubic hair characteristics and the size of the testes and the penis. For girls, Tanner stages are based on pubic hair characteristics and breast size and shape. For boys, assigning Tanner stage based on testicular and penis size is difficult because there is considerable individual variability at any given stage. Tanner staging based on pubic hair and breast size and shape is more straightforward.

For pubic hair in both boys and girls, staging is as follows:

- *Tanner 1*: prepubertal; no coarse or dark pubic hair

TABLE 7-2

PUBERTAL PROGRESSION (MEAN AGE AT ONSET IN YEARS)

Females	
Breast budding	10.9
Appearance of pubic hair	11.2
Peak height velocity	11.5
Menarche	12.7
Males	
Testicular enlargement	11.5
Appearance of pubic hair	12.0
Peak height velocity	13.5

Data from Marshall WA, Tanner JM. Variations in pubertal changes in girls. *Arch Dis Child* 1969;44: 291–303; Marshall WA, Tanner JM. Variations in the pattern of pubertal changes in boys. *Arch Dis Child* 1970;45:13–23; and Tanner JM, Davies PSW. Clinical longitudinal standards for height and height velocity for North American children. *J Pediatr* 1985;107:317–327.

- *Tanner 2*: sparse, slightly coarse pubic hair, not extending onto the mons pubis
- *Tanner 3*: darker, coarser hair extending onto the mons pubis
- *Tanner 4*: more dense hair, covering most of the external genitalia but not extending to the inner thighs
- *Tanner 5*: dense hair extending to the inner thighs

For breast development, staging is as follows:

- *Tanner 1*: prepubertal
- *Tanner 2*: breast bud with minimal breast development beyond the areola
- *Tanner 3*: breast development extending well beyond the areola
- *Tanner 4*: more breast development with elevation of the areola about the breast contour ("the double mound")
- *Tanner 5*: more breast development with loss of the double mound

In addition to gender differences, there are ethnic differences in pubertal timing. The Third National Health and Nutrition Examination Survey showed that, in the United States, African American and Mexican American girls enter puberty earlier than Caucasian girls, by 8 and 5 months on average, respectively (54).

The Breast Examination

In girls, especially, it is important to do a breast examination to look for any signs of bruising or other injury. In addition, the breast examination is an important part of Tanner staging. For boys, the breast examination offers little useful information, although gynecomastia should be noted if present. Although this can be seen with testicular tumors and marijuana use, gynecomastia is more typically a normal variation during early to mid adolescence. It happens in up to 50% of adolescent males and usually resolves within 1 year (55). It is important to assure adolescent boys that this is common and normal. This assurance may be especially important for boys who have been sexually molested.

The Female Genital Examination

The primary focus of the female genital examination is the pelvic examination. This examination has three components: the external examination, the speculum examination, and the bimanual examination. The patient should be draped appropriately and examined in the dorsal lithotomy position. The frog-leg position, used for younger patients, does not permit examination of the vaginal vault and the cervix with the speculum and is typically not used in the adolescent patient. Nonlatex gloves should be used whenever possible to avoid latex allergy reactions. If the patient has never had a pelvic examination, it is important to provide an overview of the procedure and show her the speculum before starting the examination.

While performing the external part of the pelvic examination, the examiner should note the Tanner stage and any signs of injury or infection. The external examination should begin with touching the thigh, then proceeding to the inguinal area, the perineum, and finally, the vulva. The vulva includes the mons pubis, the labia majora, the labia minora, and the vestibule. The vestibule includes the vaginal orifice, the urethral orifice, and the posterior fourchette.

The hymen should be inspected carefully. The color and the thickness of the hymen is determined by the estrogen level. The hymen in the newborn infant is typically thick and pink due to intrauterine estrogen exposure. In contrast, the hymen in girls aged 1 to 8 years is typically thin and red, reflecting the low estrogen levels in this age-group. With the increasing estrogen levels of early puberty, the hymen changes from a red to a pink color, and it thickens and becomes more distensibile. As puberty progresses, it becomes more redundant and is likely to have folds and notches (Fig. 7.5).

Usually the speculum examination is performed next. It allows the examiner to inspect the vaginal vault and the cervix and to collect laboratory samples for culture and forensic evidence. When performing a speculum examination, it is helpful to first perform a digital examination with a gloved finger, explaining to the patient that you are feeling for her cervix.

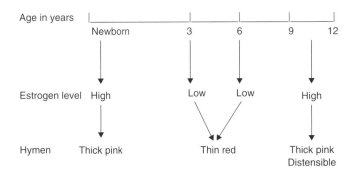

FIG. 7.5   Estrogen and the hymen.

Always ask about latex allergy and use latex-free gloves when performing this examination. This digital examination allows the examiner to assess the laxity of the vaginal opening, the length of the vagina, and the position of the cervix. Assessing the laxity of the introitus and the length of the vagina helps to determine the size of the speculum to be used. If the introitus barely admits one finger, then a speculum examination may be difficult and a vaginosope should be used.

An additional benefit of the digital examination is to ease insertion of the speculum. Before inserting the speculum, it is helpful to exert downward pressure with the examining finger, thereby helping to create a space for the speculum. As the speculum is inserted, the examining finger is removed. The position of the speculum is then adjusted on the basis of the position of the cervix as determined by the digital examination. During the digital and speculum examination, any lubrication should be achieved with water because K-Y Jelly (Johnson & Johnson, Inc.) interferes with the growth of *Neisseria gonorrhoeae*. During the speculum examination, the vaginal walls and the cervix should be examined for any signs of injury or infection, and the presence of discharge either in the vaginal vault or at the cervical os should be noted.

In providing care to the female adolescent victim of sexual abuse or sexual assault, there may be occasional circumstances in which the physician decides not to do a speculum examination. If the patient is young and sexually inexperienced or if she has significant mental retardation or developmental disabilities, attempts at the speculum insertion may be unsuccessful because of the tightness of the hymenal ring or because of the patient's resistance to the examination. In such situations, especially if there is no history of attempted vaginal penetration, no vaginal discharge, no pelvic or abdominal pain, and no vaginal bleeding, then the physician must assess how important it is to visualize the vaginal walls and the cervix and obtain endocervical cultures. If the physician decides it is important to proceed, then the two options available are the endoscopic examination using the vaginoscope or a speculum examination under conscious sedation.

After the speculum examination, the examiner should proceed to the bimanual examination. The examiner should palpate the vaginal walls and the cervix. Genital warts are sometimes more easily detected by palpation than by visualization. Cervical motion tenderness should be assessed, first by asking if there is any discomfort before moving the cervix, and then asking again while moving the cervix back and forth and up and down. Cervical motion tenderness is one of the cardinal signs of pelvic inflammatory disease and, hence, is an important part of the

physical examination. In addition, the uterus should be palpated for size and tenderness, and the adnexa should be palpated for any tenderness or masses.

The Perineal, Perianal, and Rectal Examination in the Female Patient

Following the genital examination, it is important to inspect the perineum and the perianal area and look for any signs of injury or infection. Genital warts, in particular, may be seen in either area.

The rectal examination is not typically included in the routine adolescent female examination, although in some cases it may be performed to assess uterine size and tenderness if the bimanual examination cannot be performed. However, in the patient who has been sexually victimized, the rectal examination may be quite important, particularly if there is any rectal bleeding or history of rectal trauma. In such cases, direct visualization using endoscopic techniques may be needed.

Signs of Injury in the Female Patient

Certain acute injuries, such as intravaginal tears and penetrating intra-abdominal injuries, are clear signs of forced sexual penetration. However, such injuries are not common. It is more typical for the adolescent victim to have either no injuries or minor injuries.

Minor injuries can be seen with both consensual and coercive sexual experiences. In one study, toluidine blue was applied to the vestibule of adolescent girls who had been sexually assaulted and those who had only had consensual intercourse. Minute genital lacerations were seen in the posterior fourchette for both groups and did not differ in degree or pattern (56). Tears and attenuation of the hymen are also seen with both consensual and forced sexual activity. In a study of adolescent girls without a history of sexual abuse but who were sexually active, attenuation of the hymen to less than 1 mm was found in 37% and was more common in girls who had been sexually active for more than 3 years; hymenal remnants (myrtiform caruncles) were found in 21%, and complete hymenal transections, extending through the base of the hymenal rim, were found in 84% (57). In the same study, attenuation and myrtiform caruncles were not found in girls who never had sexual intercourse (57).

In one study of sexually abused girls of ages 1 to 17 years, the most common finding following penile penetration in prepubertal and adolescent girls was a hymenal tear (58). In another study of 204 sexually abused girls aged 9 to 17 years who gave a history of penile-vaginal penetration, the most common findings were complete hymenal transections, seen in 8%, and hymenal notches (defined as sudden narrowing of the hymen to less than 1 mm in width), seen in 25%. These were most often found along the posterior rim (59).

It can be difficult to distinguish normal hymenal notches from healed tears. Those notches that extend through the base of the hymenal rim (so-called complete transactions) are strongly correlated with a history of blunt trauma and penetration, as are the deep notches near 6 o'clock (with the patient supine). Complete transactions or deep notches may be difficult to detect; it may be necessary to "run the hymen" with a Q-tip or with a distended Foley catheter (60).

The Significance of a Normal Examination in the Female Patient

As with prepubertal children, adolescents who have been sexually victimized often have normal examinations. In a study of adolescent girls with a history of penile–vaginal penetration (but no outside corroboration), 31% were normal when examined within 3 days of the assault and 85% were normal when examined more than 6 months after the assault (59). In another study of adolescent females aged 13 to 19 years, which compared those with and without a history of consensual sexual intercourse, 50% of those with a history of intercourse had intact hymens (61).

The Male Genital Examination

As with the female, the male genital examination should include Tanner staging. The approach should be systematic and include inspection and palpation of the inguinal area, the mons pubis, the testes and the scrotal sac, the shaft and glans of the penis, and the urethral meatus. The urethra should be "milked" to see if there is any urethral discharge. In the male victim, most injuries are seen near the anus and rectum (see subsequent text).

The Perineum, Perianal, and Rectum Examination in the Male Patient

In the male adolescent, examination of the perineum and perianal areas is especially important because receptive anal intercourse is more common in the male victim. As with the female, careful inspection should ascertain whether there are any signs of injury or infection. The skin and anal verge should be examined for bruising, tears, or lacerations. Reflex anal dilatation should be assessed with mild lateral traction. Excess dilatation suggests chronic abuse, although it can be seen with chronic constipation. If there is bleeding or rectal pain, a proctoscopic examination should be performed.

Laboratory Tests

The choice of specific laboratory tests is based on whether the examination is forensic in nature and on the patient's signs and symptoms. Forensic examinations are typically performed within 120 hours of the sexual assault. Various evidentiary tests may be administered as a part of the rape kit, and meticulous attention to detail and documentation are needed to maintain the "chain of evidence." (For more discussion on forensic tests, see Chapter 6 and Chapter 13.)

Testing for STIs should be considered in all patients who have been sexually abused or assaulted. The choice of lab tests will depend on what happened, whether the patient is asymptomatic, and on the time elapsed since the assault, as discussed in the next section.

Pregnancy Testing and Emergency Contraception

In adult women, the risk of pregnancy following a single sexual assault is approximately 5% (62). For adolescents, the risk is lower because anovulatory cycles are so common in the first few years following menarche. However, any female adolescent who has been sexually victimized may be at risk for pregnancy and should have a pregnancy test. This includes adolescents who have not yet had menarche, adolescents who report regular menses and no missed or late menses, and adolescents who have had vulvar coitus without vaginal penetration.

Pregnancy is diagnosed by a urine or serum test. The urine test detects pregnancy as early as 12 to 14 days after conception, whereas a serum test detects pregnancy as early as 8 days after conception. When a urine test is used, the clinician should bear in mind that a positive test result is always from a sexual encounter at least 12 to 14 days earlier. The serum test is preferred for a sexual assault examination if there is any history of a recent sexual encounter. In addition, a serum test should be performed on patients with a positive urine test and vaginal bleeding. Such patients should have a quantitative serum human chorionic gonadotropin (HCG) test, just in case of ectopic pregnancy or a threatened abortion.

Emergency contraception, also known as "the morning-after pill," should be offered to female adolescents who are seen within 5 days of a sexual assault. This method requires that the patient take a dose of hormones by mouth and repeat the dose in 12 hours. This will decrease the risk of pregnancy by up to 75%. Because nausea and emesis are common, an antiemetic should be prescribed. A urine pregnancy test should be performed prior to taking the morning-after pill and a repeat pregnancy test should be performed in 2 to 3 weeks. If emergency contraception is inadvertently taken in early pregnancy when the urine test is still negative, and the pregnancy is not interrupted, it does not appear to have adverse effects on the fetus.

Reporting Sexual Abuse and Sexual Assault

Physician reporting guidelines vary considerably from one state to the next. All states require the physician to report sexual abuse to a child protection agency, although in some states there is a statute of limitations, whereby if a specific period has elapsed since the abuse (typically more than 5–10 years), then a report is not mandated. For some states, if a teen is younger than a specified age, e.g., 12, and is diagnosed with an STI, then a report to child protection is mandatory. In other states, the physician is allowed to exercise clinical judgment in deciding when to report such cases.

Laws regarding the reporting of statutory rape vary widely. Mandatory reporting poses ethical dilemmas for the physician because making a report may jeopardize the physician–patient relationship at a time when it is especially important for the teen to have a provider she or he can trust. In a 2004 position statement on caring for the adolescent victim of sexual abuse or sexual assault, the Society for Adolescent Medicine writes the following: "Federal and state laws should allow physicians and other health care professionals to exercise appropriate clinical judgment in reporting cases of sexual activity (e.g., life-threatening emergencies, imminent harm, or suspected abuse). Ultimately, the health barriers to adolescents are so compelling that legal barriers should not stand in the way of medical care" (4).

Adolescent patients or their parents always have the option of reporting sexual abuse or sexual assault to either child protection or to the police. In general, the health care provider should not persuade or dissuade such reporting. However, in cases of acute sexual assault, the provider will typically perform a forensic examination, with its attendant "chain of evidence," even if the patient or family has not yet decided to press charges. A social work referral may help families decide how to proceed.

DIAGNOSIS AND TREATMENT OF SEXUALLY TRANSMITTED INFECTIONS

Adolescent Vulnerability to Sexually Transmitted Infections

Sexually active adolescents have higher rates of STIs than any other age-group (63,64). Up to one third of the STIs reported annually occur in adolescents,

and it is estimated that at least 25% of adolescents will develop an STI before graduating from high school (44).

Both behavioral and biologic factors contribute to these high rates of infection. Compared with several decades ago, more adolescents are now having sexual intercourse at younger ages, and more are having multiple partners. In the 2003 Youth Behavior Risk Survey conducted by the CDC, about 60% of high-school seniors reported having had intercourse by the time they were in their senior year of high school, 14% reported having at least four partners, and 37% reported nonuse of condom at the most recent sexual intercourse (6). Biologic factors also increase STI risk. Puberty causes the columnar cells lining the endocervical canal to extend onto the face of the cervix and the consequent migration of the squamocolumnar junction to the face of the cervix. *N. gonorrhoeae* and *Chlamydia* both preferentially attach to the exposed columnar epithelium (65,66); human papillomavirus preferentially attaches to the cells at the squamocolumnar junction (64). So the adolescent cervix is much more vulnerable than the prepubertal cervix to STI infection. For these reasons, the CDC recommends prophylactic STI treatment for the adolescent sexual assault victim but not for the prepubertal patient (67).

Sexually Transmitted Infection Testing and Treatment

General Considerations

Testing and treatment for STIs are a critical part of the care of the adolescent sexual assault victim (68, 69). The risk of transmission, inoculation period, and specific signs and symptoms are all important considerations in deciding when to test and when to treat for specific STIs. Specific infections are summarized in Table 7-3 and are discussed later in this section. Important general considerations are as follows:

- For the adolescent victim of sexual abuse or assault, testing for STI is as important for the asymptomatic patient as for the symptomatic patient because most infections are asymptomatic.
- The risk of transmission following potential exposure depends on such factors as the type of sexual contact, the frequency of sexual encounters, the inoculum size with each encounter, and the risk of blood or mucosal contact or exchange of bodily fluids with each encounter.
- The risk of transmission also depends on the specific organism. Some are highly infectious (e.g., *Trichomonas*, *Chlamydia*, *N. gonorrhoeae*, *Treponema pallidum*, and *Papillomavirus*) and

TABLE 7-3

CHARACTERISTICS OF SEXUALLY TRANSMITTED INFECTIONS

Disease	Transmission Risk After Sexual Assault[a]	Incubation	Percent Asymptomatic
Trichomoniasis	85%–30% (m to f > f to m)	5–28 d	Women 25%–50% Men >50%
Chlamydia	30%–70% (m to f > f to m)	7–21 d	Women 2/3 Men 1/3
Gonorrhea	20%–90% (m to f > f to m)	1–14 d	Women 20%–80% Men <20%
Syphilis	30%–60%	10–90 d (chancre) 1–6 mo (rash)	>90%
HPV	60%–70%	1.5–20 mo	>90%
HSV-2	Probably <5%	3–14 d	>90%
Hepatitis B	Probably <5%	45–160 d (average 120 d)	>90%
HIV	Probably <5%	3–6 mo	>90%

HPV, human papillomavirus; HSV, herpes simplex virus; HIV, human immunodeficiency virus.
[a]Risk depends on type of sexual activity, number of sexual acts, concurrent sexually transmitted diseases.
Data from Holmes KK, Sparling PF, March P, et al. eds. *Sexually transmitted diseases*, 3rd ed. New York: McGraw-Hill, 1999.

others are not (e.g., the human immunodeficiency virus [HIV], the herpes simplex virus [HSV], and the hepatitis B virus) (Table 7-3).

- The incubation period varies depending on the infection (Table 7-3).
- A positive test for an STI suggests prior exposure and an intervening duration of time that equals or exceeds the incubation time for that infection.
- Specific testing and treatment should be tailored to the patient's history to the extent that the history is reliable.
- In certain situations, for example, the history is deemed reliable and there has been no mucosa-to-mucosa contact or exchange of bodily fluids, the physician may decide that neither testing nor treatment for STI is necessary.
- In those situations in which mucosal contact or exchange of bodily fluids *could* have occurred, it is best to test, treat, and offer follow-up testing for certain STIs.
- STIs coexist. Finding one infection increases the likelihood that other infections are present.
- In evidentiary cases, the provider must be knowledgeable regarding the court's preference for laboratory evidence. For example, when testing for chlamydial or gonococcal infection, the provider must know whether the court will allow urine-based nonculture test results or will consider only culture results as admissible.
- For patients seen in the acute setting, the need for additional follow-up testing should be discussed. This is particularly important for infections with

long incubation periods, for example, syphilis and those caused by HIV and human papillomavirus.

Sexually Transmitted Infection Testing Following Acute Sexual Assault

- Even if mucosal contact or exchange of bodily fluids *could* have occurred, some centers advise against STI testing if patients are seen immediately following an acute sexual assault because positive results usually reflect prior sexual activity, not exposure from the sexual assault (71). This practice has not been uniformly adopted, however, because test results may influence future treatment and follow-up plans. Furthermore, evidence of prior sexual activity is no longer admissible evidence in most states (67).
- The following STI tests are usually performed after an acute sexual assault:
  - *For females*:
    - ○ Oropharynx swab for gonorrhea culture (if oral-genital contact occurred)
    - ○ Rectal swab for gonorrhea and *Chlamydia* culture
    - ○ Endocervical swab for gonorrhea and *Chlamydia* culture (urine-based testing may be substituted in certain cases)
    - ○ Wet prep of vaginal discharge to check for trichomoniasis
  - *For males*:
    - ○ Oropharynx swab for gonorrhea culture (if oral-genital contact occurred)
    - ○ Rectal swab for gonorrhea and *Chlamydia* culture

○ Urethral swab for gonorrhea and *Chlamydia* culture (urine-based testing may be substituted in certain cases)

○ Wet prep of any urethral discharge to check for trichomoniasis

• *For both females and males*:

○ Rapid plasma reagin (RPR) serologies

○ HIV screen

○ Hepatitis B serologies

Sexually Transmitted Infection Treatment Following Acute Sexual Assault

■ If a patient is seen following attempted or actual penile penetration of the mouth, vagina, or rectum, then the CDC recommends presumptive STI treatment as follows: for gonorrhea—ceftriaxone, 125 mg IM; for chlamydial infection—azithromycin, 1 gm PO, or doxycycline 100 mg PO b.i.d. for 7 days; and for trichomoniasis—metronidazole, 2 gm PO (67).

■ Some clinicians defer treatment of trichomoniasis because of an increased risk of emesis following prophylactic treatment for multiple infections. In such cases, prophylactic treatment for trichomoniasis should be offered at a follow-up visit.

■ Hepatitis B vaccine should be given if the patient has not had the hepatitis B vaccine series or if the vaccination history is unknown.

■ Although there is no effective treatment for viral sexually transmitted diseases, postexposure prophylaxis (PEP) for HIV can be offered if the patient is seen within 72 hours of the assault (see further discussion in the subsequent text).

Sexually Transmitted Infection Testing and Treatment of the Asymptomatic Patient in the Nonacute Situation

In patients who present several weeks or months after a sexual assault, testing for infection should be performed whether symptoms are present or not. For patients who are asymptomatic, treatment may be either offered or deferred pending laboratory test results. The choice will rest on the specifics of the situation, the physician's clinical judgment, and the preference of the adolescent and possibly the parent as well.

Sexually Transmitted Infection Testing and Treatment of the Symptomatic Patient

A limited number of common clinical syndromes occur in association with STIs. These syndromes and the associated infections are as follows:

■ *Vaginitis*: chlamydial infection, gonorrhea, trichomoniasis

■ *Urethritis*: chlamydial infection, gonorrhea, trichomoniasis

■ *Pelvic inflammatory disease*: chlamydial infection, gonorrhea

■ *Menorrhagia or metrorrhagia*: chlamydial infection, gonorrhea

■ *Epididymitis*: chlamydial infection, gonorrhea

■ *Ulcers*: herpes simplex, syphilis (less common: chancroid, lymphogranuloma venereum, or granuloma inguinale)

■ *Inguinal adenopathy*: herpes simplex (less common: chancroid, lymphogranuloma venereum, or granuloma inguinale)

■ *Warts*: human papillomavirus infection, syphilis

■ *Mono-like syndrome*: acute HIV infection

■ *Rash*: disseminated gonorrhea, syphilis

■ *Arthritis:*: gonorrhea and *Chlamydia*

When patients are seen with symptoms of these infections following sexual abuse or sexual assault, appropriate treatment should be offered before test results are available.

More than 30 STIs have been described (70). The more common infections are described in the text that follows.

Chlamydial and Gonococcal Infections

Epidemiology and Clinical Presentation

Both chlamydial and gonococcal infections are relatively common in adolescents, although *Chlamydia* is particularly common, with an estimated prevalence of 5% to 20% in males and 10% to 25% in females. They are similar in their clinical spectrum. Both have high rates of asymptomatic infection, although higher for females than for males, and higher for chlamydial infection than for gonorrhea. For both, the most common clinical presentation is a lower genital tract infection, manifested as a vaginal discharge or dysuria for females and as a urethral discharge or dysuria for males. Both chlamydial and gonococcal infection can cause ascending upper genital tract infection, typically manifesting as pelvic inflammatory disease in females and epididymitis in males. For females, upper tract infection, particularly with *Chlamydia*, can also lead to endometritis, which manifests as increased menstrual flow, increased intermenstrual spotting, or unusually strong menstrual cramps.

Both *Chlamydia* and *N. gonorrhoeae* can cause a perihepatitis infection, known as the Fitz-Hugh–Curtis syndrome. Typically, patients with this syndrome appear ill and have sharp, pleuritic right upper quadrant pain. Occasionally, the presentation is mild with minimal right upper quadrant tenderness.

Both *Chlamydia* and *N. gonorrhoeae* can cause proctitis in homosexual men and heterosexual women who practice receptive anal intercourse.

These patients may present with tenesmus, rectal pain, and bloody or purulent rectal discharge (72).

Chlamydial infection of the pharynx is not common, despite the high prevalence of chlamydial infection and the relative popularity of oral-genital sex (70). This type of infection appears to be self-limited and no treatment is necessary. On the other hand, gonococcal infection of the pharynx is not that uncommon, particularly in homosexual men. The pharyngitis is often mild and transient but is a primary cause of disseminated gonococcal infection. Hence, pharyngeal culture for *N. gonorrhoeae* is important if oral-genital sex has occurred.

Testing

Any body orifice subjected to attempted or actual penetration should be tested for *Chlamydia* and *N. gonorrhoeae*, the only exception being *Chlamydia* testing of the oropharynx (see preceding text). Several testing methodologies are available: culture, enzyme immunoassay (EIA), direct fluorescent antibody (DFA), nucleic acid hybridization (Gen Probe), and amplification of *Chlamydia* DNA or RNA by ligase chain reaction (LCX) or polymerase chain reaction (PCR). The EIA and DFA tests have unacceptably low sensitivities and specificities, especially in children, and the performance of the GenProbe is similar. The LCX and PCR tests have not been adequately tested for rectal or pharyngeal sites but are excellent for cervical, urethral, and urinary sites and have specificities exceeding 99%. For general STI screening, the urine-based DNA/RNA amplification tests have replaced culture methods because they do not require a speculum examination in the female or a urethral swab in the male (73,74). For forensic examinations, however, it is important to know the prevailing court opinion regarding the validity of nonculture techniques. Despite the high specificity of the newer amplified DNA or RNA tests, some courts will consider only culture results in evidentiary cases.

Treatment and Follow-up

One-dose treatments are available for both chlamydial infection and gonorrhea and are appropriate for patients who are asymptomatic or patients with only a lower tract infection, i.e., females with a vaginal discharge or males with a urethral discharge. The treatment options are azithromycin, 1 gm PO, for *Chlamydia*, and ceftriaxone, 125 mg IM, for gonorrhea. Ciprofloxacin, 500 mg PO, may also be used for gonorrhea if the patient is 18 years or older, although this is less of an option in areas reporting fluoroquinolone-resistant gonorrhea.

For patients with signs of upper tract infection, e.g., pelvic inflammatory disease, endometritis, or epididymytis, the dose of ceftriaxone is increased to 250 mg IM, and *Chlamydia* treatment should extend for 2 weeks using doxycyline at 100 mg PO b.i.d.

Depending on the situation, dual therapy for both chlamydial infection and gonorrhea may be appropriate regardless of test results. This is the standard of care for acute sexual assault. It is also recommended for patients with upper tract infection, e.g., pelvic inflammatory disease or epididymitis.

Following treatment for chlamydial or gonorrhea infection, rescreening (not test of cure) is recommended at 1 to 2 months after treatment is complete for patients at high risk of reinfection. An interval of at least a month should pass before rescreening with the nonculture methods because nonviable organisms may be present for up to a month after treatment.

Syphilis

Epidemiology and Clinical Presentation

Relative to other groups, adolescents do not have the highest rates of syphilis. The highest prevalence is found in women aged 20 to 24 and men aged 35 to 39 (75). The incidence of primary and secondary syphilis has been declining in women and in African Americans, yet pockets of infection remain, primarily among men having sex with men (76).

Most of the time, syphilis is asymptomatic. A chancre, typically painless, appears at the site of inoculation within 3 weeks of infection. This ulcer is typically 1 to 2 cm in diameter and has an indurated margin. It lasts for 3 to 6 weeks, but because it is painless and often intravaginal in women, it frequently goes unnoticed. Without treatment, the diffuse rash of secondary syphilis will appear approximately 6 weeks to several months later. This rash is typically maculopapular and often involves the palms and soles. Patients with secondary syphilis may also develop the wartlike condyloma lata lesions and systemic symptoms such as malaise, fever, sore throat, and lymphadenopathy. Without treatment, the symptoms abate and the rash disappears after 3 to 12 weeks. Early latent syphilis is diagnosed in the asymptomatic patient (i.e., "latent") who has had syphilis for less than 1 year, and late latent syphilis is diagnosed in the asymptomatic patient who has had syphilis for more than 1 year. It may be impossible to distinguish these two stages, especially if no prior serology results are available. After many years of asymptomatic infection, patients may develop the signs and symptoms of tertiary syphilis. These are not usually seen in the adolescent patient. It is important to check the HIV status of any patient with syphilis because up to 30% of HIV-infected patients who also have syphilis will have neurosyphillis by cerebrospinal fluid analysis (77).

Testing

Syphilis testing should be performed on any victim of sexual abuse or assault in which there has been mucosal contact or exchange of bodily fluids. The usual screening test is the RPR test. This is not as sensitive as the tests that measure antibody to the surface proteins of *T. pallidum* (fluorescent treponemal antibody [FTA]) or *Treponema pallidum* hemoagglutination (TPHA), so most laboratories will perform this test if the RPR is positive. The FTA becomes positive sooner than the RPR, so the patient with a chancre should have both performed. In these patients, the RPR is negative 20% of the time and the FTA is negative only 10% of the time.

The gold standard for syphilis testing is the dark-field microscope examination of the syphilitic chancre to look for the syphilitic treponemes. However, dark-field microscopes are not typically found in the emergency department (e.g., there are only two dark-field microscopes in Baltimore City), so serologic tests remain the mainstay of diagnostic testing.

Treatment and Follow-up

The definitive treatment, 2.4 million units of benzathine penicillin IM, is not usually administered in the acute phase after sexual assault unless the perpetrator is known to have syphilis or the patient has signs of primary or secondary syphilis. In the nonacute situation, benzathine penicillin, 2.4 million units IM, is recommended if the patient has positive serology results or has primary or secondary syphilis. If seroconversion cannot be documented within the prior year, then it must be assumed that the patient has a "late latent" infection, i.e., of more than 1 year's duration, and three separate weekly IM shots of benzathine penicillin should be given. If a chancre is present and syphilis is suspected, then the patient should be given penicillin without waiting for the serology results. Because the chancre is seen with primary syphilis only, one dose of penicillin should suffice. Patients with HIV are at risk for treatment failure and for neurosyphilis. An infectious disease specialist should be consulted in such cases.

Because it can take up to 3 months for antibodies to appear following exposure to syphilis, repeat testing should be considered if the initial screen was negative and the sexual assault occurred within the previous 3 months. For patients who are treated for syphilis, follow-up serologies should be repeated at 3-month intervals for at least a year to document a decrease in titers and treatment efficacy.

Human Immunodeficiency Virus

Epidemiology and Clinical Presentation

Adolescents are at substantial risk for HIV infection. Groups at special risk include men having sex with men and nonwhite adolescent women, particularly women who are the partners of men who have sex with men. HIV-infected youths are more likely to be high-school drop-outs, have older sexual partners, have more sexual partners, and have higher rates of human papillomavirus infection (45). Adolescents who engage in receptive anal intercourse are at increased risk of HIV infection; therefore, male victims of sexual assault or sexual abuse are at particularly high risk. HIV infection following receptive oral-penile sex has been reported but appears to be rare (78,79).

Most adolescents with HIV are asymptomatic. However, several weeks after the onset of infection, more than half the exposed individuals will experience an acute retroviral syndrome. This mono-like illness typically lasts for several weeks and is characterized by sore throat, malaise, weight loss, fever, and lymphadenopathy. The higher the viral load, the more severe the symptoms. As the immune system mounts a response, the viral load decreases and the symptoms abate. Patients then tend to remain asymptomatic for up to 10 years before showing signs of acquired immunodeficiency syndrome (AIDS) (66).

Many adolescents with HIV are unaware of their infection. In addition, patients who know they are positive do not always tell their partners or use condoms. Hence, asking about the partner's HIV status is important but is not an accurate means of assessing the risk of HIV exposure.

Testing

HIV testing should be considered in any adolescent victim of sexual abuse or assault. The usual screen for asymptomatic HIV infection is the enzyme-linked immunoabsorbent assay (ELISA). Following HIV exposure, the ELISA will be negative for several weeks, and often for several months. By 6 months, it will be positive in 95% of patients. Not all positive ELISA results indicate HIV infection, so a confirmatory Western Blot must be performed. Occasionally the Western Blot results are indeterminate and the patient will need repeat tests over several months to determine the true status.

For patients who present with signs and symptoms of the acute retroviral syndrome, both the ELISA and the HIV RNA PCR (viral load) should be checked. Patients at this stage of the illness may not yet have mounted the antibody response that makes the ELISA positive, yet they will have a high viral load.

HIV screening is not always performed in the emergency department setting because of the difficulties in ensuring that the patient will return for the results and follow-up counseling. However, because the adolescents and young adults who are most at risk may not have a primary care provider, it is important to offer HIV testing and provide for follow-up counseling. In patients who present to the emergency department with possible acute retroviral syndrome, testing should be performed to expedite early diagnosis and possible initiation of treatment.

HIV testing requires written informed consent in most states and should be performed with appropriate pretest counseling. It should not be performed in patients who are suicidal. In most cases, the adolescent patient is considered competent to provide this consent. However, clinical judgment should be exercised, particularly for the younger adolescent, in deciding whether or not to include the parent in the pretest counseling and the consent process. If the adolescent is tested as HIV positive, considerable emotional support is needed, and parental support may be crucial. On the other hand, particularly for the older adolescent, requiring parental consent may dissuade the adolescent from getting tested. This situation is highlighted by the experience in Connecticut. At one point, the State of Connecticut required parental consent for HIV testing of adolescent patients. Then the law was changed, dropping the parental consent requirement. Subsequently, there was a doubling in the number of adolescent requests for HIV testing (80).

Treatment and Follow-up

In the acute care setting, two specific clinical situations warrant consideration of HIV treatment: (a) PEP for patients presenting immediately following an assault and (b) treatment for patients who present with acute retroviral syndrome.

PEP for HIV exposure can be quite effective when used appropriately and has become the standard of care for occupational HIV exposure (76). Postexposure HIV prophylaxis should also be considered for all acute sexual assault victims (79,81). The State of New York has established guidelines recommending that HIV prophylaxis be offered to all victims of acute sexual assault; although elsewhere many recommend a risk assessment before initiating therapy. HIV PEP should be offered if the perpetrator is known to be HIV positive (82). It also should be offered if the area has a high prevalence of HIV and the patient has ulcerative genital lesions, because these markedly increase the risk of transmission. A final consideration is patient preference. If a patient wants HIV prophylaxis, it should be offered. In one study of adult women survivors of rape, 40% feared contracting HIV (83).

Important barriers to effective PEP include prompt initiation of therapy following the exposure (within 2 hours is best), the need for strict adherence to the recommended dosing regimens on a daily basis for 4 weeks, and, finally, the incidence of side effects, most commonly fatigue and mild gastrointestinal upset. These barriers are problematic for all patients, but especially for the adolescent patient. For these reasons, universal PEP for all acute adolescent sexual assault victims has not been advocated (84,85).

In patients who have documented acute retroviral syndrome, some suggest initiating aggressive long-term antiretroviral therapy as soon as possible (86). However, an HIV specialist should be consulted because there are no definitive studies supporting this approach. For adolescents, specifically, initiating long-term antiretroviral therapy in this setting may be ill-advised given the multiple drugs, their side effects, and the strict need for adherence.

Follow-up testing is particularly important for HIV infection because the incubation period is so long. By 6 months after exposure, 95% of patients will have antibodies detectable by the ELISA screen. Hence, if initial serology results are negative, follow-up ELISA screens are recommended at 6, 12, and 24 weeks after the assault.

Trichomoniasis and Bacterial Vaginosis

Epidemiology and Clinical Presentation

In one review of adult female victims, trichomoniasis and bacterial vaginosis were the most commonly acquired infections following sexual assault (68). Both infections are commonly asymptomatic and are confined to the lower genital tract.

Trichomoniasis is asymptomatic more than half the time. The incubation period following initial infection is 5 to 28 days, and the most common symptoms in females are dysuria or a frothy vaginal discharge and, in males, dysuria or urethral discharge.

Bacterial vaginosis is also asymptomatic most of the time. It is found only in females and the specific etiologic agent has yet to be identified. It is more common in sexually active adolescents, but it is also seen in patients who have never had sexual intercourse (87). The clinical signs of bacterial vaginosis are a fishy vaginal odor and a thin, homogeneous, grey-white vaginal discharge. Patients with mild bacterial vaginosis may not have a discharge but complain of a fishy odor, especially after sexual intercourse. (The alkaline pH of the semen will cause the bacteria to release the distinctive amines.)

Testing

The wet prep is the principal diagnostic test for both trichomoniasis and bacterial vaginosis, but for trichomoniasis it has a sensitivity of only 60%. *Trichomonas vaginalis* can also be found in urine. Spun urine may show *T. vaginalis* when the wet prep is negative (88). For bacterial vaginosis, the diagnosis is supported if there is a fishy odor when potassium hydroxide is applied or when a significant percentage of the epithelial cells (>20%) are clue cells.

Blake et al. (89) found that patient-administered vaginal swabs were as good as physician-administered swabs using a speculum for the recovery of samples that could be tested for both trichomoniasis and bacterial vaginosis.

Treatment and Follow-up

Prophylactic treatment for trichomoniasis is usually offered to the acute sexual assault victim. A single dose of metronidazole, 2 gm PO, is usually sufficient. This may induce nausea, so some care providers will offer it during the 2-week follow-up visit instead of during the acute visit, when other prophylactic medications are given. Also, some prefer a 7-day course of metronidazole at 500 mg PO b.i.d. This is as effective for trichomoniasis and more effective for bacterial vaginosis. Follow-up testing for either trichomoniasis or bacterial vaginosis is based on clinical signs and symptoms. If the patient remains symptom-free, then follow-up testing is optional.

Human Papillomavirus

Epidemiology and Clinical Presentation

Human papillomavirus (HPV) is the most common STI in the United States (64). In a review of the medical literature from 1988 to 1998 related to STIs in sexually abused children and adolescents, one of the most significant findings was an increase in the diagnosis of genital warts (condyloma acuminatum) and HPV infection during that period (90).

Most HPV transmission occurs through receptive vaginal or anal intercourse. Both complete and attempted penetration poses a significant risk for transmission. It is not known whether condoms prevent the transmission of HPV, although infection is correlated with the number of sexual partners and early age of sexual debut.

The incubation period following acute infection is up to 3 months. Most infections are asymptomatic, even at 3 months. A small percentage of female patients have abnormal Papanicolaou (Pap) smears following HPV exposure, and an even smaller number have genital warts. Cancer can develop following many years of infection with specific "high-risk" HPV serotypes. Fortunately, this is not common in the adolescent patient. In most cases, HPV infection actually regresses over time (91,92).

Testing

In males, there are no routine screening tests for HPV infection. In females, the Pap smear is the principal screening test. In this test, a sample of cells is taken from the cervical squamocolumnar junction and sent for histologic examination. If the Pap smear is abnormal, HPV serotyping may be performed to assess the risk of progression. In patients with significantly abnormal Pap smears, referral is made to gynecology, where colposcopy and biopsy may be performed.

Screening for human papillomavirus is not typically performed in the acute care setting because arranging and monitoring follow-up care for abnormal Pap smears is time intensive and more suited to the primary care office. This is particularly important in light of recent studies that showed that once adolescent patients have abnormal Pap smears, up to 90% will revert to normal over the next 3 years (92). This has led to a revision of the U.S. Preventive Task Force guideline on screening for cervical cancer to include postponing the first Pap smear until 3 years after the first sexual intercourse or by age 21 (93). These guidelines do not address the needs of the adolescent who was sexually abused as a child, and many practitioners feel that these adolescents should have Pap smears sooner. In addition, the adolescent who seeks care immediately after a sexual assault is often very concerned about STI exposure and may want to have a follow-up Pap smear. For such patients the Pap smear should be performed at the primary care office 3 to 6 months after the assault.

Patients who present with genital warts should be tested for other STIs, especially syphilis, because the condyloma lata of secondary syphilis can occasionally look like genital warts.

Treatment and Follow-up

There is no prophylaxis for HPV exposure. Patients who present with condyloma acuminatum can be treated with patient-applied imiquimod cream (Aldara), or the provider can apply trichloroacetic acid (TCA) or topical podophyllin. Because podophyllin should not be used during pregnancy, Aldara and TCA are preferred treatments for adolescent patients. Follow-up and retreatment may be needed on a weekly or biweekly basis for up to 6 weeks. If there is no response to treatment, the patient should be referred for cryosurgery or laser treatment. Topical treatment is often ineffective if the condyloma is large, and patients with this condition should be referred directly to gynecology.

Patients with an abnormal Pap smear should have follow-up Pap smears at 3- to 6-month intervals until the Pap smear reverts to normal. Those patients who have persistent mildly abnormal Pap smears (atypical cells of undetermined significance [ASCUS] or low-grade squamous intraepithelial lesion [LGSIL]) or moderately abnormal Pap smears (high-grade squamous intraepithelial lesions [HGSIL]) should be referred to gynecology for colposcopy and possible biopsy.

Herpes Simplex

Epidemiology and Clinical Presentation

HSV type 1 usually causes oral infection and HSV type 2 usually causes genital infection. The incidence of HSV type 1 genital infection seems to be increasing, possibly reflecting more oral–genital sexual behavior. In the past 30 years, the prevalence of genital herpes has increased markedly for the population as a whole and for adolescents specifically.

The incubation period following transmission of HSV is 2 to 10 days. Some patients do not develop any symptoms with this initial infection; others have painful genital ulcers plus malaise and fever. Typically, ulcers regress and disappear after a week or two. The subsequent clinical course is characterized by variable symptom-free periods plus episodic recurrence of the ulcers. The frequency of outbreaks tends to decrease over time. With recurrent disease, there are often minimal local prodromal symptoms, such as itching, followed by the appearance of vesicular lesions, which then progress to shallow painful ulcers that in turn heal over a period of several days. The highest risk of transmission is when there are genital ulcers, although shedding of the virus occurs several days before the ulcer appears and several days after it heals.

Testing

The usual test for HSV infection is viral culture. Ideally, the culture is taken from the base of the ulcerative lesion when it is still moist. Serologic tests also may be helpful, particularly when trying to establish if the ulcers are primary or secondary because immunoglobulin M (IgM) antibodies will be elevated in primary, and not secondary, outbreaks.

Although herpes simplex is the most common agent causing genital ulcers, other STI agents should also be considered. Most important of these is syphilis. Testing for syphilis should be considered for any patient with new-onset genital ulcers. Other infections such as chancroid, granuloma inguinale, and lymphogranuloma venereum are much less common and should be considered only if there is significant lymphadenopathy or ulcers that persist for several weeks or longer.

Treatment and Follow-up

The primary treatment for genital herpes is acyclovir. Dosing regimens differ for acute and recurrent disease and are summarized in the CDC's STI treatment guidelines (67). Treatment shortens the duration of symptoms and, perhaps, viral shedding, but it does not cure the infection. It is most effective if offered within 48 hours of the ulcer first appearing. No specific follow-up tests are needed following HSV infection.

Hepatitis B

Epidemiology and Clinical Presentation

Although hepatitis A, B, and C can be transmitted sexually, by far the most common following sexual abuse and sexual assault is hepatitis B. Hepatitis B is highly infectious and can be transmitted with a small inoculum. It is most often transmitted by percutaneous or mucosal exposure; it can also be transmitted sexually. Most cases are asymptomatic, although up to one third are associated with a self-limited acute hepatitis that appears 40 to 100 days after transmission. One percent of these patients develop acute hepatic failure, and of these 75% will die. Chronic hepatitis B occurs in approximately 5% of cases, and this in turn can develop into primary carcinoma of the liver. Following initial transmission, it can take up to 6 months for the infection to resolve or become chronic.

Testing

Universal hepatitis B vaccination has been recommended for several years. Fortunately, most children and young adults have been immunized and thus are protected if they are exposed to the virus. Nonetheless, it is standard practice to perform hepatitis B serologic tests on all sexual assault victims. These tests will indicate passive immunity if the patient has received hepatitis vaccines in the past, and they will distinguish acute, subacute, resolved, and chronic infections if the patient has never received the hepatitis B vaccinations. The adolescent who has been immunized will have the hepatitis B surface antibody but not the hepatitis B core antibody or the hepatitis B surface antigen. The adolescent who has cleared a prior infection will have the hepatitis B surface and core antibodies but not the hepatitis B surface antigen. And the adolescent who is a chronic carrier will have the hepatitis B surface antigen and the hepatitis B core antibody but not the hepatitis B surface antibody.

Treatment and Follow-up

The hepatitis B vaccine affords excellent protection against hepatitis B and should be given following acute sexual assault if the victim has either not received the complete set of hepatitis B vaccinations or has an unknown vaccination status. Patients should also be given hepatitis B immune globulin if the offender is known or suspected to have hepatitis B. Patients who receive vaccinations should have follow-up titers drawn at 3 and 6 months.

MENTAL AND SOCIAL CONSEQUENCES OF SEXUAL ASSAULT AND SEXUAL ABUSE

The mental, behavioral, and psychosocial consequences of child and adolescent sexual victimization are far reaching (Fig. 7.4). The more significant ones include the need for immediate crisis-intervention in the acute situation, long-standing depression and anxiety, and an array of high-risk behaviors as discussed in the subsequent text.

Acute Mental Health Needs

Crisis counseling should be offered to all adolescent victims following acute sexual assault. It should also be offered to the parents of the adolescent. Studies have shown that the adolescent's most immediate concern following rape are fears of bodily harm, shame, and fears of pregnancy and STIs (64,94). These should be addressed during the visit, as should any legitimate concerns with safety. If the adolescent is suicidal, she or he should be admitted if at all possible. If the patient is discharged from the emergency department, a follow-up phone call should be made within 24 hours and a follow-up visit should be scheduled within 1 to 2 weeks.

Depression

Sexual assault victims are at increased risk for depression and anxiety, and at least 50% will experience significant depression in the year following the assault (95). Adolescents, specifically, are at a significantly increased risk of depression and suicidality if they have a history of a coercive sexual experience. This can manifest as more subtle problems such as increased somatization, inability to concentrate, and problems at school or work. Adolescents who were sexually abused as children are also at increased risk for similar mental health problems that may appear several years after the abuse has ended (96,97).

Many studies link depression to sexual victimization. In a study of attempted suicide in gay and bisexual youth, Remafedi et al. found that suicide attempters were more likely to have a history of sexual abuse (98). In the 1997 Commonwealth Fund Survey of Adolescent Girls, it was found that adolescent girls with a history of physical or sexual abuse were twice as likely to have depressive symptoms or low self-esteem (13). In a study of 5,780 students in the 7th through 12th grades, self-reported physical or sexual abuse was associated with an increased risk of considering or attempting suicide (99). In an anonymous survey, high-school students with a history of sexual abuse were more than three times likely to attempt suicide (100).

Eating Disorders

Adolescents with a history of sexual abuse may present with eating disorders (13,99,101). This includes not only excess weight loss but also excess weight gain as a means of distancing themselves from the perpetrator.

High-risk Sexual Activity and Coercive Sexual Behavior

Many studies have linked high-risk sexual behavior with a history of childhood sexual victimization (96, 102–104). One survey also showed that high-school students with a history of sexual abuse were $3\frac{1}{2}$ times as likely to be sexually active (100), and another showed that condom negotiation skills were weak in teens who had been sexually abused (105). In a study of 9th through 12th graders in a midwestern state, Lodico et al. (106) found a striking correlation between a history of abuse and subsequent victimization. Self-reported sexual aggression was twice as common in adolescents who had been sexually abused, and self-reported sexual victimization was six times as common.

Teen Pregnancy

Many studies have shown an increased risk of pregnancy in adolescents with a history of sexual abuse (106–108). A study of 535 young mothers in Washington state found that two thirds had been sexually abused, 42% had been victims of attempted rape, and 44% had been raped (109). Another study found that adolescent girls with a history of abuse were more likely to try to conceive or pressure their boyfriends in helping them conceive and had more concerns about fertility (110). At least two studies have shown that adolescent males with a history of forced sexual intercourse are more likely to be fathers (111,112).

Teen pregnancy is associated with statutory rape and is more commonly seen with older partners. In the 1995 National Survey of Family growth, the Alan Guttmacher Institute found that for women under 18, having a partner who was 6 or more years older increased the risk of pregnancy 3.7 times, compared with having a partner only 2 years older (113).

Substance Abuse

Substance abuse in adolescents not only leads to an increased risk of sexual victimization but also is clearly associated with a history of childhood sexual abuse and a history of sexual assault or coercive sexual experiences (13).

Juvenile Delinquency

Adolescent boys who have been sexually victimized are less likely to internalize their feelings and more likely to exhibit antisocial and externalizing behaviors. Problems with the law and involvement with the juvenile justice system may follow (114). Fortunately, a good probation officer can provide much-needed guidance and direction.

Teen Runaways and Prostitution

For both adolescent girls and boys, there is a very strong association between runaway behavior and sexual abuse histories (114,115). Prostitution is also linked to childhood sexual abuse (116). The peak age for entering prostitution is 14 or younger, and in most cases runaway behavior precedes the prostitution.

Sex Offender Status

Adolescents are the perpetrators in at least 20% of child sexual abuse cases (117). In addition, up to 80% of adult sex offenders began their sexually aggressive behavior in adolescence (118). More than half the adolescent child molesters were themselves sexually abused as children (119), and a substantial number of imprisoned child molesters have a history of being victims of sexual abuse as children (120). Hence, sexual victimization is a cycle, and the victim often becomes the victimizer.

SUMMARY

Adolescence offers unique and difficult challenges in the identification and treatment of sexual victimization. More often than not, sexual victimization is linked to antecedent and subsequent high-risk behaviors, and the adolescent comes to medical attention because of these behaviors and not the act of actual sexual victimization. Effective intervention requires an understanding of how the adolescent processes information; how this is affected by emotion, stress, and life experience; and how their sexual behavior, risk-taking, and identity formation are all entwined during the adolescent years. When an adolescent who has been sexually assaulted seeks care in an urgent care setting, there are tremendous time constraints. Moreover, this may be the first and

last time the care provider cares for that patient. Nonetheless, the intensity of the visit provides the physician a window of opportunity to offer help, guidance, and redirection. The compassion and care provided during the visit may be critical in shaping the adolescent's recovery from victimization. If the urgent care physician can mobilize assistance from social work groups and communicate with the primary care physician, then the multiple long-term comorbidities associated with sexual abuse and sexual assault will have been addressed and the cycle of sexual violence can be interrupted.

REFERENCES

1. American Academy of Pediatrics Committee on Adolescence. Care of the adolescent sexual assault victim. *Pediatrics* 2001;107:1476–1479.
2. Olson DE, Rickert VI, Davidson LL. Identifying and supporting young women experiencing dating violence: what health practitioners should be doing now. *J Pediatr Adolesc Gynecol* 2004;17:131–136.
3. Irwin CE Jr, Rickert VI. Coercive sexual experiences during adolescence and young adulthood: a public health problem. *J Adolesc Health* 2005;36:359–361.
4. American Academy of Family Physicians. Protecting adolescents: ensuring access to care and reporting sexual activity and sexual abuse. Position paper of the American Academy of Family Physicians, the American Academy of Pediatrics, the American College of Obstetricians and Gynecologists, and the Society for Adolescent Medicine. *J Adolesc Health* 2004;35:420–423.
5. Stewart D. Adolescent sexual abuse, sexual assault, and rape. In: Hofmann AD, Greydanus DE, eds. *Adolescent medicine*, Stamford, CT: Appleton and Lange, 1997.
6. Centers for Disease Control and Prevention. Youth risk behavior surveillance—United States 2003. *MMWR* 2004;53(ss-2):1–29.
7. Finkelhor D. The victimization of children: a developmental perspective. *Am J Orthopsychiatry* 1995;65(2):177–193.
8. Kendall-Tackett KA, Simon AF. Molestation and the onset of puberty: data from 365 adults molested as children. *Child Abuse Negl* 1988;12:73–81.
9. Jones JS, Rossman L, Wynn BN, et al. Comparative analysis of adult versus adolescent sexual assault: epidemiology and patterns of anogenital injury. *Acad Emerg Med* 2003; 10:872–877.
10. Langan PA, Harlow CW. *Crime data brief: child rape victims 1994*, U.S. Department of Justice, Bureau of Justice Statistics, NCJ-147001, 1994.
11. Rennison CM. *Criminal victimization 1998*. U.S. Department of Justice, Bureau of Justice Statistics, HCJ 176353, 1999.
12. Kaestle C, Halpern CT. Sexual intercourse precedes partner violence in adolescent romantic relationships. *J Adolesc Health* 2005;36:386–392.
13. The Commonwealth Fund. *Survey on the health of adolescent girls*. New York: The Commonwealth Fund, 1997.
14. Finkelhor D, Dziuba-Leatherman J. Children as victims of violence: a national survey. *Pediatrics* 1994;94:413–420.
15. Koss MP, Gidycz CA, Wisniewski N. The scope of rape: incidence and prevalence of sexual aggression and victimization in a national sample of higher education students. *J Consult Clin Psychol* 1987;55:162–170.
16. Greenfeld LA. *Sex offenses and offenders: an analysis of data on rape and sexual assault*. NCJ-163392, U.S. Department of

Justice, 1997. Available at http://www.ojp.usdoj.gov/bjs/pub/pdf/soo.pdf. Accessed on October 21, 2005.

17. Adolescent Acquaintance Rape. ACOG committee opinion: Committee on Adolescent Health Care Number 122—May 1993. *Int J Gynaecol Obstet* 1993;42:209–211.

18. Scarce M. Same-sex rape of male college students. *J Am Coll Health* 1997;45(4):171–173.

19. Hanson RF, Kievit LW, Saunders BE, et al. Correlates of adolescent reports of sexual assault: findings from the National Survey of Adolescents. *Child Maltreat* 2003;8:261–272.

20. Kellogg ND, Huston RL. Unwanted sexual experiences in adolescents: patterns of disclosure. *Clin Pediatrics* 1995;34:306–312.

21. Monroe LM, Kinney LM, Weist MD, et al. The experience of sexual assault: findings from a statewide victim needs assessment. *J Interpers Violence* 2005;20:767–776.

22. Berliner L, Conte JR. The process of victimization: the victims' perspective. *Child Abuse Negl* 1990;14:29–40.

23. Kershner R. Adolescent attitudes about rape. *Adolescence* 1996;31(121):29–33.

24. Blumberg ML, Lester D. High school and college students' attitudes towards rape. *Adolescence* 1991;26(103):727–729.

25. Koval JE. Violence in dating relationships. *J Pediatr Health Care* 1989;3:298–304.

26. Wiemann CM. Rohypnol—the "date-rape" drug. *NASPAG News* 1998;12:1–5.

27. Finkelson L, Oswalt R. College date rape: incidence and reporting. *Psychol Rep* 1995;77(2):526.

28. Davis TC, Peck GQ, Storment JM. Acquaintance rape and the high school student. *J Adolesc Health* 1993;14:220–224.

29. Herman-Giddens ME, Slora EJ, Wasserman RC, et al. Secondary sexual characteristics and menses in young girls seen in office practice: a study from the Pediatric Research in Office Settings Network. *Pediatrics* 1997;99:505–512.

30. Duke PM, Carlsmith JM, Jennings D, et al. Educational correlates at early and late sexual maturation during adolescence. *J Pediatr* 1982;100(4):633–637.

31. Duncan PD, Ritter PL, Dornbusch SM, et al. The effects of pubertal timing on body image, school behavior, and deviance. *J Youth Adolesc* 1985;14:227–235.

32. Ponton LE. *The romance of risk: why teenagers do the things they do*. New York: Basic Books, 1997.

33. Rutter M, Graham P, Chadwick OF, et al. Adolescent turmoil: fact or fiction? *J Child Psychol Psychiatry* 1976;7:35–36.

34. Offer D, Ostrov E, Howard KI. Adolescence: what is normal? *Am J Dis Child* 1989;143:731–736.

35. Council on Scientific Affairs, American Medical Association. Adolescents as victims of family violence. *JAMA* 1993;270:1850–1856.

36. Cheng TL, Savageau JA, Sattler AL, et al. Confidentiality in health care: a survey of knowledge, perceptions, and attitudes among high school students. *JAMA* 1993;269:1404–1407.

37. Marks A, Malizio J, Hock J, et al. Assessment of health needs and willingness to utilize health care resources of adolescents in a suburban population. *J Pediatr* 1983;102:456–460.

38. AMA Council on Scientific Affairs. Confidential health services for adolescents. *JAMA* 1993;269:1420–1424.

39. American Academy of Pediatrics. *Confidentiality in adolescent health care*. Policy statement. AAP News, 1989.

40. Morrissey JD, Hofmann AD, Thorpe JC. *Consent and confidentiality in the health care of children and adolescents: a legal guide*. New York: Free Press, 1986.

41. English A. Treating adolescents: legal and ethical considerations. *Med Clin North Am* 1990;74:1092–1112.

42. Newacheck PW, McManus MA, Brindis C. Financing health care for adolescents: problems, prospects, and proposals. *J Adolesc Health* 1990;11:398–403.

43. Klein JD. Adolescence, the health care delivery system, and health care reform. In: Brindis C, Irwin C, Langlykke K, et al. eds. *Health care reform: opportunities for improving adolescent health*. Washington, DC: Bureau of Maternal and Child Health, 1994.

44. Ozer EM, Brindis CD, Millstein ST, et al. *America's adolescents: are they healthy?* San Francisco: University of California, San Francisco, National Adolescent Health Information Center, 1997.

45. Ellickson PC, Collins RL, Bogart LM, et al. Scope of HIV risk and co-occurring psychosocial health problems among young adults: violence, victimization, and substance abuse. *J Adolesc Health* 2005;36:401–409.

46. Mohler-Kuo M, Dowdall GW, Koss MP, sfxet al. Correlates of rape while intoxicated in a national sample of college women. *J Stud Alcohol* 2004;65:37–45.

47. Ferguson DM, Horwood LH, Lynsbey MT. Childhood sexual abuse, adolescent sexual behaviors, and sexual revictimization. *Child Abuse Negl* 1997;21:789–803.

48. Humphrey JA, White JW. Women's vulnerability to sexual assault from adolescence to young adulthood. *J Adolesc Health* 2000;27:419–424.

49. Cinq-Mars C, Wright J, Cyr M, et al. Sexual at-risk behaviors of sexually abused adolescent girls. *J Child Sex Abuse* 2003;12:1–18.

50. Tharinger D, Horton CB, Millea S. Sexual abuse and exploitation of children and adults with mental retardation and other handicaps. *Child Abuse Negl* 1990;134:301–312.

51. Chamberlain A, Rauh J, Passer A. Issues in fertility control for the mentally retarded female adolescents: sexual activity, sexual abuse, and contraception. *Pediatrics* 1984;73:445–450.

52. Small SA, Kerns D. Unwanted sexual activity among peers during early and middle adolescence: incidence and risk factors. *J Marriage Family* 1993;55:941–952.

53. Hook SM, Elliot DA, Harbison SA. Penetration and ejaculation: forensic aspects of rape. *NZ Med J* 1992;105:87–89.

54. Wu T, Mendola P, Buck GM. Ethnic differences in the presence of secondary sex characteristics and menarche among US girl: The Third National Health and Nurition Examination Survey, 1988–1994. *Pediatrics* 2002;110:752–757.

55. Neinstein LS. Gynecomastia. In: Neinstein LS, ed. *Adolescent health care: a practical guide*, 3rd ed. Chapter 10. Baltimore, MD: Williams & Wilkins, 1996.

56. McCauley J, Gorman RL, Guzinski G. Toluidine blue in the detection of perineal lacerations in pediatric and adolescent sexual abuse victims. *Pediatrics* 1986;78:1039–1043.

57. Emans SJ, Woods ER, Allred EN, et al. Hymenal findings in adolescent women: impact of tampon use and consensual sexual activity. *J Pediatr* 1994;125:153–160.

58. Muran D. Child sexual abuse: relationship between sexual acts and genital findings. *Child Abuse Negl* 1989;13:211–216.

59. Adams JA, Knudson S. Genital findings in adolescent girls referred for suspected sexual abuse. *Arch Pediatr Adolesc Med* 1996;150:850–857.

60. Jones JS, Dunnuck C, Rossman L, et al. Adolescent Foley catheter technique for visualizing hymenal injuries in adolescent sexual assault. *Acad Emerg Med* 2003;10:1001–1004.

61. Adams JA, Botash AS, Kellogg N. Differences in hymenal morphology between adolescent girls with and without a history of consensual sexual intercourse. *Arch Pediatr Adolesc Med* 2004;158:280–285.

62. Hampton HL. Care of the woman who has been raped. *N Engl J Med* 1995;332:234–237.

63. Cates W. The epidemiology and control of sexually transmitted diseases in adolescents. *Adolesc Med: State Art Rev* 1990;1:409–427.

64. American Academy of Pediatrics Committee on Adolescence. Sexually transmitted diseases. *Pediatrics* 1994;94:568–572.

65. Stamm WE. Chlamydia trachomatis infections of the adults. In: Holmes KK, Sparling PF, March P, et al. eds. *Sexually transmitted diseases*. 3rd ed. Chapter 29. New York: McGraw-Hill, 1999.

66. Berman SM, Hein K. Adolescents and STDs. In: Holems KK, Sparling PF, March P, et al, eds. *Sexually transmitted diseases*, Chapter 9. 3rd ed. New York: McGraw-Hill, 1999.

67. Centers for Disease Control and Prevention. Sexually transmitted diseases treatment guidelines 2002. *MMWR* 2002;51(RR-6):1–78.

68. Jenny C, Hooton TM, Bowers A, et al. Sexually transmitted diseases in victims of rape. *N Engl J Med* 1990;322(11):713–716.

69. Glaser JB, Schachter J, Benes S, et al. Sexually transmitted diseases in postpubertal female rape victims. *J Infect Dis* 1991;164:726–730.

70. Holmes KK, Sparling PF, March P, et al. eds. *Sexually transmitted diseases*, 3rd ed. New York: McGraw-Hill, 1999.

71. LeDray L. Sexual assault evidentiary exam and treatment protocol. *J Emerg Nurs* 1995;21:355–359.

72. Rompalo AM. Diagnosis and treatment of sexually acquired proctitis and protocolitis: an update. *Clin Infect Dis* 1999;28(Suppl 1):S84–S90.

73. Joffe A. Amplified DNA testing for sexually transmitted diseases: new opportunities and new questions. *Arch Pediatr Adolesc Med* 1999;153:111–113.

74. Shafer JA, Pantell RH, Schachter J. Is the routine pelvic examination needed with the advent of urine-based screening for sexually transmitted diseases? *Arch Pediatr Adolesc Med* 1999;153:119–125.

75. Centers for Disease Control and Prevention. Primary and secondary syphilis—United States, 2000–2001. *MMWR* 2002;51:971.

76. Centers for Disease Control. Updated US public health guidelines for the management of occupational exposures to HBV, HCV, and HIV and recommendations for postexposure prophylaxis. *MMWR* 2001;50(RR-11):1–42.

77. Malone JL, Wallace MR, Hendrick BB, et al. Syphilis and neurosyphilis in a human immunodeficiency virus type-1 seropositive population: evidence for frequent serologic relapse after therapy. *Am J Med* 1995;99:55–63.

78. Lifson AR, O'Malley PM, Hessol NA, et al. HIV seroconversion in two homosexual men after receptive oral intercourse with ejaculation: implications for counseling concerning safe sexual practices. *Am J Public Health* 1990;80:1509–1511.

79. Katz MH, Gerberding JL. Postexposure treatment of people exposed to the human immunodeficiency virus through sexual assault or IV drug use. *N Engl J Med* 1997;336:1097–2000.

80. Meehan TM, Hansen H, Klein WC. The impact of parental consent on the HIV testing of minors. *Am J Public Health* 1997;87:1338–1341.

81. Bamberger JD, Waldo CR, Gerberding JL, et al. Postexposure prophylaxis for human immunodeficiency virus (HIV) infection following sexual assault. *Am J Med* 1999;106:323–326.

82. Goston LO, Lazzarini A, Alexander D, et al. HIV testing, counseling, and prophylaxis after sexual assault. *JAMA* 1994;271:1436–1444.

83. National Victim Center, Crime Victims Research and Treatment Center. *National women's study*, reports in Rape in America: A Report to the Nation, 1992.

84. Merchant RC, Keshavarz R. Human immunodeficiency virus postexposure prophylaxis for adolescents and children. *Pediatrics* 2001;108:E38.

85. American Academy of Pediatrics Committee on Pediatric AIDS. Postexposure prophylaxis in children and adolescents for nonoccupational exposure to human immunodeficiency virus. *Pediatrics* 2003;111:1475–1489.

86. Perlmutter BL, Glaser JB, Oyugi SO. How to recognize and treat acute HIV syndrome. *Am Fam Physician* 1999;60:535–546.

87. Bump RC, Bueschin WJ. Bacterial vaginosis in virginal and sexually active adolescent females: evidence against exclusive sexual transmission. *Obstet Gynecol* 1988;158:935–939.

88. Blake DR, Duggan A, Joffe A. Use of spun urine to enhance detection of Trichomonas vaginalis in adolescent women. *Arch Pediatr Adolesc Med* 1999;12:1222–1225.

89. Blake D, Duggan A, Quinn T. Evaluation of vaginal infections in adolescent women: can it be done without a speculum? *Pediatrics* 1998;102:939–944.

90. Beck-Sague CM, Solomon F. Sexually transmitted diseases in abused children and adolescent and adult victims of rape: review of selected literature. *Clin Infect Dis* 1999;28(Suppl 1):S74–S83.

91. Moscicki AB, Shiboski S, Hills NK, et al. Regression of low-grade squamous intra-epithelial lesions in young women. *Lancet* 2004;364(9446):1678–1683.

92. Moscicki AB, Shiboski S, Broering J, et al. The natural history of human papillomavirus infection as measured by repeated DNA testing in adolescent and young adult women. *J Pediatr* 1998;132(2):277–284.

93. Screening for Cervical Cancer. U.S. Preventive Services Task Force, January 2003. Available at http://www.ahrq.gov/clinic/uspstf/uspscerv.htm. Accessed on October 21, 2005.

94. Mann EM. Self-reported stresses of adolescent rape victims. *J Adolesc Health Care* 1981;2:29–33.

95. Moscarello R. Psychological management of victims of sexual assault. *Can J Psychiatry* 1990;35:25–30.

96. Gerlina D. The persisting negative effect of incest. *Psychiatry* 1983;46:312–332.

97. Brand EF, King CA, Olson E, et al. Depressed adolescents with a history of sexual abuse: diagnostic comorbidity and suicidality. *J Am Acad Child Adolesc Psychiatry* 1996;35(1):34–41.

98. Remafedi G, Farrow JA, Deisher RW. Risk factors for attempted suicide in gay and bisexual youth. *Pediatrics* 1991;87:869–875.

99. Hibbard RA, Ingersoll GM, Orr DP. Behavioral risk, emotional risk, and child abuse among adolescents in a non-clinical setting. *Pediatrics* 1990;86:896–901.

100. Riggs S, Alario AJ, McHorney C. Health risk behaviors and attempted suicide in adolescents who report prior maltreatment. *J Pediatr* 1990;116:815–821.

101. Wonderlich SA, Crosby RD, Mitchell JE, et al. Eating disorders and sexual trauma in childhood and adolescence. *Int J Eat Disord* 2001;30:401–412.

102. Nagy S, Adcock AG, Nagy MC. A comparison of risky health behaviors of sexually active, sexually abused, and abstaining adolescents. *Pediatrics* 1994;93:570–575.

103. Polit DF, White CM, Morton TD. atlChild sexual abuse and premarital intercourse among high-risk adolescents. *J Adolesc Health Care* 1990;11:231–234.

104. Zierler S. Adult survivors of childhood sexual abuse and subsequent risk of HIV infection. *Am J Public Health* 1991;81:572–575.

105. Beckman LJ, Harvey SM. Factors affecting the consistent use of barrier methods of contraception. *Obstet Gynecol* 1996;88(3 Suppl):65S–71S.
106. Lodico MA, Gruber E, DiClemente RJ. Childhood sexual abuse and coercive sex among school-based adolescents in a midwestern state. *J Adolesc Health* 1996;18:211–217.
107. Kenny JW, Reinholtz C, Angelini PJ. Ethnic differences in childhood and adolescent sexual abuse and teenage pregnancy. *J Adolesc Health* 1997;21:3–10.
108. Fiscella K, Kitzman HJ, Cole RE, et al. Does child abuse predict adolescent pregnancy? *Pediatrics* 1998;101:620–624.
109. Boyer D, Fine D. Sexual abuse as a factor in adolescent pregnancy and child maltreatment. *Fam Plann Perspect* 1992;24:4–16, 19.
110. Rainey DY, Stevens-Simm C, Kaplan DW. Are adolescents who report prior sexual abuse at higher risk for pregnancy? *Child Abuse Negl* 1995;19:1283–1288.
111. Pierre N, Shrier LA, Emanns SJ, et al. Adolescent males involved in pregnancy: associations of forced sexual contacts and risk behaviors. *J Adolesc Health* 1998;26:364–369.
112. Anda RF, Felitti VJ, Chapman DP, et al. Abused boys, battered mothers, and male involvement in teen pregnancy. *Pediatrics* 2001;107:E19.
113. Darroch JE, Landry DJ, Oslak S. Age difference between sexual partners in the United States. *Fam Plann Perspect* 1999;31:160–167.
114. Famularo R, Kinscherff R, Fento T, et al. Child maltreatment histories among runaway and delinquent children. *Clin Pediatr* 1990;29:713–718.
115. Stiffman AR. Physical and sexual abuse in runaway youths. *Child Abuse and Neglect* 1989;13:417–426.
116. Schetky DH, Green AH. *Child sexual abuse: a handbook for health care and legal professionals.* New York: Brunner/Mazel, 1988.
117. American Medical Association. *Diagnostic and treatment guidelines on child sexual abuse.* Chicago: American Medical Association, 1992.
118. Myers JEB. *Legal issues in child abuse and neglect practice.* Thousand Oaks, CA: Sage Publications, 1999.
119. Deisher RW, Wenet GA, Paperny DM, et al. Adolescent sexual offense behavior: the role of the physician. *J Adolesc Health Care* 1982;2:279–286.
120. Greenfield LA. *Child victimizers: violent offenders and their victims.* Office of Juvenile Justice and Delinquency Prevention. U.S. Department of Justice, NCJ-153258, 1996.

THE ACUTE ASSESSMENT

8

■ MARY-THERESA L. BAKER

A child who has been sexually assaulted requires examination by the most competent medical provider available in an appropriately timely manner. Such referral to the most experienced examiner will reduce trauma to the patient, eliminate repeated examinations, preserve forensic evidence, and facilitate treatment and appropriate referrals for services. Until recently, cases presenting to a health care provider were considered acute if less than 72 hours had elapsed since the assault. Changes at the federal level have now extended the time for collection of forensic evidence such as DNA to up to 120 hours. In this sense, "forensic evidence" refers to cervical specimens for sperm and/or semen from *postpubertal* patients. For prepubertal children and in suspected fondling cases, 72 hours remains the general cutoff for acute assessments.

Being prepared to care for sexually assaulted children means being ready for anything from a completely normal examination, to a trying, emotion-laden examination, to victims/patients with significant or even life-threatening injuries. Because of this range of presentations, most jurisdictions conduct acute evaluations in an emergency department (ED). A local child advocacy center or child abuse center (CAC) may be preferable, as long as it has ready access to resources such as radiology, surgery, and inpatient care. Obviously, a child who comes in calmly holding a supportive parent's hand can be seen in a setting different from one used for a child who arrives by ambulance with suspected closed head injury and genitorectal bleeding. Some jurisdictions provide different examination sites, which are used on the basis of the child's presentation.

TRIAGE

The acute evaluation should be categorized as urgent or semiurgent. Waiting times should not exceed 1 hour for the appropriate medical care provider to be available. Consideration should be given to providing a victim/family waiting area that is separate from that used by the general ED population. Emotional support can begin as soon as the case is recognized, utilizing resources such as the ED's social worker, a child protection worker, or a rape crisis worker, particularly for teenage victims. Some programs can provide separate support personnel for the patient and the family member.

Child sexual abuse victims are still pediatric patients. Routine triage should include at least an accurate measurement of weight, for use in calculating drug doses. The rest of the basic vital signs should be collected according to existing ED protocols.

HISTORY

A detailed medical history is necessary for the proper assessment of an alleged child sexual abuse case. Starting with familiar medical history collection can ease the patient or family into the details of the alleged incident. When very small children are

150

involved, the parent's knowledge of the incident is generally all that is available. If possible, the parent's comments should be collected at a place that is out of the hearing range of the child. The routine history can be collected and a review of systems conducted with parent and child together so that both may contribute; the practitioner then has the option of asking the parent to step out of the room so that details about the abuse incident can be ascertained from the child. Some children want to keep the accompanying parent in their sight at all times, so each case must be handled individually.

When possible, the child should be alone when asked by the examiner for details about the abuse. The child should never be questioned in the presence of the alleged abuser. Open-ended questions (such as, "Why are you here?") should be asked whenever possible.

It is not completely clear what level of history collection will be exempted from hearsay rulings and what will not. What patients say to medical care personnel to obtain appropriate medical care is usually protected from hearsay exceptions. What is said to the first medical personnel encountered by the victim after the incident will likely be exempted from hearsay as well, but unfortunately these providers are not necessarily experienced in interviewing young children.

Information about the incident is needed to correctly assess and treat the patient. The time of initial presentation and disclosure is often when the child is most willing to talk about the incident. Children who are freely giving verbal narratives should be allowed to talk, and everything should be documented carefully. Some other children may not want to speak at all in the acute setting, and their wishes should be respected. The practitioner should record the child's actual words in quotes and, ideally, the question that elicited the response.

NOTIFICATION

In all states, physicians are mandated by law to report cases of suspected child sexual abuse. If sexual abuse is not the presenting complaint but a physical symptom has made the family suspicious (e.g., blood in the underwear, vaginal discharge, "it looks funny down there"), then child protection authorities would be notified only if something in the examination corroborates this suspicion (genital trauma, a sexually transmitted disease [STD] [Table 8-1], disclosure by the child). Professionals who examine children for evidence of sexual abuse must be aware of variants of normal conditions and conditions that mimic sexual abuse. Examples are urethral prolapse, which can cause blood stains in the underwear and vaginal

TABLE 8-1

SEXUAL AND NONSEXUAL TRANSMISSIONS OF INFECTIOUS ORGANISMS

Organisms Transmitted Sexually

Neisseria gonorrhoeae needs to be reported (transmission at birth through an infected birth canal has been reported; symptoms can manifest as late as 28 days after birth)

Chlamydia trachomatis needs to be reported (neonatal transmission can result in carriage up to 29 months)

Trichomonas vaginalis needs to be reported (transmission at birth through an infected birth canal has been reported)

Treponema pallidum (syphilis)

Human immunodeficiency virus

Organisms Transmitted Both Sexually and Nonsexually

Gardnerella vaginalis

Human papillomavirus (condyloma acuminatum) needs to be reported, workup is necessary (transmission at birth through an infected birth canal has been reported)

Herpes simplex types 1 and 2 need to be reported, workup is necessary (transmission at birth through an infected birth canal has been reported)

Organisms Transmitted through the Placenta and Amniotic Fluid

Treponema pallidum (syphilis)

Human immunodeficiency virus

discharge, which can be caused by the onset of puberty at as young as 8 or 9 years of age. In 1996, Kini et al. associated clinical indicators with appropriate levels of concern for use during the physical examination of children in whom sexual abuse is suspected (1) (Table 8-2). Even in the absence of physical symptoms or findings, if the family expresses reasonable concern about sexual abuse, the case should be reported to child protective services. It is reasonable suspicion of assault or abuse, not medical certainty, that is required for making a report to authorities.

REVIEW OF SYSTEMS

The key components of the review of systems are skin, gastrointestinal, genitourinary, and behavioral. Chronic skin conditions that may mimic abuse should be identified (Table 8-3) and any recent injuries should be noted. It is not useful to ask if the child bruises easily, as almost all parents and caretakers say "yes." The caretaker should be asked about unusual amounts or patterns of bruising and about marks or lumps different from those typically seen in active children of similar age. Anal fissures,

TABLE 8-2

CLINICAL INDICATORS AND LEVEL OF CONCERN

No Concern
Normal physical examination or the following features:
  Anatomic
        Anterior, midline anal skin tags
        Perianal erythema
        Labial adhesions or imperforate hymen
        Smooth, anterior hymenal concavities
        Periurethral bands or ridges
        Perineal erythema or erythema of the vestibule
        Normal hymen variants
  Nonanatomic
        Diaper region erythema
        Diaper dermatitis (irritant or related to *Candida*)
Some Concern
    Anal dilatation >2 cm (with stool in ampulla)
    Anal fissures outside the infant age-group
    Perianal bruising
    Friable posterior fourchette
    Presence of labial friability or adhesions in girls
        outside the diaper age-group
Serious Concern
    Anal scars outside the midline
    Hymenal border disruptions, such as thinning or
        absence of hymenal tissue posteriorly if confirmed
        in knee–chest position
    Anal tags outside the midline
    Posterior concavities, scars, or transections
    Anal dilatation >2 cm (without stool in the ampulla)
    Obvious genital injury, such as avulsion, laceration,
        or contusion
Grave Concern
    Pregnancy
    Any sexually transmitted disease that is not perina-
        tally acquired
    Presence of semen, sperm, or acid phosphatase
    Obvious extensive anogenital injury

From Kini WJ, Brady S, Lazoritz N. Evaluating child sexual abuse in the emergency department: clinical and behavioral indicators. *Acad Emerg Med* 1996;3:966–976.

rectal bleeding, and even rectal prolapse can be caused by recent or frequent bouts of diarrhea or by constipation and therefore are not necessarily related to sexual assault. A sudden onset of incontinence is suspicious in a toilet-trained child. The presence of blood in the stool is a significant finding if the alleged abuser had access to the child recently. Urinary symptoms such as dysuria, pain not associated with urination, discharge, blood, frequency, urgency, prior procedures, and unintentional injuries should be noted. Any history of vaginal irritation, redness, pain, discharge, or blood should be documented.

TABLE 8-3

SKIN CONDITIONS THAT MIMIC SEXUALLY TRANSMITTED DISEASES

Behçet's syndrome
Bowenoid papulosis
Bullous pemphigoid
Candida albicans infection
Contact dermatitis
Crohn's disease
Epidermal nevus
Hemangioma of infancy
Kawasaki's syndrome
Langerhans cell histiocytosis
Labial adhesions
Lichen sclerosus et atrophicus
Molluscum contagiosum
Pemphigus vulgaris
Perianal pseudoverrucous papules and nodules
Perianal streptococcal dermatitis
Pinworms
Posttraumatic injuries
Psoriasis
Seborrheic dermatitis
Vulvovaginitis

From Siegfried EC, Frasier LD. Anogenital skin diseases of childhood. *Pediatr Ann* 1997;26:321–331.

The clinician should look for behavioral changes related to the abuse. Acting out sexually with other children is always worrisome. A sudden change in personality such as depression, withdrawal, clinging, outbursts of anger, or out-of-control aggression may pinpoint the onset of the abuse. Regressive behaviors should also be noted, such as bed-wetting once the child has been dry for 6 months, refusal to sleep alone, stool withholding, daytime wetting, or incontinence. Acquiring new fears of people or particular places, sleep walking, or excessive nightmares and nighttime awakenings may be related to abuse. In teenagers, the onset of delinquent behavior such as running away, taking drugs, getting in fights, being suspended from school, having a drop in grades, early initiation of sexual activity, pregnancy, and STDs may all stem from sexual abuse.

PHYSICAL EXAMINATION

Children should never be forced to have an examination. They should be offered choices and made aware of what the examination will entail. When an examination is medically necessary and a child cannot or will not cooperate (e.g., a mentally retarded teenager or a small child in pain), sedation may be needed.

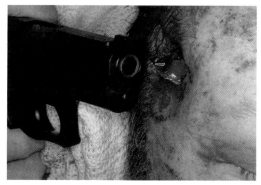

FIG. 4.9b   Forceful expansion of the skin overlying the right temple resulted in a muzzle contusion from the barrel of a 9-mm semiautomatic handgun.

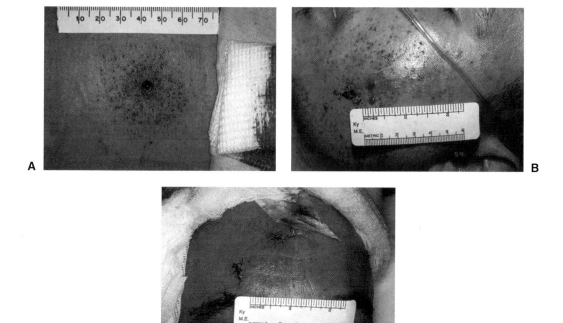

A

B

C

FIG. 4.12   **A:** "Tattooing" is the result of partially burned or unburned gunpowder making contact with the skin. The "tattoos" are punctate abrasions associated with an intermediate-range gunshot wound. Tattooing has been seen with wounds as close as 1 cm and as far away as 1 m. **B:** This patient stated he was shot with a .22 caliber handgun at a distance of 12 in. His cheek exhibited punctate abrasions or "tattooing" associated with intermediate-range gunshot wounds. **C:** Forehead "tattooing" from an intermediate-range gunshot wound. The patient reported he was shot with a .38 caliber revolver from a distance of 18 in .

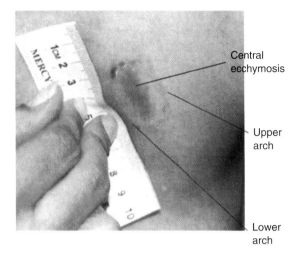

Central
ecchymosis

Upper
arch

Lower
arch

FIG. 6.5 Bite mark on the breast.

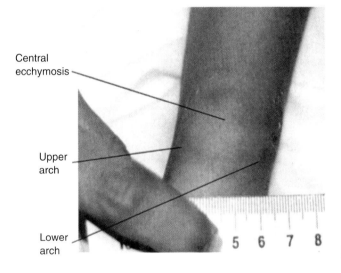

Central
ecchymosis

Upper
arch

Lower
arch

5 6 7 8

FIG. 6.6 Bite mark on the wrist.

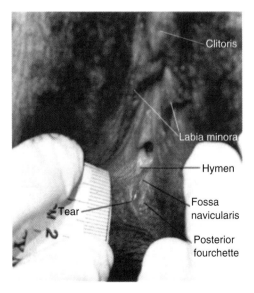

Clitoris

Labia minora

Hymen

Tear

Fossa
navicularis

Posterior
fourchette

FIG. 6.7 Tear to posterior fourchette.
Female Tanner 4 sexual assault patient.

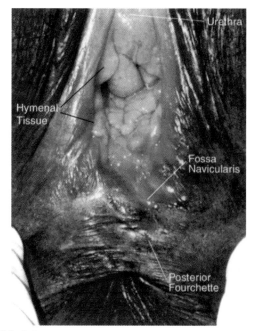

FIG. 6.8   Female sexual blue dye testing.

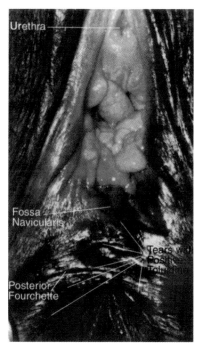

FIG. 6.9   Female sexual assault victim Tanner 5 after
toluidine blue dye testing.

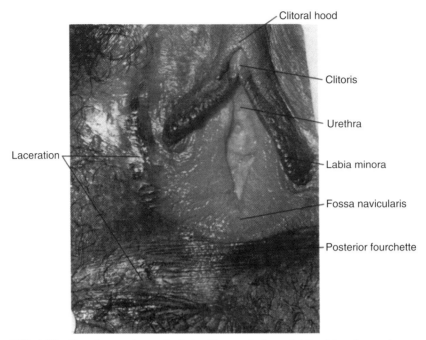

FIG. 6.10 Female sexual assault victim Tanner 5 after toluidine blue dye testing.

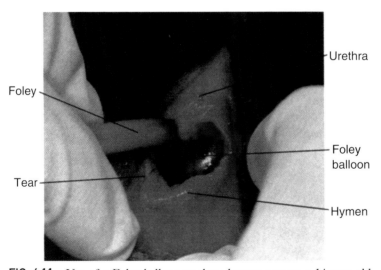

FIG. 6.11 Use of a Foley balloon to show hymen tear on a 14-year-old sexual assault patient.

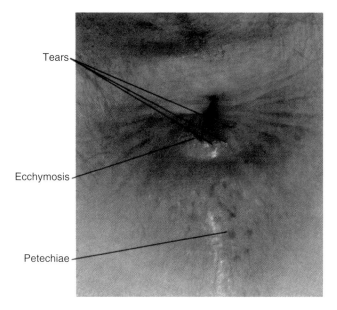

Tears

Ecchymosis

Petechiae

FIG. 6.12 Anal trauma in a female with a history of anal penetration.

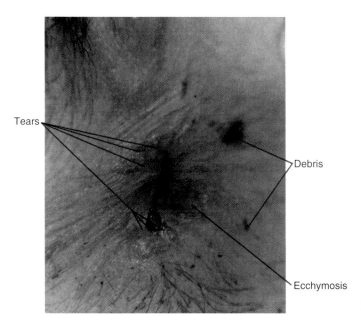

Tears

Debris

Ecchymosis

FIG. 6.13 Anal trauma in a female with history of anal penetration.

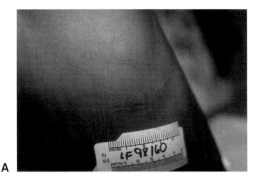

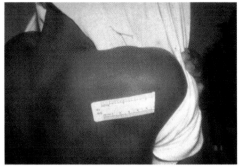

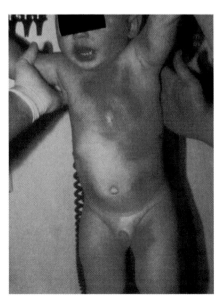

FIG. 9.1 Pattern injuries. **A:** A looped-belt injury. **B:** Another looped-belt injury. **C:** A fly-swatter injury. Note the square pattern produced from two overlapping blows through a diaper. (Courtesy of Chief Medical Examiner's Office, Louisville, Kentucky.)

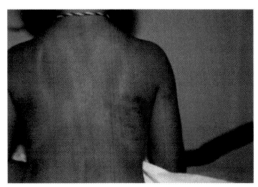

FIG. 9.2 Hand-slap mark. Note parallel linear contusions with central sparing that highlight the imprint of fingers. (Courtesy of Dr. William Smock, University of Louisville School of Medicine.)

FIG. 9.3 A V-shaped scald burn caused by hot liquid cooling as it poured down this child's body. This scald caused both first- and second-degree burns. (Courtesy of Chief Medical Examiner's Office, Louisville, Kentucky.)

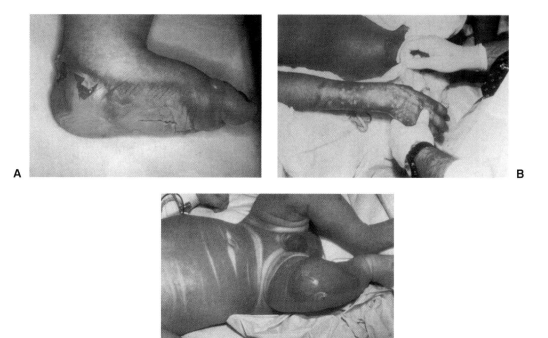

FIG. 9.4 Immersion burns. **A:** Immersion or "dunk" burn caused by dipping foot in hot liquid. Note the clear delineation of burned and normal skin along with the uniform degree of burn (here a second-degree burn) throughout the burn distribution. **B:** Immersion burn caused by dipping infant in hot liquid. **C:** Note where skin folds protect underlying tissue from serious burn. (Courtesy of Dr. William Smock, University of Louisville School of Medicine.)

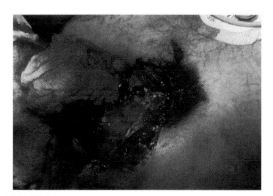

FIG. 17.2 The soot on this close-range shotgun wound is short lived. It will be removed when the wound is scrubbed in preparation for debridement and closure.

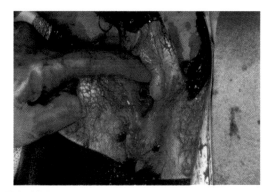

FIG. 17.7 A large vaginal laceration resulting from sexual assault. The presence of blood and the graphic nature of the injury resulted in the judge ruling the photograph inflammatory and not admissible.

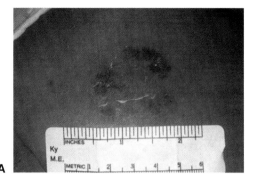 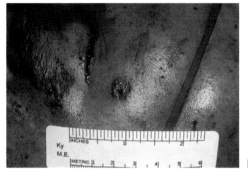

A   B

FIG. 17.13   Good use of ring-flash lighting on injuries. **A:** Healing bite mark on breast. **B:** Gunshot entrance wound with the associated abrasion collar.

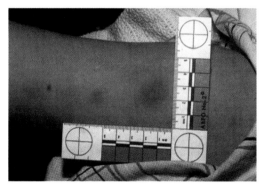

FIG. 17.22   A photograph with a scale and without perspective distortion permits accurate measurement of a wound. These fingertip contusions on the upper left arm are from a domestic assault.

The physical examination should include a complete head-to-toe assessment, with particular attention given to the mouth and nasal area and to the genital and anal region. Most abusers have no desire to harm their victims because they want to continue the abuse. Therefore, the lack of physical signs of abuse does not mean that abuse has not occurred.

When evaluating the head and neck of an infant, the clinician should remember that babies have a natural reflex to suck. Therefore, the mouth, the nose, and the eyes should be examined for the presence of sperm or discharge, and these areas should be swabbed, as should the fat folds of the neck and the external ear. Tears to the frenulum and mucosal petechiae should be documented. The entire body should be examined for suck marks and bite marks. The extremities should be checked for bruises caused by grasping, pinching, or tying.

GENITAL EXAMINATION

The genital examination is mandatory in alleged child sexual abuse scenarios. Even if the allegation is "only oral sex" at the time of presentation, a genital examination is warranted because, as cases evolve, additional allegations can come to light later. The best opportunity for detection of abnormalities and collection of forensic samples is at the time of initial presentation. Basic standard equipment for a genital examination consists of a good source of light and some level of magnification. Several systems (e.g., Second Opinion software, colposcopes, The Medscope, digital camera) are available to aid the practitioner in documenting the findings of the child sexual abuse examination.

The standard of care in this area requires some sort of photographic documentation. This makes it possible to review the findings any number of times without subjecting the child to a repeat examination. It allows comparison as healing occurs, and, in some cases, the observation of a change toward abnormal after another alleged assault. Conscientious providers of child sexual assault examinations regularly review their case photographs or tapes with other experts in the field. This provides the opportunity to improve the technique and learn from others. Any equipment to be used should be introduced to the patient in a sensitive manner.

When evaluating the hymen and genital area of the female, it is important to remember how these organs change with age. From birth to approximately 2 years of age, the hymen and vagina are influenced by the presence of estrogen. Estrogen causes the hymen to be thick, pale, and fluffy, with some elasticity to it and to the vagina. Glycogen is present, supporting the growth of beneficial organisms such as lactobacilli.

Physiologic discharge will also be present and is usually clear to white. There can be a normal withdrawal bleed from about 4 to 10 days of age in the newborn.

As estrogen leaves the system, the vaginal epithelium thins and the hymen becomes delicate, reddened, and very painful to touch. Similar vaginal changes are associated with menopause. Glycogen and lactobacilli are no longer present. The urethra is the food site, so culture swabs of this area are frequently more productive than are vaginal swabs. When puberty begins, estrogen again causes thickening and elasticity of the hymen and vagina. In prepubertal children, *Neisseria gonorrhea* and *Chlamydia trachomatis* rarely produce ascending infection that leads to pelvic inflammatory disease or infectious arthritis.

Adequate written documentation is essential, because any case could be taken to court. The documentation should include an explanation of what made the examination findings unusual or abnormal. Drawings made on a template that is part of the paperwork are very useful. Pertinent things to include are gender, age, and the Tanner stage of the child. It should be ascertained whether there are bites, bruises, scratches, abrasions, rashes, lacerations, surgical changes, foreign matter, or erythema of the pudendum, inner thighs, buttocks, or external genitals. The presence of pubic lice or human papillomavirus (HPV) lesions should be documented. For females, the hymenal configuration (usually annular, crescentic, or fimbriated) and hymenal defects, erythema, discharge, scratches, lacerations, abrasions, petechiae, bruising, or bleeding should be noted, with an indication as to where on the hymen they occurred, based on a clock-face description (e.g., complete defect at 6 o'clock). Variations such as urethral prolapse, septate or imperforate hymen, cysts, masses, midline thickenings, labial adhesions, or midline variations should be recorded. In the male, marks, bruises, rashes, discharge, surgical changes, scratches, lacerations, abrasions, or patterned injuries should be noted.

Adult rape kits are frequently adapted for use in the pediatric patient. Only those parts indicated for the specific case should be used; many items provided in the adult rape kit will not apply to scenarios involving children. The paperwork in the rape kit is also not specific for the examination of children, but it provides a step-by-step reminder of what to document. Many areas and centers have prepared their own forms, including check boxes that simplify documentation and pediatric-type drawings. If the record-keeping mechanism is consistent and standardized, clinicians will spend less time filling them out and will find it easier to defend them in court. The State of Maryland, through the Maryland Coalition Against Sexual Assault (MCASA), is preparing a pediatric rape kit adapted from the Massachusetts kit, the only pediatric rape kit currently available.

TESTING

Selective culturing is used in child sexual abuse cases (2 [pp 159–167 and 713], 3). Most cases require no testing at all. Cultures are not required when fondling is alleged and the child has a normal prepubertal examination.

Genital cultures should be considered if (a) discharge is present, (b) genital-to-genital and/or genital-to-anal contact is alleged, (c) body fluid contact is disclosed, (d) the examination findings are suspicious or abnormal, or (e) the patient is beyond Tanner stage III development. Blood testing is recommended if (a) body fluid exposure is alleged, (b) genital-to-genital and/or genital-to-anal contact is disclosed, (c) STD or pregnancy is found, (d) the perpetrator is over 14 years age, (e) multiple perpetrators are alleged, and/or (f) the perpetrator has a history of HIV/AIDS. If the perpetrator has ever been incarcerated, blood testing is also warranted, and hepatitis C testing should be considered as well. Blood should be tested for human immunodeficiency virus (HIV), rapid plasma reagin (RPR), hepatitis B, and, if indicated, β-human chorionic gonadotrophin or hepatitis C. If the victim or a member of the victim's family expresses a desire for testing, it should be done.

Group A β-streptococci should be suspected in the prepubertal female with sudden onset of discharge and erythema or irritation. Streptococcal proctitis presents similarly in males. The test for *Trichomonas* involves immediate wet prep by an experienced individual or culture if discharge is noted. An examination for yeast may reveal the cause of a discharge and has no implications for sexual abuse. If herpes lesions are suspected, a culture must be obtained. Visual diagnosis is not sufficient, because other viruses mimic this disease.

NUCLEIC ACID AMPLIFICATION TESTS VERSUS TRUE CULTURES

There are advantages and disadvantages to nucleic acid amplification tests (NAATs) and true cultures. The NAAT components have a long shelf storage life prior to use and excellent sensitivity and usually call for noncontact collection methods (e.g., urine first void). Their disadvantage is that they are not approved by the U. S. Food and Drug Administration (FDA) for prepubertal patients. A court case based only on a positive NAAT is more difficult to present and win. True cultures

have the advantage of being the gold standard for court presentations, and they are approved by the FDA for use in children. Unfortunately, the rate of false-negative culture results, particularly for *Chlamydia*, is cause for concern.

Ideally, the clinician would request both types of cultures at the same time and receive the same results for each. In the real world, however, there will be times that the NAAT is positive and the true culture does not grow. This circumstance is frequently encountered when a screening NAAT is positive at an outside center and the child is treated before being referred for a sexual abuse examination. Also, in some areas of the country, true culture for *Chlamydia* is not available. In both cases, a second NAAT should be performed, focusing on a different part of the genome, to confirm the diagnosis in prepubertal children. A positive NAAT is normally confirmed by true culture before treating a prepubertal child. In cases that yielded a positive NAAT but a negative true culture, the practitioner's testimony in a court proceeding would have to reflect this.

TREATMENT

In situations associated with high risk for STDs, prophylaxis should be offered. Such scenarios include penetrating genital contact, abnormal examination findings, a sibling or another child in the same household with an STD, or exposure to body fluid or blood during the assault. If indicated, pregnancy prophylaxis should also be considered. At present, the data on the efficacy and safety of postexposure HIV prophylaxis among children and adults following sexual assault (2 [pp 380–381]) are inconclusive. The risk of HIV transmission from a single sexual assault is low, but not zero. The treatment protocols of medical facilities should state whether patients presenting within 72 hours of high-risk contact should receive prophylaxis.

FOLLOW-UP

Repeat cultures may be needed. The finding of an STD on initial presentation of a sexually assaulted child may represent preexisting infection. Retesting for incubating infection should be done about 2 weeks later. Patients given ceftriaxone for gonorrhea or azithromycin or doxycycline for *Chlamydia* infection do not need repeat testing. Patients given any other medication should be followed up for test of cure at about 3 weeks.

The American Academy of Pediatrics' *Red Book* (2) recommends follow-up blood testing at 6, 12, and 24 weeks for HIV and syphilis. If the child has been immunized against hepatitis B, follow-up is not needed. If the child has not been immunized, initiation of the hepatitis B series is recommended, including an IgM test for hepatitis B on initial blood tests. If the IgM test is negative, no further follow-up is needed.

In reality, most families will not return to the ED three times for blood draws. Referral to a CAC at the location most convenient for the family will increase the likelihood of repeat testing and allow coordination of follow-up examinations. If a CAC is not available, the child can be seen for follow-up with the family physician. Discharge information should include the recommended follow-up schedule, individualized to each case.

A formal forensic interview can be very therapeutic for the child. An interview conducted by an expert trained in forensic interview techniques, in conjunction with or after the physical examination, is recommended. This session may occur immediately after the clinical examination or it can be scheduled at a later date that accommodates everyone involved in the investigation. This type of interview is usually conducted at a CAC, but some jurisdictions have other arrangements. There should be clear lines of referral and existing agreements in place as to where and who will do the interview and follow-up. The medical personnel performing the sexual assault examination should not have to create new protocols on the spot.

Every child involved in a suspected case of sexual assault needs to be referred for counseling and therapy. The discharge information should include contact information for these resources for the victim and the family.

Cooperation between all entities involved in investigation of these cases is essential. Law enforcement, social work services, and the prosecutor's office as well as the examining medical care provider must work together to protect patients and treat all aspects of alleged child sexual abuse.

REFERENCES

1. Kini WJ, Brady S, Lazoritz N. Evaluating child sexual abuse in the emergency department: clinical and behavioral indicators. *Acad Emerg Med* 1996;3:966–976.
2. Pickering LK, ed. *Red book: 2003 report of the committee on infectious diseases*, 26th ed. Elk Grove Village, Ill: American Academy of Pediatrics, 2003.
3. U.S. Department of Health and Human Services. Centers for disease control and prevention. 1998 Guidelines for treatment of sexually transmitted diseases. *Morbid Mortal Weekly Rep* 1998;47(No. RR-1):108–114.

9

■ RICHARD LICHENSTEIN
■ ADRIENNE H. SUGGS

Child maltreatment is an unfortunate aspect of clinical forensic medicine. Caffey (1) first described child abuse in 1946, when he recognized that some patients with long-bone fractures also had subdural hematomas. Kempe et al. (2) elaborated and coined the term "battered-child syndrome" in 1962. Since then, health care professionals have become increasingly aware of child abuse and its manifestations, and laws have been enacted that mandate reporting of suspected child abuse by health care professionals, educators, and human service workers.

Although definitions vary by state, physical child abuse is usually defined as the physical injury of a child by a parent, a household or family member, or another person who has permanent or temporary custody or responsibility for supervision of that child. Other forms of child maltreatment include neglect, sexual abuse, and emotional abuse.

The National Clearinghouse on Child Abuse and Neglect Information statistics for 2003, document an estimated 2.9 million referrals to child protective services for investigation of child maltreatment (3). Of these, more than two-thirds were accepted for investigation, and approximately 30% were substantiated, translating to a victimization rate of 12.4 per 1,000 children. Of substantiated cases, more than 60% (63.2%) suffered neglect, and almost one fifth (18.9%) suffered physical abuse. Approximately 10% were victims of sexual abuse, 5% suffered psychological or emotional abuse, and 2.3% suffered medical neglect. Seventeen percent were victims of more than one type of abuse. An estimated 1,500 children died of abuse and neglect, translating to a fatality rate of 2 per 100,000 children in the general population.

Victimization rates continue to be the highest for the youngest children (0–3 years of age), at 16.4 per 1,000 children nationally, and decline with increasing age. Girls are slightly more likely to be victims than boys. Pacific Islanders, American Indians/Alaska Natives, and African Americans have the highest victimization rates at 21.4, 21.3, and 20.4 per 1,000 children, respectively. These rates are almost twice those of whites and Hispanics, at 11.0 and 9.9 per 1,000 children (3).

Although perpetrators of child maltreatment tend to be female, perpetrators of physical and sexual abuse tend to be male. Most perpetrators of child maltreatment are parents (84%) or other relatives (6%). Fewer than 1% are day-care providers or facility staff. However, when looking at sexual abuse alone, nearly 76% of perpetrators are friends or neighbors, 30% are other relatives, and <3% are parents (3).

Pediatricians and emergency department physicians must maintain a high level of suspicion when children present with injuries highly specific for abuse or when children have injuries not consistent with the history provided. The physician must be aware of the many risk factors for abuse and must be able to identify clues in the history that raise the suspicion for abuse. More than half of the physical abuse cases have no physical manifestations (4). Factors that increase the likelihood of being a victim of physical abuse and neglect include prematurity, chronic illness, mental retardation, and difficult temperament. Caretaker and environmental risk factors include young parents, abuse of the caretaker as a child, previous removal of a child by protective services, substance abuse, mental illness, lack of family support, and low socioeconomic status (3–6). Clues that suggest abuse include an account not consistent with the injury or the developmental age of the child, changing or inconsistent histories, a history of abuse, delay in seeking treatment, projection of blame onto a third-party (such as a sibling), and aggressiveness of the caretaker (3–6).

Physicians must maintain a high degree of suspicion if the history suggests physical abuse, and caretakers who do not fit the profile should not fool them. For example, Jenny et al. reported that young age of the child, white race, less severe symptoms, and an "intact" family were key features that led to missed diagnoses of abusive head trauma (AHT) (see subsequent text) (7).

HEAD TRAUMA/CENTRAL NERVOUS SYSTEM INJURY

Inflicted head trauma constitutes the leading cause of nonaccidental death associated with child abuse (8,9). When caregivers provide a history that is inadequate to explain the extent of head injury, child abuse must be considered. In a population-based study, Keenan et al. documented an incidence of traumatic brain injury among children younger than 2 as 17 per 100,000 (95% CI, 13–21 per 100,000 year); the incidence was seven times greater for children younger than 1 year of life (10). Perpetrators of nonaccidental head trauma are usually male (in decreasing frequency: father, stepfather, and mother's boyfriend). Mothers and female babysitters have also been implicated (11,12). Risk factors for AHT are similar to those for child abuse in general. The child may be premature or have a difficult temperament or chronic illness (6). The family may have the stressors of poverty, drug abuse, parental depression, low education level, or other males (stepfathers and boyfriends) living in the home (13).

Shaken baby syndrome (SBS) is classically described as occurring in infants younger than 6 months, with minimal or no external signs of trauma, subdural hematomas, and retinal hemorrhages (6). It usually presents as a spectrum of findings, including intracranial, cervical cord, intraocular, skeletal, and cutaneous injuries. Caretakers may be unaware of the specific injuries that can be caused by shaking, but it is reported that the act of shaking or slamming can be so violent that competent individuals observing the shaking would recognize it as dangerous (14). SBS has also been called *shaken impact syndrome*, based on the combination of autopsy findings in infants who were fatally abused and of biomechanical studies not performed on humans. The study concluded that severe head injuries require impact, not shaking alone (15). However, most authors claim that impact is not needed. Most also agree that inflicted head trauma encompasses a constellation of findings, with or without impact (6), thereby producing the general terms of *nonaccidental head trauma, inflicted head trauma*, or *AHT*.

It is important to distinguish between accidental and inflicted head injuries. Most short vertical falls in infants, usually less than 4 feet (most childhood falls), result in minor injury or no injury at all. Although falls from low heights may cause linear, unilateral skull fractures without intracranial injury, significant force is required to sustain depressed, stellate, complex, bilateral, or basilar skull fractures. Other than the rare reported cases of epidural hemorrhage, falls from low heights do not cause significant intracranial pathology, including subdural or subarachnoid hemorrhage, or retinal hemorrhage (15–18). Child abuse must be considered in children with intracranial injuries but without a history of motor vehicle trauma, falls from heights greater than 4 feet, or head impact from a moving object.

In AHT there may be an absence of external findings to implicate nonaccidental trauma (19). The degree of injury depends on the force or severity of the shake or impact and the time elapsed from the event. Symptoms may be vague and occur intermittently, which may be misleading to evaluating physicians (20). The range of manifestations includes poor feeding, vomiting, lethargy, irritability, colic, apnea, seizures, and death (6). Children in one study were seen and diagnosed by physicians with other conditions 2.8 times before being diagnosed with inflicted head injury (7).

Intracranial pathology encountered in AHT includes, most commonly, subdural hemorrhages along with parenchymal injuries, including diffuse axonal injury (DAI). During shaking, because the infant's head is heavy and the neck muscles are weak, intracranial bleeding results from a tearing of cortical bridging veins, which stretch and shear as the head is subjected to rotational forces. These same inertial forces and rotational acceleration forces also permit tearing of axons in the child's incompletely myelinated brain, resulting in DAI, contusions, parenchymal tears, and cerebral edema (21). Other intracranial pathology includes subarachnoid hemorrhage and cerebral contusions. Contusions and lacerations are proportional to the contact forces applied. Skull fractures are seen in these cases but can also be seen with unintentional trauma. In general, because there may be similarities in the types of skull fractures in unintentional and intentional injury, abuse should be suspected if the injury does not correlate with the history and the physical examination findings. Multiple bilateral skull fractures should be reviewed carefully as to a possible abusive source but may be explained by some types of unintentional injury (22). Parenchymal injury is also seen secondary to hypoxia and ischemia (23). The incidence of epidural hematoma is low (6–8). On the basis of a study of head-injured children younger than 3 years of age, Wells et al. (24) reported that 78% of epidural hemorrhages were felt to be unintentional compared with 18% associated with abuse.

Shaken infants are also at risk for cervical cord injury because of the infant's large head-to-torso ratio and weak neck musculature. Spinal cord contusions and subdural and epidural hematomas at the cervicomedullary junction may lead to morbidity and mortality (6).

Retinal hemorrhages are associated with extraordinary force and are rare occurrences in minor unintentional trauma (25–27). Unilateral or bilateral retinal hemorrhages are present in 75% to 95% of cases of AHT (20). Retinal hemorrhages do occur with unintentional trauma, birth trauma, bleeding disorders, and glutaric aciduria type I, for example, but diffuse and severe retinal hemorrhages are considered specific for AHT. In AHT, retinal hemorrhages usually involve the multiple layers of the retina and extend outside the posterior pole to the periphery and oro serrata, to the periphery of the retina (28). Retinal folds or detachment may also develop (5). In children with birth trauma, retinal hemorrhages may be seen (in approximately 30% of newborns), but they resolve by the age of 4 weeks (6). Retinal hemorrhage after cardiopulmonary resuscitation (CPR) has been reported (rarely), but not in the absence of previous head trauma or abnormal coagulation and platelet studies. When such hemorrhage is found, it tends to be morphologically different from that associated with AHT (29,30).

The interval between head injury and symptom onset may help identify a perpetrator. Determining whether a lucid interval has occurred can be difficult because perpetrators may not be telling the truth (31). Gilliland found that neurologic changes and severe symptoms, such as difficult breathing, unresponsiveness, and respiratory collapse, occurred less than 24 hours after head injury in most of the incidents. Of note, whenever information was supplied by someone other than the perpetrator, the child was not described as normal during the period (32). Starling et al., studying perpetrators, found that 97% of convicted perpetrators who admitted to inflicting head trauma were with the child at the time of onset of symptoms, suggesting that symptoms occur soon

after the abuse, as opposed to emerging over hours or days (11). In a more recent study of perpetrator admissions, perpetrators said symptoms appeared immediately after the abuse (33). In a retrospective review of 95 unintentional fatalities involving head injury, only one patient, with an epidural hematoma, had a lucid interval (34).

Another controversy is the theory of rebleeding, after minor or no trauma, into chronic or subacute subdural hemorrhages. This theory has implications in identifying a perpetrator. After reviewing the literature in 1999, Block concluded that "there is no evidence to support the current concept that rebleeding of an organizing subdural hemorrhage can occur from a subsequent trivial injury and cause severe neurologic impairment or death" (29). However, there have been rare reports that led investigators to continue to examine the issue. In 2002, Hymel et al. published two case reports involving indoor, unintentional, and pediatric closed head trauma that resulted in intracranial rebleeding. Both impacts occurred in medical settings and were witnessed by medical personnel (35).

Physicians should be aware that intentional head trauma is often associated with extracranial signs of abuse, although physical findings such as cutaneous bruising may or may not be present (12). Posterior rib fractures can occur because of squeezing the infant's chest while shaking the infant (36). Long-bone fractures may be present. In one review, 32% of the victims had long-bone fractures because of repetitive abuse (36). The physician should perform a careful search for other physical signs of abuse or neglect.

ABDOMINAL AND THORACIC INJURY

Both solid and hollow organs are at risk for injury in thoracoabdominal trauma. Abdominal trauma is the second most common cause of child abuse deaths (37, 38). Although motor vehicle crashes (MVCs) are the leading cause of major abdominal trauma in children, child abuse poses a greater risk of subsequent death. In fact, compared with unintentional injuries, including MVC, the mechanism of child abuse increases the likelihood of death from traumatic abdominal injuries sixfold (39). Unfortunately, children who sustain severe abdominal trauma from child abuse often present late for medical attention (39). Generally, their presentation is in response to the pathology that results from abdominal injury rather than to the injury itself (40). Blunt abdominal trauma can result in no external evidence of injury, even if there is severe organ and tissue damage (39–41). Initial manifestations may be nonspecific and include abdominal pain and distention, nausea, vomiting, and fever. Peritonitis and associated sepsis may become evident within hours to days after abdominal injury, whereas hematoma and subsequent intestinal obstruction usually take longer, possibly days, to diagnose. Multiple injuries are seen in 18% to 37% of children with inflicted abdominal trauma (37).

Sometimes older children can describe the causative event. In the case of a younger child, diagnosis of abdominal trauma may rest on the history provided by the caretaker or on the suspicion of the physician. As with head trauma, the absence of any history, or the report of a minor injury despite evidence of serious trauma, should raise suspicion that the injury may have been inflicted.

Nonaccidental blunt thoracic trauma can result in rib fractures and injury to underlying structures. Lower rib fractures may lacerate the spleen or liver. Rib fractures can cause pneumothorax or pneumomediastinum. Direct blunt anterior trauma can lead to esophageal perforation, pneumomediastinum, or mediastinitis.

The spleen and the liver can sustain damage when the lower ribs are fractured. Blunt abdominal trauma may cause contusions of these organs as well. Liver injury can range from small, asymptomatic contusions to fractures that lead to significant blood loss and death. Delay in evaluation of severe liver injury increases pediatric mortality. Diagnosis of liver injury may be determined by a history of blunt abdominal trauma, abdominal pain and tenderness, elevated aspartate aminotransferase/alanine aminotransferase, and computed tomography findings. Elevated liver enzymes can be helpful in evaluating occult liver injuries, even when there is no report of abdominal trauma or clinical evidence of abdominal injury (38). The spleen can be injured in both unintentional and intentional trauma scenarios, but inflicted injury should be suspected when the patient is an infant who is not yet able to walk.

In general, pancreatic injury is not common in childhood (38), but when present it may be the result of inflicted trauma. In addition to MVCs, incidents involving impact against seat belts or bicycle handlebars may damage this potentially volatile organ. Injury to the pancreas requires deep abdominal wall indentation (37). In a recent review of pancreatic trauma in children, as with abdominal trauma in general, MVC was the leading cause of pancreatic injury. Child abuse was the third most common cause of injury and the second most common cause of death in children with pancreatic injuries (42).

Injury to either or both kidneys can result from blunt thoracoabdominal trauma. The kidneys are generally well protected by the lower ribs but are not completely protected from blunt or penetrating trauma.

The abdominal viscera are also at risk of injury from blunt trauma associated with child abuse. In general, the small intestine is protected from blunt abdominal trauma, but the fixed retroperitoneal course of the duodenum renders it vulnerable (43). The duodenum is the abdominal structure most frequently injured in MVCs. The second most frequent mechanism is child abuse (44). Most children with duodenal injuries have associated trauma, including bruises, acute and healing rib fractures, and long-bone fractures. The most common form of duodenal injury from blunt trauma is intramural hematoma, resulting in partial obstruction, nausea, and vomiting. In some cases, the duodenum is ruptured and/or transected. Because delay in seeking treatment is common after abdominal trauma resulting from child abuse, peritonitis may be significant when the child is brought to the emergency department.

The ileum and jejunum are less prone to injury from blunt trauma. Ileal and jejunal injuries manifest as hematoma or perforation (37).

The colon and rectum can be injured by blunt mechanisms, usually resulting in bruising or perforation. In addition, pelvic trauma may lead to rectal injury, as can anal penetration. Substantial blunt force is required to injure these organs. Absence of plausible history and delay in seeking treatment are indicators of abuse.

CUTANEOUS MANIFESTATIONS OF CHILD ABUSE

Skin Lesions

The cutaneous markings of child abuse are many, some subtler than others. Injuries involving the skin are the most prevalent injuries seen in child abuse—bruises are the most frequent type of child abuse injury reported (45). The skin is a remarkable recorder. Many types of trauma, including blunt trauma from objects and burns, produce specific injury patterns. However, as noted previously, more than half of abused children have no physical findings (4).

Contusions are the result of blunt trauma and, in many cases, take the shape of the instrument used to inflict them (e.g., hand-slap, belt, and loop cord) (Fig. 9.1). A hand-slap mark may consist of parallel, linear contusions with central clearing, giving the appearance of skin having been struck repeatedly with a linear, cylindrical object (Fig. 9.2). If blunt trauma is reported, it is important for the clinician to understand the nature of the contusion that can result to determine if the physical findings are consistent with the history.

As with fractures, a general rule is that "those who don't cruise rarely bruise" (46). Bruises are rare in infants who do not yet "cruise" (e.g., walk by holding onto furniture) but become common among

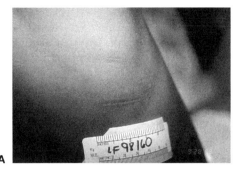
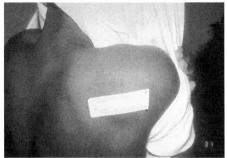
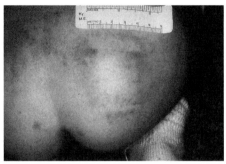

FIG. 9.1   Pattern injuries. **A:** A looped-belt injury. **B:** Another looped-belt injury. **C:** A fly-swatter injury. Note the square pattern produced from two overlapping blows through a diaper (see color plate). (Courtesy of Chief Medical Examiner's Office, Louisville, Kentucky.)

walkers. Bruises in infants younger than 9 months who have not yet begun to walk should prompt investigation into the cause (46).

Some parts of the body are prone to routine superficial traumas. In active children, the extensor surfaces of the arms and legs may sustain incidental bruises from minor, unintentional trauma. The protruding bony surfaces of the face, such as the chin, cheekbones, and forehead, are often the recipients of minor blunt trauma from falls and other accidental

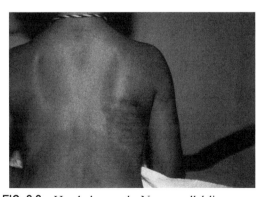

FIG. 9.2   Hand-slap mark. Note parallel linear contusions with central sparing that highlight the imprint of fingers (see color plate). (Courtesy of Dr. William Smock, University of Louisville School of Medicine.)

incidents. On the other hand, certain parts of the body are routinely "protected" during minor falls or injuries: the inner arms, submental or throat area, abdomen, lower back, and inner thighs. When cutaneous injuries in these protected areas are evident, a careful history must be taken to delineate the nature of their cause.

One frequently asked question is whether bruises can be dated to determine when they were inflicted. Accurate dating of bruises may indeed direct investigators to possible perpetrators. However, formal dating of bruises is difficult because there are many variables from patient to patient and within each patient. Many factors can determine a bruise's appearance, including depth, location, amount of bleeding into the tissues, and the circulatory status of the bruised area (47). Depth of injury may determine how soon a bruise will appear. Superficial injuries may show skin discoloration sooner than deep injuries, which may not appear for more than 24 hours. Bruise location can affect the timing of the bruise appearance as well. Areas of the body with loose tissue (e.g., periorbital) may show bruising sooner than denser regions (e.g., bony prominences). In addition, the patient's skin color may enhance or mask the appearance of bruises. Children with fair skin will display contusions from small impacts, whereas extensive contusions may be obscured in dark-skinned children.

Bruises show multiple color changes as they age. They are red or purple when fresh, then progress to blue, then to brown or yellow or green. Although these color changes can help distinguish "early" (recent) from "late" (older) bruises, color should not be the only determinant of a bruise's age and implication in abuse (48).

Bruises should always be documented in the medical record to create a lasting record for future reference long after the wound has healed. The measurements of bruises can be recorded in a medical report; the bruises can be sketched and diagrammed on the report, and they can be photographed to provide prints or slides as a depiction of the injury. It must be recognized, however, that photographic representation depends on lighting and technique and may not always portray bruises accurately.

Burns

Burning is a significant form of child abuse. Burns may be inflicted by hot liquids, flames, contact with hot objects, or caustic agents. Children's skin is thinner than adult skin and less resistant to thermal trauma; therefore, children are burned more deeply and by less heat, and the burns often involve more body surface area and more scarring. Burning can account for 10% to 25% of child abuse injuries (49–51). Abusive burns tend to be more severe, deeper, and larger than unintentional burns (50). And abusive burns are more fatal than burns not caused by abuse (49). Distinguishing inflicted burns from unintentional burns is a critical duty of the pediatrician or emergency physician evaluating infants and children after thermal injury.

Patterns of burns from hot liquid can help determine whether the burn was unintentional or inflicted. A common unintentional scenario involves a toddler reaching up to pull a cup or a pan of hot liquid from a table edge or stove. As the hot liquid spills down over the child, it can soak through clothes, leaving a characteristic burn pattern. This scald burn pattern typically has irregular, sometimes indistinct, margins. There may be areas of both superficial and partial-thickness involvement. Satellite splash lesions may also be noted. In some cases, the burn has a typical V-shaped pattern, in which the burn diminishes distally on the child's body, representing cooling of the liquid as it descends (50) (Fig. 9.3).

An inflicted burn from hot liquid may be the result of scalding or immersion. Typically, scald burns in abuse involve simultaneous burns of both lower extremities and of the buttocks or perineal areas (52). With immersion burns, children's buttocks or limbs are dipped into hot water. When burns have a stocking- or glovelike (circumferential) pattern or bilateral/mirror image distribution, abuse must be

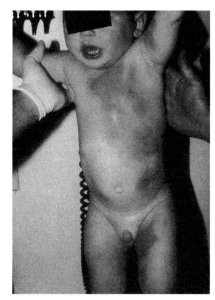

FIG. 9.3 A V-shaped scald burn caused by hot liquid cooling as it poured down this child's body. This scald caused both first- and second-degree burns (see color plate). (Courtesy of Chief Medical Examiner's Office, Louisville, Kentucky.)

considered. Features of immersion burns include distinctly clear margins between burned tissue and intact skin (50), a uniform degree of burn (e.g., second-degree) throughout the wound, and a circumferential distribution. Satellite splash marks are generally absent, and areas of skin pressed against the tub or the container of liquid, as well as skin folds, are spared (50) (Fig. 9.4). Hot tap water can cause severe scald burns, especially if the water heater setting is excessively high (53). For example, water at 111°F requires 6 hours to produce thermal skin injury, whereas water at 130°F requires only 10 seconds to cause second- and third-degree scald burns. At 140°F, the burn can occur after 1 second (50,51).

Contact with hot objects (e.g., curling irons, cigarettes, or chemicals) can also result in thermal injury. Specific hot objects making contact with skin produce pattern burns. Differentiation between unintentional and inflicted burns may depend on reconstruction of the event based on the child's story, the caretaker's story, and the pattern itself. Generally, inflicted burns result when rigid objects hot enough to produce at least a second-degree burn are pressed against the skin (50). The burn degree is usually uniform throughout the wound. Unintentional burns may have variability in appearance, resulting from the victim's pulling away from the hot object.

Single burns from steam irons or curling irons must be evaluated carefully in relation to burn

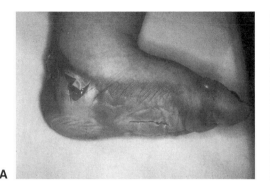
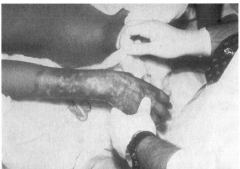
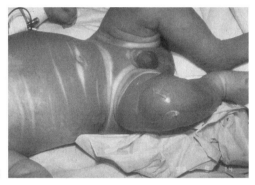

FIG. 9.4   Immersion burns. A: Immersion or "dunk" burn caused by dipping foot in hot liquid. Note the clear delineation of burned and normal skin along with the uniform degree of burn (here a second-degree burn) throughout the burn distribution. B: Immersion burn caused by dipping infant in hot liquid. C: Note where skin folds protect underlying tissue from serious burn (see color plate). (Courtesy of Dr. William Smock, University of Louisville School of Medicine.)

location (e.g., buttocks or perineum), the age of the burn, the age of the child, and the history given (53–55). Cigarette burns (that typically measure 8 mm in diameter) should spark the investigator's curiosity because lit cigarettes are not common childhood hazards (55,56).

Multiple burns are rarely accidental (55,57). Suspicion should also be raised when burns coexist with other injuries or with neglect (55,57,58). A grasp of burn injuries and their identification and evaluation is a powerful tool for assessing the truthfulness of a caretaker's history (50,55).

Bite Wounds

Bite wounds can be located on any body surface. The investigator must first determine if the wound is indeed a bite mark, whether the bite is human or animal, and whether another child or an adult inflicted the bite. Humans have four incisors in each dental arch and short canines. The incisors leave rectangular marks, and the canines leave triangular marks. Dogs have six incisors and possess canine teeth that protrude and create puncture marks, separate from the other smaller teeth, and tear tissue (59).

The upper and lower arches help define a human bite wound. They create an oval wound (if both arches are involved) or an arc-shaped wound if only one arch was used. Bite injuries result from the force of the teeth leaving their imprint in the skin, producing contusions or abrasions. A bite wound may have a central area of ecchymosis, caused by either positive pressure while closing the teeth or negative pressure from suction (60).

Both adults and children can inflict bite wounds. To determine if a bite wound was created by adult jaws, the distance between the canine teeth marks should be measured. The normal distance between the maxillary canine teeth in adult humans is 2.5 to 4 cm. If the intercanine distance is less than 2.5 cm, a child may have caused the bite. If the distance is 2.5 to 3 cm, the bite is likely from a child or small adult. A distance greater than 3 cm indicates the perpetrator was likely an adult (60).

Bite wounds should be diagrammed, with measurements recorded as well as photographed, if possible. A measuring indicator, such as a ruler, should be included in the photograph to aid in further evaluations. In some cases, when a bite wound induces significant swelling, the measurements and photographs can be repeated 24 hours later for clarity.

Bite wounds can be contaminated with human saliva (see Chapter 6). Blood group antigens can be secreted in saliva, and DNA is present in epithelial cells from the mouth and may be deposited in bites. Even if the wound is dry, a sample can be collected on a sterile moistened cotton swab (60).

Intraoral Soft-Tissue Injuries

Intraoral soft-tissue injuries are frequently accidental in mobile children but can be seen in the setting of child abuse, particularly in young infants. They can occur when significant external force is applied to the child's mouth. A common example is a contusion or laceration of the mucosal surface of the lip, produced when the child's own teeth imprint on the soft-tissue. This may occur from a direct blow or from putting a hand over the child's mouth in an attempt to quiet or suffocate him/her. If the external force produces severe distortion of the upper or lower lips, the delicate frenula of the lip may tear partially or completely. The frenulum of the tongue is less likely to be torn by external force but may be injured by objects thrust into the mouth, such as a bottle or spoon. Objects forced into the mouth can lead to direct trauma of the buccal mucosa, the hard and soft palates, the posterior oropharynx, and the tonsillar pillars. A careful oral examination should be included in the assessment of child abuse (47,61,62).

SKELETAL MANIFESTATIONS OF CHILD ABUSE

Fractures are the second most common injury in abused children presenting to an emergency department. The reported frequency varies between 11% and 55% (62). Although the incidence varies between studies, 30% to 40% of victims of child abuse who present to an emergency department have fractures (63,64), with or without associated injuries. Caffey's early work identified the connection between long-bone fractures and intracranial bleeding and paved the way for child abuse investigations (1). Fifty-five percent to 70% of fractures attributed to child abuse are in victims younger than 1 year, and 80% are in victims younger than 18 months. Only 2% of fractures in this age-group are unintentional (62).

Although some fractures are highly specific for child abuse, no single fracture is pathognomonic. First the clinician must understand the types of fractures seen in children (Table 9-1). Understanding the forces that result in particular fractures can aid in deciding whether a presented history explains the fracture (65).

When evaluating children with fractures, the physician must consider the history given, as

TABLE 9-1

TYPES AND CAUSES OF FRACTURES SEEN IN CHILDREN

Fracture	Mechanism
Spiral	Torsional forces
	Often assumed to be secondary to child abuse, but they can result from intentional incidents, such as when a child trips while running
Buckle	Axial loading at the metaphyseal/diaphyseal junction
	Common unintentional injuries, such as from a fall onto an outstretched hand
	Can be associated with abuse, particularly in a child <9 mo old
Transverse and greenstick	Tensile or bending loads
	May be caused by direct blows to an extremity
Completed transverse (nongreenstick)	Usually a result of high-energy events, e.g., collision with a car or fall from a great height
Oblique	Combination loading, e.g., compression with rotation
Metaphyseal (classic metaphyseal lesions)	Shearing injury through newly formed bone just beyond the epiphysis
	Typical causes: shaking and yanking
	Highly suspicious for abuse
	Appear on radiograph film as a corner or bucket-handle configuration
	In rare cases, this fracture can result from a nonintentional event.

Based on Pierce MC, Bertocci GE, Vogeley E, et al. Evaluating long-bone fractures in children: a biomechanical approach with illustrative cases. *Child Abuse Negl* 2004;28(5):505–524.

well as fracture types, location, number, age, and developmental level of the child. Fractures in nonambulatory children are extremely rare and should raise the possibility of abuse (22,66).

Fractures of the extremities are the most common fractures seen in association with child abuse. The clavicle is the most commonly fractured bone in childhood, occurring in 2% to 10% of children, and such a fracture may be accidental or inflicted. The middle third is the most frequently fractured portion. Fractures in the lateral third may be more suggestive of abuse, although not diagnostic (67).

After the extremities, the second most commonly fractured bone in child abuse is the skull. Often, but not always, a scalp hematoma is present at the site of impact (67). The most common skull fracture, whether due to abuse or accident, is a linear fracture of the parietal bone (68). A simple, single, linear, and nondisplaced fracture of one bone of the skull suggests accidental trauma, especially if there are no findings of intracranial injury. Multiple fractures that are comminuted or involve more than one bone are often a result of child abuse or significant forceful trauma, such as a high-speed motor vehicle collision. The probability of child abuse is increased when there is associated intracranial bleeding. As mentioned earlier, vertical falls from heights of less than 4 feet are not likely to produce substantial injury (16–18).

Rib fractures are highly specific for child abuse, accounting for 5% to 27% of abuse-related injuries (67). A recent literature review confirms that rib fractures in children younger than 3 years are highly predictive of nonaccidental injury, and that among children with rib fractures, the likelihood of nonaccidental injury decreases with increasing age (69). One study calculated a positive predictive value (PPV) of 95% for nonaccidental trauma in rib fractures in children younger than 3 years of age. When children with a defined history of accident and/or disease were excluded, the PPV rose to 100% (70).

Rib fractures can result from thoracic compression (squeezing) or blunt injury to the chest (22). In child abuse they are often multiple and most frequently located posteriorly, at the costovertebral angles; however, they can also occur laterally and at the costochondral junction in abused infants. Typically, they are the result of shaking an infant or young child while holding him or her about the torso. Acute rib fractures can be difficult to detect initially and may not be evident on a radiograph. It may not be until callous formation, at around 2 weeks after injury, that the fracture becomes radiologically evident.

Femur fractures account for approximately 20% of the fractures seen in abused children. They are not pathognomonic for child abuse. Femur fractures are more likely because of abuse in infants than in older children. In abuse, fractures usually occur because of violent twisting or swinging of the leg. Femur fractures can be accidental when a major force is encountered; however, trivial injury is unlikely to cause a femur fracture in a healthy infant. Therefore, the clinician must make a careful determination of whether the history is consistent with the injury.

The humerus is a frequently injured bone in abused children. Such fractures are typically diaphyseal or distal metaphyseal, unlike supracondylar fractures found commonly in nonabusive situations. The mechanism includes pulling, swinging, or jerking the arm, resulting in a range of fractures, including oblique or spiral fractures.

Tibial fractures represent less frequent abuse than other fractures. One must be aware of the "toddler's fracture," a nondisplaced oblique fracture of the distal tibia that can occur with a trivial mechanism in toddlers who are learning to walk (between the ages of 9 months and 3 years). However, spiral fractures can signal abuse, so a careful history must be elicited and correlated with the injury.

Additional fractures related to child abuse are vertebral fractures (71) (occurring after severe hyperflexion, often at the thoracolumbar junction), facial fractures (<2% of child abuse injuries), and sternal fractures. Scapular and pelvic fractures, also rare, require a significant amount of force; therefore, the clinician must maintain a high level of suspicion for abuse when these types of injury are detected (67). Kleinman (72) reviewed the specificity of fractures as they relate to child abuse (Table 9-2).

Bones progress through predictable stages of healing: resolution of soft-tissue injury, subperiosteal new bone formation (SPNBF), loss of fracture line definitions, soft callus, hard callus, and remodeling. However, the onset and completion of these phases vary, depending on the age of the patient. In general, the younger the infant the more rapidly their bones will heal. Kleinman provides guidelines for dating fractures but points out that the ability to date fractures based on radiographs is inexact (72). However, when reviewing fractures of the appendicular skeleton the emergency physician can consider several reasonable facts. A shaft fracture without SPNBF is usually less than 7 to 10 days old and is rarely 20 days old. A fracture with definitive but slight SPNBF may have occurred as recently as 4 to 7 days ago. A 20-day-old fracture will almost always have well-defined SPNBF. A fracture with a large amount of SPNBF or callus is more than 14 days old. And a loss of marginal sharpness of the fracture line definition occurs somewhat later than SPNBF and may be delayed for as long as 14 to 21 days (72).

A skeletal survey is the method of choice for global skeletal imaging in cases of child abuse (73).

TABLE 9-2

SPECIFICITIES OF FRACTURES AS TO INDICATION OF CHILD ABUSE

High specificity
  Classic metaphyseal lesions
  Rib fractures (especially posterior)
  Scapular fractures
  Spinous process fractures
  Sternal fractures
Moderate specificity
  Multiple fractures, especially bilateral
  Fractures of different ages
  Epiphyseal separations
  Vertebral body fractures and subluxations
  Digital fractures
  Complex skull fractures
Low specificity
  Subperiosteal new bone formation
  Clavicular fractures
  Long-bone shaft fractures
  Linear skull fractures

Based on Kleinman PK. *Diagnostic imaging of child abuse*, 2nd ed. St. Louis, MO: Mosby, 1998.

Abbreviated skeletal surveys in which a few images encompass the infant's entire body have no role, as they fail to provide the necessary contrast and spatial resolution to detect subtle, but highly specific, bony abnormalities. The American Academy of Pediatrics recommends that a complete skeletal survey be performed in all children younger than 2 years who are suspected of being victims of physical abuse (73). This should strongly be considered in all children younger than 1 year with significant skin or skeletal injury.

A skeletal survey should also be considered in patients with head injury or other injuries associated with abuse and in their siblings, who are also at risk. Children between 2 and 5 years of age can be handled individually. A skeletal survey has little value in children above the age of five (73). A follow-up skeletal survey 2 weeks after the initial evaluation may aid in dating injuries or detect healing fractures not visualized on initial films (73,74). The follow-up should be done when abuse is strongly suspected. Bone scan may be performed as a complement to the skeletal survey. In fact, bone scans show greater sensitivity than the skeletal survey for the detection of acute rib fractures, subtle shaft fractures, and areas of early periosteal elevation (73,75), but radiography shows greater sensitivity for classic metaphyseal lesions (CMLs) (75). However, it is not practical to replace the skeletal survey with a bone scan. A scan

may require sedation and is difficult to obtain in the emergency department setting. For the child who is in a safe environment, a 2-week repeat skeletal survey may provide the necessary information (73).

MUNCHAUSEN SYNDROME BY PROXY

In 1951, Asher used the term *Munchausen syndrome* to describe a series of patients whose fanciful descriptions of their fictitious illnesses and medical histories led to numerous surgeries and hospitalizations (76). In 1977, Meadow introduced the term *Munchausen syndrome by proxy* (MSBP) in pediatrics for children presenting with unfathomable illnesses that require extensive diagnostic evaluations, including invasive tests, surgeries, or hospitalizations (77). MSBP is relatively uncommon: based on a 2-year prospective study, McClure et al., in the United Kingdom, estimated that it occurs at a rate of 0.4 per 100,000 in children younger than 16 years of age and 2 per 100,000 in children younger than 1 year (78). Those investigators also noted that the average age of the child at diagnosis was 20 months. The true incidence is unknown, because it is probably underdiagnosed and underreported (79). MSBP is found throughout the world, and boys and girls are equally affected, with a wide spectrum of severity. The caregiver responsible for the deception is the child's mother in 94% to 99% of cases (80). Although Munchausen syndrome is a psychiatric illness, MSBP is psychiatric illness that implies child abuse. As defined by the American Professional Association of Child Abuse (APSCA), MSBP has two components: the adult perpetrator and the child victim who has the falsification of a pediatric medical illness or symptom. MSBP is classified as a factitious disorder in the *Diagnostic and Statistical Manual of Mental Disorders*, 4th edition (81), although the mother herself may or may not have a history (carry the diagnosis) of Munchausen syndrome. A child is used as a means of obtaining attention, often to the point of enforcing the child's invalidism to increase the degree of instability and therefore the amount of medical attention paid to the caregiver. Other characteristics of the caregiver in MSBP are variable. The caregiver (usually the mother) will be compliant, will be familiar with medical knowledge, and will bond with the hospital staff (82,83). She is able to describe signs and symptoms, such as apnea, seizures, or bleeding that initiate further medical investigation. The caretaker can fabricate illness by lying or by actual poisoning, suffocation, or manipulation of specimens or medical records.

Some cases of MSBP can *simulate* illness. For example, Meadow (77) described mothers who submitted false histories of illness in their children and submitted contaminated urine for examination. In general, simulated illness is faked in its description but does not harm the child. Alternatively, persons with MSBP can *produce* illness. For example, in the same report, large amounts of salt were fed to a child, producing hypernatremia. A produced illness is one in which the caregiver inflicts injury on the child to create the signs of disease, such as scratching the child to generate a rash or injecting saliva into the intravenous line to cause sepsis (76,77). Both simulated and produced illnesses lead to multiple medical procedures and testing. Since Meadow's description, there have been numerous reports of MSBP, including presentations of the child or reporting by the mother of seizures (84), cystic fibrosis (85), and bleeding (86,87). Rosenberg's review of 117 cases (80) includes these presentations as well as central nervous system depression, apnea, diarrhea, vomiting, fever, and rash. Suffocation, poisoning, or other mechanisms can bring on actual illness in MSBP. Many types of agents have been used to poison children, including ipecac, laxatives, anticonvulsants, opiates, benzodiazepines, acetaminophen, antihistamines, insulin, and chloral hydrate (80,88). In McClure's prospective series (70), the anticonvulsant carbamazepine was the most common single drug used.

Morbidity associated with MSBP may be short term or long term. Long-term morbidity leaves permanent disfigurement; it occurs in 8% of patients (80). Morbidity associated with MSBP includes failure to thrive, nonaccidental injury, poisoning, neglect, and developmental delay. The mortality associated with MSBP is 6% to 8% (80). Repetition of abuse in siblings is common—50% for suffocation and 40% for poisoning cases (89). Children may die from injury or illness inflicted by a caregiver. Fatal outcomes are associated with poisoning, suffocation, or complications resulting from medical investigative procedures and hospitalizations.

MSBP should be suspected when bizarre symptoms of an illness appear only when the mother is present. The primary "diagnosis" tends to be a very rare disorder, and the results of laboratory investigations do not concur with the child's appearance. The child may have multiple, recurrent serious medical problems and/or a family history of an unexplained sibling death, including sudden infant death syndrome (SIDS). Treatments are often not tolerated (vomiting and intravenous line dislodgment), and the child's symptoms and signs are not present when the mother is absent (77).

The diagnosis of MSBP may be difficult to confirm. In most cases, hospital admission will protect the child and facilitate the medical evaluation (88). Toxicologic screens and assays of blood, gastric contents, and intravenous fluids may be helpful

for certain types of MSBP associated with poisoning (80). In some circumstances, court orders can be obtained to videotape the child in a controlled setting (90). A multidisciplinary team, including social workers experienced in MSBP, law enforcement personnel, child protective services, and the hospital legal department, can provide advice about how to observe the parents (91). The child's medical records from other institutions should be reviewed for documentation of day-to-day observations by staff members (92).

If MSBP is suspected, a court order is needed to separate the parent from the child. This can be diagnostic and therapeutic, as the child improves when the mother is not present. Moreover, all children in the home should be examined and have their medical data reviewed. A pediatric social worker and the hospital child protection team can investigate and evaluate the home setting. The current and future health of the child is the focus in MSBP, as is seeking help for the perpetrator, who may have a mental illness.

CONDITIONS THAT MIMIC CHILD ABUSE

Mistakes can occur when reporting cases of child abuse. Suspected child abuse must be reported, so the clinician should be reasonably certain that the history, physical examination, and laboratory studies support evidence of abuse while ruling out other causes. An incorrect diagnosis of child abuse may trigger an awkward investigation (93,94). Unintentional injuries, cutaneous manifestations of systemic illness, skeletal disorders, cultural and racial factors, and SIDS can be mistaken for child abuse by an untrained eye.

Child abuse can be confused with unintentional injury. In distinguishing the two, it is important to consider the nature of the injury, the caretaker's explanation of how it occurred, and the presence or absence of previous injuries. The child's developmental level should also be assessed to determine if the account of injury is plausible. The child's nutritional status, hygiene, and overall health should be assessed as well.

Skin lesions are the most common presenting sign of child abuse. However, certain skin manifestations can be confused with child abuse. Mongolian spots, present from birth, can be mistaken for bruises. They may appear gray–blue in dark-skinned children and may be found over the back and buttocks. Mongolian spots are differentiated from bruising in that they are not tender and fade over months to years. Bruising or persistent bleeding can also be seen secondary to acquired or congenital coagulopathies, such as hemophilia or von Willebrand's disease.

Acquired causes of bruising or bleeding include idiopathic thrombocytopenic purpura, neuroblastoma and leukemia, and vitamin K deficiency. In these instances, a complete blood count with platelets, prothrombin (PT) time, partial thromboplastin (PTT) time, bleeding time, Platelet Function Analyzer 100 or von Willebrand factor antigen test, and factor level assays, in conjunction with history and physical examination findings, may be necessary for the correct diagnosis (95). A detailed history, physical examination, and selected laboratory evaluation should help distinguish a bleeding disorder from abuse.

Some ingestions can be associated with bruising and bleeding. Salicylate ingestion causes subconjunctival and skin petechiae and purpura from increased platelet capillary permeability and decreased platelet adhesiveness. In addition, there are other clinical manifestations, such as vomiting and hyperventilation, as well as abnormal laboratory studies (anion gap metabolic acidosis and positive salicylates in a toxicology screening). Warfarin-type anticoagulants can cause bruising and bleeding by interfering with vitamin-K–dependent clotting factors. PT will be prolonged with significant ingestions of these substances (96).

Easy bruising can also be seen with the Ehlers–Danlos syndrome, a rare autosomal dominant connective tissue disorder characterized by eight subtypes of varying severity. Skin in this syndrome is described as "cigarette paper thin" and is associated with hyperelasticity, bruisability, and fragility. Joint hypermobility, dislocation, and kyphoscoliosis are also seen. Children with Ehlers–Danlos may present with gaping lacerations and a history of poor wound healing (97).

Vasculitis can be associated with bruising and therefore be confused with child abuse. In individuals with Henoch–Schönlein purpura, the legs and buttocks become bruised; in addition, arthritis, nephritis, and gastrointestinal bleeding may be seen. Erythema multiforme is present on the extensor surfaces of the hands, arms, feet, legs, palms, and soles. Lesions can be macular, papular, nodular, urticarial, or vesicobullous. Intradermal hemorrhage or petechiae may be present. The clinical features of the rash can help the physician make the diagnosis (98).

Pediatric skin disorders that cause blistering can be confused with burns, a common presentation of child abuse. Impetigo is a *superficial* skin infection caused by streptococcal and staphylococcal species (98). Skin lesions, seen on the trunk, face, and extremities, appear as blisters that can rupture, leaving red circular ulcers resembling cigarette burns (98). Cigarette burns appear as *deep* symmetric craters (8 mm) with purple crusts and with heaped-up borders if found on the dorsum of the hand, foot, or face. They heal slowly and leave a scar. Cigarette burns are usually third-degree, compared with impetigo lesions, which are flat and crusted.

Phytophotodermatitis is a skin reaction characterized by erythema and bullae that denudate in streaking patterns, resembling a caustic burn. This occurs when the skin is exposed first to limes, lemons, or plants that contain furocoumarins and then to the sun. The furocoumarins induce cross-linking of DNA strands on exposure to ultraviolet light (99). The reaction may be delayed for 2 to 3 days; therefore, its cause may not be evident.

The hair tourniquet syndrome occurs when a hair or thread wraps tightly around an infant's digit. Distal to the hair, the digit is edematous, painful, and discolored, and the injury may resemble a burn (100).

Skeletal defects that simulate child abuse may be secondary to congenital, metabolic, or nutritional disorders. They may also be caused by infection or drugs. Osteogenesis imperfecta (OI), also known as brittle bone disease, is a group of rare inherited disorders characterized by frequent fractures, blue sclerae, large fontanel, excessive joint laxity, easy bruisability, short stature, abnormal dentition, and hearing loss (101). Spiral or transverse fractures through the diaphyses are commonly seen; however, metaphyseal fractures resulting from child abuse have been reported (102). The disease is caused by a defect in the synthesis of type I collagen (103). There are four major categories of OI, which result from autosomal dominant inheritance or a spontaneous mutation. Type I OI is the most common, accounting for 80% of cases, and has an incidence of 1 per 30,000 births. It is less severe than the other forms, with fractures occurring between the ages of 2 and 3 years and again between the ages of 10 and 15 years. Other findings include otosclerosis, dentinogenesis imperfecta, enamel fractures of the frontal incisors, and radiographic evidence of bell-shaped crowns and wide pulp chambers (104,105). Type II OI is a lethal, perinatal form, which occurs in 1 per 60,000 births. It is characterized by extreme bone fragility, crumpled femurs, blue sclerae, and intrauterine or early infant death (106). Type III OI is similar to type II but less severe. In these cases, sclerae may not be blue, and a progressive bowing deformity is usually noted. Type IV OI is very rare and characterized by moderate impaired growth and sclerae, which may be blue in childhood and become white in adulthood (106). Wormian bones of the skull are seen in most patients with type III OI and in one-third of patients with type I and type IV OI. Osteopenia in patients with type I and type IV OI results from the immobilization used to treat fractures, rather than causing the initial fracture (107). If the history and physical examination are accurate, the physician is unlikely to miss the diagnosis of OI. If blue sclerae or progressive deformity is absent, and there is a negative family history, the likelihood of abuse in an infant who presents with a spiral femur fracture attributed to minor trauma is much greater than the presence of OI (108). Skin fibroblast culture allows analysis of collagen for questionable cases, but these tests are expensive and time consuming (106).

A deficiency of copper can also cause bony deformities similar to those associated with child abuse. This element may be deficient in malnourished infants with chronic diarrhea, severely premature infants with low hepatic stores of copper, and children with Menkes syndrome, also known as kinky-hair disease, which is an X-linked, inherited disorder characterized by defective intestinal absorption of copper (108). Copper deficiency is also associated with hematologic, neurologic, dermatologic, and skeletal anomalies. Sideroblastic anemia, leukopenia, neutropenia, as well as distended weak tortuous vessels may be present secondary to defective production of elastin (109). Neurologic manifestations (more severe with Menkes syndrome) may include intracranial hemorrhage, hypotonia, psychomotor retardation, seizures, failure to thrive, and progressive neurologic deterioration from vascular insufficiency (110). Dermatologic manifestations include thin, coarse, brittle hair and horizontal eyebrows. The bony changes induced by copper deficiency are secondary to abnormal collagen formation. Osteopenia is seen early and progresses with metaphyseal sickle-shaped spurs at the ends of long-bones as well as periosteal reaction along the diaphyses. Fractures through the metaphyseal bone spurs can be mistaken for the metaphyseal–epiphyseal fractures seen with child abuse.

Deficiencies in vitamins D and C can produce bone deformities similar to those associated with child abuse. Vitamin D deficiency, the cause of rickets, becomes evident in infants who are covered and therefore receive little exposure to sunlight and are given no supplemental vitamin D. It also occurs in premature infants being given total parenteral nutrition without adequate calcium or phosphorus replacement. It can also be seen in children with seizure disorders who are maintained long term on phenobarbital or phenytoin (111). In advanced rickets, serum calcium and phosphorus concentrations are low, and the alkaline phosphatase level is elevated. Radiographic findings include cupping, fraying of the metaphyseal bones, separation of the metaphyses from the epiphyses, bone demineralization, and cortical thinning (111). Children with advanced rickets, unlike those with active rickets, tend to have normal bone density and frayed metaphyseal fractures; in contrast, fractures in abused children have sharply delineated fragments. In healing rickets, noncalcified osteoid between the zone of provisional calcification and the main shaft can be mistaken for a metaphyseal fracture. Increased periosteal reaction can be mistaken for a healing shaft fracture.

Vitamin C deficiency, or scurvy, can be seen in breast-fed infants of mothers with vitamin-C–deficient diets and in infants who have received boiled juice or milk without vitamin supplementation (112). Vitamin C is needed for collagen formation. Clinical findings of vitamin C deficiency include bleeding, swelling of the extremities from subperiosteal hemorrhage, poor wound healing, recurrent fever, and megaloblastic anemia (113). Radiographic changes seen with vitamin C deficiency include generalized osteopenia; the epiphyses are outlined with dense sclerotic rings, and the zones of provisional calcification become thickened, well-calcified lines adjacent to the radiolucent spongiosa. Fractures may be seen through the zones of provisional calcification and metaphyses. With healing, elevated periosteum may become calcified (112). The complete clinical picture, including dietary history, should help differentiate scurvy from child abuse.

Congenital syphilis is an infection that causes bony changes and may mimic abuse. The clinical constellation of symptoms of syphilis includes acral mucocutaneous rash, snuffles, hepatosplenomegaly, lymphadenopathy, recurrent fever, and failure to thrive. One fourth of the children with congenital syphilis have skeletal changes. Many infants with congenital infection present with pseudoparalysis of an extremity, secondary to osteomyelitis. Destructive lesions resulting from osteomyelitis in the metaphysis or diaphysis can vary from small corner separations to large cortical lesions and pathologic fractures. Syphilis can be confirmed with serologic testing (112).

Skeletal reactions similar to those seen in child abuse can occur secondary to side effects of certain medications. Prostaglandin E, sometimes used for treatment of congenital heart disease, may be associated with cortical proliferation along the ribs similar to posttraumatic periostitis. Vitamin A toxicity can produce hard, tender, swollen areas on the extremities that appear as periosteal reaction of the diaphysis without fracture. It can also cause widening of the cranial sutures secondary to increased intracranial pressure (114).

Hereditary sensorineuropathy is a rare autosomal recessive disorder that can be confused with child abuse. Patients are unable to feel pain and temperature, so they present to health care providers with multiple and repeated bruises, burns, lacerations, and skeletal deformities. Skeletal injuries may be undetected, leading to complications such as epiphyseal slips, aseptic necrosis, and chronic metaphyseal osteomyelitis (115). The diagnosis is made with a detailed history, sensory neurologic examination, nerve conduction studies, and nerve biopsy.

Certain cultural practices produce patterned skin lesions that may be mistaken for child abuse. When cultural practices injure a child, it is important to analyze the context of the therapy before accusing the caretaker of abuse.

Cupping is a common practice between Mexican and Eastern European immigrants, whereby a small amount of alcohol is placed in a cup and lit. The cup is inverted and placed on the skin. With cooling, a vacuum is created that leaves a circular ecchymotic lesion. Cupping is believed to decrease pain and inflammation by drawing the deep-seated offending agent to the surface (116).

Coining (cao gio, which means "scratch the wind") is practiced in Southeast Asia and Vietnam as a treatment for headache, chills, and fever. The process is thought to release illness causing "bad winds" from the body. The back or chest is initially massaged with mentholated oil; then the edge of a coin is rubbed against the skin until petechiae or purpura emerge (117). Lesions are usually self-limited, although a case of renal contusion with microscopic hematuria has been reported (118).

Spooning (quat cha) is similar to coining and practiced in China to relieve headache and fever. Water or saline is applied to the neck, back, shoulder, chest, or forehead; the area is pinched or massaged until it becomes reddened. It is then scratched with a porcelain spoon until ecchymotic lesions appear. It is believed that this practice also helps rid the body of "bad winds causing illness" (119).

Moxibustion is a form of acupuncture practiced in Southeast Asia. The moxa herb is burned on the skin with a piece of yarn, incense, or a cigarette near the area of pain to draw out the illness. Consequently, partial- or full-thickness burns are seen as discrete circular lesions (120).

Maquas is a practice of Bedouins, Arabs, Druses, Russians, and Oriental Jews, whereby hot metal spits are used to produce burns near the region of disease or pain. It is believed that when pus oozes from the burn, the primary disease drains out (121).

Salting is an ancient Asian custom, whereby the skin is salted in the neonatal period to produce healthier skin. However, in one instance, the salt was absorbed through denuded skin, leading to hypernatremia and intracranial hemorrhage (122).

A sunken fontanel (mollera caida) is believed in some Mexican American communities to be the cause of vomiting, diarrhea, and lethargy. Treatment of mollera caida may include shaking the baby upside down, which can lead to retinal and intracranial hemorrhage. Applying garlic to the skin of an infant is a naturopathic remedy that may cause burns (123).

It is important to realize that many conditions can, at first, mimic abuse. Although a detailed history and physical examination can diagnose most of these mimickers, the degree of investigation required can sometimes be difficult to achieve in the emergency department. Early involvement of a pediatrician or child abuse expert is essential.

SIDS has many of the markings of death resulting from abuse. The American Academy of Pediatrics estimates that less than 1% to 5% of apparent SIDS deaths are abuse-related (124). Parents of infants with apparent life-threatening events have been observed to harm or even suffocate their infants (91). Investigation of all unexpected deaths among children should include a thorough death scene investigation, a complete forensic autopsy, a review of all medical records, and the involvement of a child-death review team (125). Therefore, referral to the medical examiner and child protective services is appropriate in all unexplained infant deaths.

NEGLECT

Child neglect can present in many ways, some overt and some subtle. Neglect is the most common form of child abuse. Over 500,000 cases were reported in 2003 (3). Child neglect is responsible for more than half of the cases reported to child protection services but still may represent only the tip of the iceberg because signs and symptoms are not usually as flagrant as those seen in physical or sexual abuse (126). Child neglect remains underdiagnosed and underreported, despite statutes that mandate reporting. Unless neglect leads to threatening medical problems or death, it is seldom addressed directly by health care practitioners. The emergency department has become the primary source of health care for many impoverished families. Neglect may be overlooked during an emergency department evaluation because of more severe, acute medical conditions.

The definition of neglect may include all instances in which the major needs of children—food, shelter, protection, clothing, health care, education, and emotional support—are not met (127). Neglect can be physical, social, medical, or emotional. Indications of physical neglect include the lack of appropriate clothing for the weather, fatigue, lack or absence of food, poor hygiene, and lack of protection. Children may have signs such as severe diaper rash from poor hygiene and injuries resulting from poor supervision. Social neglect ensues from the failure to ensure that the child's educational needs are met. Medical neglect is seen when obvious medical/physical problems have been unattended (missed appointments, absence of appropriate dental care, absence of necessary health aids such as eyeglasses or hearing aid) and failure to thrive. Emotional neglect can be insidious and is demonstrated when there is inadequate love or emotional support in the family, which can lead to mental health problems. If children are not stimulated and early lapses in language skills or hearing deficits are not identified, additional developmental delay may compound social problems and difficulties in school. Lack of emotional support and developmental stimulation constitutes a common cause of neglect and may be associated with depression, anxiety, sleep disturbances, aggressive or listless behavior, and impaired peer group and interpersonal relationships (128).

Determining if a child is at risk for *potential* harm should be included in the assessment of neglect. For example, a small child left unsupervised for any length of time is at risk for injury from trauma or toxic substance ingestion. Most cases are not clear-cut, and experience and reason may help practitioners determine whether neglect is present. The occasional missed pediatric office visit or clinic visit may simply be noncompliance, but refusal to provide formal health care, ensure that immunizations are up-to-date, and seek rapid medical attention for significant injuries are more consistent with neglect and abuse. Neglect may manifest as a pattern of omissions or as behavior that repeatedly subjects a child to actual or potential harm (127).

Child neglect is related to family factors (child and parent) and community factors (129). Maternal depression or drug or alcohol abuse may contribute to neglect and abuse of children. Family dysfunction, domestic violence, and poverty are other risk factors. Poverty is frequently associated with chaotic and high-risk conditions in neighborhoods where drugs, guns, and violence are widespread. Even well-meaning parents may have inferior child-rearing skills. There may be only one parent in such households and they may be working several jobs to make ends meet, so the child-rearing may fall to someone outside the household. The child may have a particularly difficult or complex medical condition that needs to be treated and managed. These factors, coupled with poor education and lack of societal resources, foster neglect and abuse.

The evaluation of neglect begins with the patient's medical history, the family history for potential sibling abuse, and whether the child has had the standard "medical upkeep" (i.e., meeting developmental milestones; receiving immunizations as recommended; and having regular checkups, including dental care). Trends can be charted, such as the child's height and growth progress, cognitive development, and any evidence of failure to thrive. Compliance with medical follow-up appointments should be noted. The patient's social development, including progress in school, is also

an important element to investigate. A careful physical examination can assess physical development, hydration and nutrition status, as well as overt or subtle marks of abuse. Laboratory tests should be performed if failure to thrive may have an organic cause. Parent–child interactions and how the parent demonstrates feelings toward the child should be explored. If simple problems are noted (such as poor dental hygiene or diaper rash), counseling the parents may prevent further problems.

All states have laws requiring physicians to report child neglect to a child protective services agency (129). Hospitalization is warranted if the child may be at continued risk, for example, in cases of chronic neglect, under high-risk conditions such as near drowning or ingestion, and when interactions between the parent and child, and therefore the parent's ability/willingness to care for the child, are questioned by the clinician (124). Referral to outside agencies may help the parents improve their parenting skills and their ability to meet the child's needs, such as providing a nutritious diet. A referral to a social worker may be necessary to enable the parents to apply for Medicaid or state benefits for their children.

CONCLUSION

Once child abuse or neglect is suspected, steps must be taken to protect the child from further abuse. Although not required, it is usually recommended that the family be informed before a report is filed. This helps maintain a positive and constructive relationship with the family, even if they are the perpetrators. The clinician should remind the parents that they have the child's best interest and safety in mind. If the child is discharged, it must be to a safe environment pending investigation, which could include placement with other family members or emergency foster or shelter care. Child protective services will decide on appropriate placement. Other children in the household are also at risk for abuse and neglect and require timely assessment.

Many state laws require any person who suspects that a child has been subject to abuse or neglect to make a report to child protective services or local law enforcement. Mandated reporters (health practitioners, police officers, educators, and human service workers) who knowingly fail to make a required notification of abuse may be subject to professional or legal sanctions.

Emergency physicians *must* consider child abuse or neglect as a potential source of injury or illness and make appropriate referrals when necessary. The determination of child abuse or neglect will be based on a number of factors, resulting in investigations by child protective services, a hospital child protection team, social workers, and police. The burden of responsibility for the diagnosis does not rest on the emergency physician alone. Although the diagnosis of child abuse can be difficult, especially in the emergency department setting, the emergency clinician may be the only person who can intervene and save a child from a life-threatening situation.

ACKNOWLEDGMENT

The authors thank Scott Krugman and Wendy Lane for reviewing the chapter.

REFERENCES

1. Caffey J. Multiple fractures in long bones suffering from chronic subdural hematoma. *AJR Am J Roentgenol* 1946;56(2):163–173.
2. Kempe CH, Silverman FN, Steele BF, et al. The battered-child syndrome. *JAMA* 1962;181:17–24.
3. Administration on Children, Youth and Families: Child Maltreatment 2003. Reports from the States to the National Child Abuse and Neglect Data System. Washington, DC: U.S. Government Printing Office, 2005.
4. Trocme N, MacMillan H, Fallon B, et al. Nature and severity of physical harm caused by child abuse and neglect: results from the Canadian Incidence Study. *Can Med Assoc J* 2003;169(9):911–915.
5. Duhaime AC, Christian CW, Rorke LB, et al. Nonaccidental head injury in infants–the "shaken-baby syndrome". *N Engl J Med* 1998;338(25):1822–1829.
6. Conway EE Jr. Nonaccidental head injury in infants: the shaken baby syndrome revisited. *Pediatr Ann* 1998;27(10):677–690.
7. Jenny C, Hymel KP, Ritzen A, et al. Analysis of missed cases of abusive head trauma. *JAMA* 1999;281(7):621–626.
8. Lancon JA, Haines DE, Parent AD. Anatomy of the shaken baby syndrome. *Anat Rec* 1998;253(1):13–18.
9. American Academy of Pediatrics: Committee on Child Abuse and Neglect. Shaken baby syndrome: rotational cranial injuries—technical report. *Pediatrics* 2001;108:206–210.
10. Keenan HT, Runyan DK, Marshall SW, et al. A population-based comparison of clinical and outcome characteristics of young children with serious inflicted and noninflicted traumatic brain injury. *Pediatrics* 2004;114(3):633–639.
11. Starling SP, Holden JR, Jenny C. Abusive head trauma: the relationship of perpetrators to their victims. *Pediatrics* 1995;95(2):259–262.
12. King WJ, MacKay M, Sirnick A. Shaken baby syndrome in Canada: clinical characteristics and outcomes of hospital cases. *Can Med Assoc J* 2003;168(2):155–159.
13. Stiffman MN, Schnitzer PG, Adam P, et al. Household composition and risk of fatal child maltreatment. *Pediatrics* 2002;109(4):615–621.
14. American Academy of Pediatrics Committee on Child Abuse and Neglect. Shaken baby syndrome: inflicted cerebral trauma. *Pediatrics* 1993;92(6):872–875.
15. Duhaime AC, Gennarelli TA, Thibault LE, et al. The shaken baby syndrome: a clinical, pathological, and biomechanical study. *J Neurosurg* 1987;66(3):409–415.
16. Tarantino CA, Dowd MD, Murdock TC. Short vertical falls in infants. *Pediatr Emerg Care* 1999;15(1):5–8.
17. Duhaime AC, Alario AJ, Lewander WJ, et al. Head injury in very young children: mechanisms, injury types, and ophthalmologic findings in 100 hospitalized patients younger than 2 years of age. *Pediatrics* 1992;90(2 Pt 1):179–185.
18. Reece RM, Sege R. Childhood head injuries: accidental or inflicted? *Arch Pediatr Adolesc Med* 2000;154(1):11–15.
19. Tzioumi D, Oates RK. Subdural hematomas in children under 2 years: accidental or inflicted? A 10-year experience. *Child Abuse Negl* 1998;22(11):1105–1112.
20. Krous HF, Byard RW. Shaken infant syndrome: selected controversies. *Pediatr Dev Pathol* 1999;2(6):497–498.
21. Case ME, Graham MA, Handy TC, et al. Position paper on fatal abusive head injuries in infants and young children. *Am J Forensic Med Pathol* 2001;22(2):112–122.
22. Leventhal JM, Thomas SA, Rosenfield NS, et al. Fractures in young children: distinguishing child abuse from unintentional injuries. *Am J Dis Child* 1993;147(1):87–92.
23. Gilles EE, Nelson MD Jr. Cerebral complications of nonaccidental head injury in childhood. *Pediatr Neurol* 1998;19(2):119–128.
24. Wells RG, Vetter C, Laud P. Intracranial hemorrhage in children younger than 3 years: prediction of intent. *Arch Pediatr Adolesc Med* 2002;156(3):252–257.
25. Hadley MN, Sonntag VK, Rekate HL, et al. The infant whiplash-shake injury syndrome: a clinical and pathological study. *Neurosurgery* 1989;24(4):536–540.
26. Kanter RK. Retinal hemorrhage after cardiopulmonary resuscitation or child abuse. *J Pediatr* 1986;108(3):430–432.
27. Johnson DL, Braun D, Friendly D. Accidental head trauma and retinal hemorrhage. *Neurosurgery* 1993;33(2):231–235.
28. Levin A. Retinal hemorrhages and child abuse. In: David T, ed. *Recent advances in pediatrics*, Vol 18. London: Churchill Livingstone, 2000:151.
29. Block RW. Child abuse–controversies and imposters. *Curr Probl Pediatr* 1999;29(9):249–272.
30. Odom A, Christ E, Kerr N, et al. Prevalence of retinal hemorrhages in pediatric patients after in-hospital cardiopulmonary resuscitation: a prospective study. *Pediatrics* 1997;99(6):E3.
31. Swenson J, Levitt C. Shaken baby syndrome: diagnosis and prevention. *Minn Med* 1997;80(6):41–44.
32. Gilliland MG. Interval duration between injury and severe symptoms in nonaccidental head trauma in infants and young children. *J Forensic Sci* 1998;43(3):723–725.
33. Starling SP, Patel S, Burke BL, et al. Analysis of perpetrator admissions to inflicted traumatic brain injury in children. *Arch Pediatr Adolesc Med* 2004;158(5):454–458.
34. Willman KY, Bank DE, Senac M, et al. Restricting the time of injury in fatal inflicted head injuries. *Child Abuse Negl* 1997;21(10):929–940.
35. Hymel KP, Jenny C, Block RW. Intracranial hemorrhage and rebleeding in suspected victims of abusive head trauma: addressing the forensic controversies. *Child Maltreat* 2002;7(4):329–348.
36. Lazoritz S, Baldwin S, Kini N. The whiplash shaken infant syndrome: has Caffey's syndrome changed or have we changed his syndrome? *Child Abuse Negl* 1997;21(10):1009–1014.
37. Cameron CM, Lazoritz S, Calhoun AD. Blunt abdominal injury: simultaneously occurring liver and pancreatic injury in child abuse. *Pediatr Emerg Care* 1997;13(5):334–336.
38. Coant PN, Kornberg AE, Brody AS, et al. Markers for occult liver injury in cases of physical abuse in children. *Pediatrics* 1992;89(2):274–278.
39. Trokel M, DiScala C, Terrin NC, et al. Blunt abdominal injury in the young pediatric patient: child abuse and patient outcomes. *Child Maltreat* 2004;9(1):111–117.
40. Spitz WU, Spitz DJ, Fisher RS. *Spitz and Fisher's medicolegal investigation of death: guidelines for the application*

of pathology to crime investigation, 4th ed. Springfield, IL: Charles C Thomas Publisher, 2004.

41. American College of Surgeons. *Advanced trauma life support, instructors manual*. Chicago, IL: American College of Surgeons, 2003.

42. Jacombs AS, Wines M, Holland AJ, et al. Pancreatic trauma in children. *J Pediatr Surg* 2004;39(1):96–99.

43. Champion MP, Richards CA, Boddy SA, et al. Duodenal perforation: a diagnostic pitfall in non-accidental injury. *Arch Dis Child* 2002;87(5):432–433.

44. Gaines BA, Shultz BS, Morrison K, et al. Duodenal injuries in children: beware of child abuse. *J Pediatr Surg* 2004;39(4):600–602.

45. Keshavarz R, Kawashima R, Low C. Child abuse and neglect presentations to a pediatric emergency department. *J Emerg Med* 2002;23(4):341–345.

46. Sugar NF, Taylor JA, Feldman KW. Puget Sound Pediatric Research Network. Bruises in infants and toddlers: those who don't cruise rarely bruise. *Arch Pediatr Adolesc Med* 1999;153(4):399–403.

47. The American Academy of Pediatrics. *The visual diagnosis of child physical abuse*, 2nd ed. Elk Grove Village, IL: The American Academy of Pediatrics, 2003.

48. Schwartz AJ, Ricci LR. How accurately can bruises be aged in abused children? Literature review and synthesis. *Pediatrics* 1996;97(2):254–257.

49. Purdue GF, Hunt JL, Prescott PR. Child abuse by burning–an index of suspicion. *J Trauma* 1988;28(2):221–224.

50. Lenoski EF, Hunter KA. Specific patterns of inflicted burn injuries. *J Trauma* 1977;17(11):842–846.

51. Hight DW, Bakalar HR, Lloyd JR. Inflicted burns in children: recognition and treatment. *JAMA* 1979;242(6):517–520.

52. Daria S, Sugar NF, Feldman KW, et al. Into hot water head first: distribution of intentional and unintentional immersion burns. *Pediatr Emerg Care* 2004;20(5):302–310.

53. Chadwick DL. The diagnosis of inflicted injury in infants and young children. *Del Med J* 1997;69(7):345–354.

54. Feldman KW, Schaller RT, Feldman JA, et al. Tap water scald burns in children. *Pediatrics* 1978;62(1):1–7.

55. Keen JH, Lendrum J, Wolman B. Inflicted burns and scalds in children. *Br Med J* 1975;4(5991):268–269.

56. Stone NH, Rinaldo L, Humphrey CR, et al. Child abuse by burning. *Surg Clin North Am* 1970;50(6):1419–1424.

57. Ayoub C, Pfeifer D. Burns as a manifestation of child abuse and neglect. *Am J Dis Child* 1979;133(9):910–914.

58. Rosenberg NM, Marino D. Frequency of suspected abuse/neglect in burn patients. *Pediatr Emerg Care* 1989;5(4):219–221.

59. Fischer H, Hammel PW, Dragovic LJ. Images in clinical medicine: human bites versus dog bites. *N Engl J Med* 2003;349(11):e11.

60. American Academy of Pediatrics. Committee on Child Abuse and Neglect. American Academy of Pediatric Dentistry. Ad Hoc Work Group on Child Abuse and Neglect. Oral and dental aspects of child abuse and neglect. *Pediatrics* 1999;104(2 Pt 1):348–350.

61. Kempe CH. Uncommon manifestations of the battered child syndrome. *Am J Dis Child* 1975;129(11):1265.

62. Reece R, Ludwig S, eds. *Child abuse: medical diagnosis and management*, 2nd ed. Philadelphia, PA: Lippincott Williams & Wilkins, 2001.

63. Hyden PW, Gallagher TA. Child abuse intervention in the emergency room. *Pediatr Clin North Am* 1992;39(5):1053–1081.

64. Calmar E, Vinci R. Orthopedic emergencies: the anatomy and physiology of bone fracture and healing. *Clin Pediatr Emerg Med* 2002;3(2):85–93.

65. Pierce MC, Bertocci GE, Vogeley E, et al. Evaluating long bone fractures in children: a biomechanical approach with illustrative cases. *Child Abuse Negl* 2004;28(5):505–524.

66. Johnson T. Updates and current trends in child protection. *Clin Pediatr Emerg Med* 2004;5:270–275.

67. Kleinman PK, Nimkin K, Spevak MR, et al. Follow-up skeletal surveys in suspected child abuse. *AJR Am J Roentgenol* 1996;167(4):893–896.

68. Rao P, Carty H. Non-accidental injury: review of the radiology. *Clin Radiol* 1999;54(1):11–24.

69. Williams RL, Connolly PT. In children undergoing chest radiography what is the specificity of rib fractures for non-accidental injury? *Arch Dis Child* 2004;89(5):490–492.

70. Barsness KA, Cha ES, Bensard DD, et al. The positive predictive value of rib fractures as an indicator of nonaccidental trauma in children. *J Trauma* 2003;54(6):1107–1110.

71. Levin TL, Berdon WE, Cassell I, et al. Thoracolumbar fracture with listhesis–an uncommon manifestation of child abuse. *Pediatr Radiol* 2003;33(5):305–310.

72. Kleinman PK. *Diagnostic imaging of child abuse*, 2nd ed. St. Louis, MO: Mosby, 1998.

73. American Academy of Pediatrics. Section on radiology: diagnostic imaging of child abuse. *Pediatrics* 2000;105(6):1345–1348.

74. Worlock P, Stower M, Barbor P. Patterns of fractures in accidental and non-accidental injury in children: a comparative study. *Br Med J (Clin Res Ed)* 1986;293(6539):100–102.

75. Mandelstam SA, Cook D, Fitzgerald M, et al. Complementary use of radiological skeletal survey and bone scintigraphy in detection of bony injuries in suspected child abuse. *Arch Dis Child* 2003;88(5):387–390.

76. Asher R. Munchausen's syndrome. *Lancet* 1951;1(6):339–341.

77. Meadow R. Munchausen syndrome by proxy: the hinterland of child abuse. *Lancet* 1977;2(8033):343–345.

78. McClure RJ, Davis PM, Meadow SR, et al. Epidemiology of Munchausen syndrome by proxy, non-accidental poisoning, and non-accidental suffocation. *Arch Dis Child* 1996;75(1):57–61.

79. Ayoub CC, Alexander R, Beck D, et al. Position paper: definitional issues in Munchausen by proxy. *Child Maltreat* 2002;7(2):105–111.

80. Rosenberg DA. Web of deceit: a literature review of Munchausen syndrome by proxy. *Child Abuse Negl* 1987;11(4):547–563.

81. American Psychiatric Association. Factitious disorder by proxy. *Diagnostic and statistical manual of mental disorders*, 4th ed. Washington, DC: American Psychiatric Association, 1994.

82. Souid AK, Keith DV, Cunningham AS. Munchausen syndrome by proxy. *Clin Pediatr (Phila)* 1998;37(8):497–503.

83. Meadow R. Munchausen syndrome by proxy. *Arch Dis Child* 1982;57(2):92–98.

84. Guandolo VL. Munchausen syndrome by proxy: an outpatient challenge. *Pediatrics* 1985;75(3):526–530.

85. Orenstein DM, Wasserman AL. Munchausen syndrome by proxy simulating cystic fibrosis. *Pediatrics* 1986;78(4):621–624.

86. Malatack JJ, Wiener ES, Gartner JC Jr, et al. Munchausen syndrome by proxy: a new complication of central venous catheterization. *Pediatrics* 1985;75(3):523–525.

87. Clark GD, Key JD, Rutherford P, et al. Munchausen's syndrome by proxy (child abuse) presenting as apparent autoerythrocyte sensitization syndrome: an unusual presentation of polle syndrome. *Pediatrics* 1984;74(6):1100–1102.

88. Hettler J. Munchausen syndrome by proxy. *Pediatr Emerg Care* 2002;18(5):371–374.

89. Davis P, McClure RJ, Rolfe K, et al. Procedures, placement, and risks of further abuse after Munchausen syndrome by proxy, non-accidental poisoning, and non-accidental suffocation. *Arch Dis Child* 1998;78(3):217–221.

90. Hall DE, Eubanks L, Meyyazhagan LS, et al. Evaluation of covert video surveillance in the diagnosis of Munchausen syndrome by proxy: lessons from 41 cases. *Pediatrics* 2000;105(6):1305–1312.

91. Southall DP, Plunkett MC, Banks MW, et al. Covert video recordings of life-threatening child abuse: lessons for child protection. *Pediatrics* 1997;100(5):735–760.

92. Meadow R. Management of Munchausen syndrome by proxy. *Arch Dis Child* 1985;60(4):385–393.

93. Meadow R. Unnatural sudden infant death. *Arch Dis Child* 1999;80(1):7–14.

94. Christoffel KK, Zieserl EJ, Chiaramonte J. Should child abuse and neglect be considered when a child dies unexpectedly? *Am J Dis Child* 1985;139(9):876–880.

95. Bays J. Conditions mistaken for child abuse. In: Reece R, ed. *Child abuse: medical diagnosis and management.* Philadelphia, PA: Lea & Febiger, 1994:358–385.

96. Haddad LM, Winchester JF, ed. *Clinical management of poisoning and drug abuse.* Philadelphia, PA: WB Saunders, 1990.

97. Owen SM, Durst RD. Ehlers-danlos syndrome simulating child abuse. *Arch Dermatol* 1984;120(1):97–101.

98. Cohen B. *Pediatric dermatology.* St. Louis, MO: Mosby, 1999.

99. Coffman K, Boyce WT, Hansen RC. Phytophotodermatitis simulating child abuse. *Am J Dis Child* 1985;139(3):239–240.

100. Poole SR. The infant with acute, unexplained, excessive crying. *Pediatrics* 1991;88(3):450–455.

101. Carty H. Brittle or battered. *Arch Dis Child* 1988;63(4):350–352.

102. Astley R. Metaphyseal fractures in osteogenesis imperfecta. *Br J Radiol* 1979;52(618):441–443.

103. Edwards MJ, Graham JM Jr. Studies of type I collagen in osteogenesis imperfecta. *J Pediatr* 1990;117(1 Pt 1):67–72.

104. Wright JT, Thornton JB. Osteogenesis imperfecta with dentinogenesis imperfecta: a mistaken case of child abuse. *Pediatr Dent* 1983;5(3):207–209.

105. Gahagan S, Rimsza ME. Child abuse or osteogenesis imperfecta: how can we tell? *Pediatrics* 1991;88(5):987–992.

106. Paterson CR, McAllion SJ. Osteogenesis imperfecta in the differential diagnosis of child abuse. *BMJ* 1989;299(6713):1451–1454.

107. Taitz LS. Child abuse and osteogenesis imperfecta. *Br Med J (Clin Res Ed)* 1987;295(6606):1082–1083.

108. Danks DM, Campbell PE, Stevens BJ, et al. Menkes's kinky hair syndrome: an inherited defect in copper absorption with widespread effects. *Pediatrics* 1972;50(2):188–201.

109. Ashkenazi A, Levin S, Djaldetti M, et al. The syndrome of neonatal copper deficiency. *Pediatrics* 1973;52(4):525–533.

110. Levy Y, Zeharia A, Grunebaum M, et al. Copper deficiency in infants fed cow milk. *J Pediatr* 1985;106(5):786–788.

111. Zeiss J, Wycliffe ND, Cullen BJ, et al. Radiological case of the month. Simulated child abuse in drug-induced rickets. *Am J Dis Child* 1988;142(12):1367–1368.

112. Brill P. Diagnostic imaging of child abuse. In: Kleinman PK, ed. *Differential diagnosis of child abuse.* Baltimore, MD: Williams & Wilkins, 1987:221–224.

113. Stewart GM, Rosenberg NM. Conditions mistaken for child abuse: Part I. *Pediatr Emerg Care* 1996;12(2):116–121.

114. Radkowski MA. The battered child syndrome: pitfalls in radiological diagnosis. *Pediatr Ann* 1983;12(12):894–903.

115. Spencer JA, Grieve DK. Congenital indifference to pain mistaken for non-accidental injury. *Br J Radiol* 1990;63(748):308–310.

116. Asnes RS, Wisotsky DH. Cupping lesions simulating child abuse. *J Pediatr* 1981;99(2):267–268.

117. Yeatman GW, Shaw C, Barlow MJ, et al. Pseudobattering in vietnamese children. *Pediatrics* 1976;58(4):616–618.

118. Longmire AW, Broom LA. Vietnamese coin rubbing. *Ann Emerg Med* 1987;16(5):602.

119. Leung A. Ecchymosis from spoon scratching simulating child abuse. *Clin Pediatr (Phila)* 1986;25:98.

120. Feldman KW. Pseudoabusive burns in Asian refugees. *Am J Dis Child* 1984;138(8):768–769.

121. Rosenberg L, Sagi A, Stahl N, et al. Maqua (therapeutic burn) as an indicator of underlying disease. *Plast Reconstr Surg* 1988;82(2):277–280.

122. Yercen N, Caglayan S, Yucel N, et al. Fatal hypernatremia in an infant due to salting of the skin. *Am J Dis Child* 1993;147(7):716–717.

123. Garty BZ. Garlic burns. *Pediatrics* 1993;91(3):658–659.

124. American Academy of Pediatrics, Committee on Hospital Care and Committee on Child Abuse and Neglect. Medical necessity for the hospitalization of the abused and neglected child. *Pediatrics* 1998;101(4 Pt 1):715–716.

125. Reece RM. Fatal child abuse and sudden infant death syndrome: a critical diagnostic decision. *Pediatrics* 1993;91(2):423–429.

126. Wang CT, Daro D. Current trends in child abuse reporting and fatalities: the results of the 1997 annual fifty state survey. *Paper presented at: Prevent Child Abuse America*, Chicago, IL, 1998.

127. Dubowitz H. Child neglect. In Reece RM, ed. *Child abuse: medical diagnosis and management.* Philadelphia, PA: Lea & Febiger, 1994:279–297.

128. Cicchetti D. How research on child maltreatment has informed the study of child development: perspectives from developmental psychopathology. In: Cicchetti D, Carlson V, ed. *Child maltreatment.* New York: Cambridge University Press, 1984:377–432.

129. Dubowitz H, Giardino A, Gustavson E. Child neglect: guidance for pediatricians. *Pediatr Rev* 2000;21(4):111–116.

10

■ ADAM J. GEROFF
■ JONATHAN S. OLSHAKER

When I was a laddie
I lived with my granny
And many a hiding ma granny di'ed me.
Now I am a man
And I live with my granny
And do to ma granny
What she did to me.
Anonymous traditional rhyme (1)

The abuse or mistreatment of an elderly person constitutes actions that many consider to be as heinous as the abuse of a child. Indeed, state and federal laws exist specifically to protect elder Americans from such activity, just as child-abuse statutes protect our youth. Great strides have been made over the past three decades in the more widely popularized areas of domestic violence—child abuse and spousal or partner abuse—in terms of research, education, intervention, and overall funding. However, elder abuse, although present in society for centuries, has received attention in the medical literature only recently. Despite the appearance of an increasing number of studies, articles, and books on the subject, there are few national authorities and a relative paucity of research in comparison with other forms of domestic violence. The research that does exist is inconsistent with regard to form, methods, and even definition of simple terms. Certain authors include forms of abuse, such as self-neglect or financial abuse, that others do not. This situation makes a review and comparison of the literature difficult and confusing at times. It parallels the clinical aspect of this problem: many providers simply cannot recognize, will

not report, and do not intervene appropriately in cases of elder abuse or mistreatment.

Elder maltreatment is a problem that crosses all lines and knows no boundaries. Senior citizens of all racial, ethnic, and socioeconomic groups can be victims. Their abusers, while most commonly a close family member such as a spouse or adult child, may also be professional caregivers in a domestic or institutionalized setting. There have been risk factors identified that can stratify those elders at greatest risk for abuse or neglect. However, these individuals are often the hardest to reach and most difficult to evaluate because of isolation, impairment, or dependence. This chapter will delineate the salient features of elder abuse and mistreatment. These points include history, definition of terminology, epidemiologic factors, and a review of specific types of abuse and neglect. Characteristics of abusers and victims will be examined and risk factors elucidated. Clinical aspects will also be discussed, including the varied presentations to health care providers, reporting obligations and issues, and intervention techniques and recommendations. In addition, a review of some of the legal terminology and medicolegal and ethical aspects of elder abuse and maltreatment will be presented.

Ultimately, using this guide as a tool, awareness of this problem can be heightened among providers to identify this type of domestic violence. Once this first step of recognition is achieved, continuing education in this field should follow. This will allow these providers to approach victims of elder abuse or mistreatment in a specialized manner, utilizing appropriate hospital, community, and government resources in a multidiscipliined, coordinated effort to achieve positive results for elders, their families, and their caregivers.

HISTORY

Elder abuse and mistreatment, like all other types of domestic violence, has been an unfortunate part of human existence since ancient times. Greek mythology and literature relate stories of the slaying of parents, called *parricide*, to gain power (2). Some primitive societal customs have involved killing, abandoning, or encouraging the ritual suicide of the less productive tribal elderly to promote the common welfare of the group in times of scarcity (2). In early American history, witch-hunt victims who were tortured or burned at the stake were often postmenopausal women (3). Elder mistreatment, like all forms of family violence, was traditionally regarded as a private matter and was historically excused from outside scrutiny (2,4). Despite the incidence of elder abuse throughout history, it was not until 1975 that this subject, called *granny battering*, was introduced in two British journals published one month apart (5,6). Sporadic reports appeared in the United States soon after, and before the end of the decade, the U.S. Senate Special Committee on Aging reported on mistreatments in nursing homes (7) and on domestic parental battering (8). Since then, there has been more extensive research worldwide (9–17). Research has led to provider awareness, dedication of resources, and appropriation of funds.

In the United States, congressional hearings on this issue first took place in the late 1970s and early 1980s. As a result, in 1987 the amendments to the Older Americans Act (OAA) sought to define terms for purposes of problem recognition. Following these, the Department of Health and Human Services established an Elder Abuse Task Force in 1990 to expand the scope of federal involvement in elder mistreatment. In so doing, the federal government identified elders in the community as well as residents of institutions as victims in need of aid. A year later, the Elder Care Campaign undertaken by the U.S. Administration on Aging created a National Aging Resource Center on Elder Abuse (NARCEA), currently called the National Center on Elder Abuse (NCEA). At about the same time, the Joint Commission on Accreditation of Healthcare Organizations (JCAHO) included elder abuse among other forms of domestic violence in its mandate for improvements in the recognition and management of these maladies (7,8,18). Since then, more states have jumped on the bandwagon to pass legislation regarding elder abuse and mistreatment.

The relative explosion of interest and preliminary research that arose where virtually none had existed before prompted some experts to designate the 1980s the decade devoted to eradicating elder abuse (19). Slowly, health care providers, politicians, and other advocates are becoming more aware of this health issue as it is revealed from behind the closed doors that, until relatively recently, obscured our awareness of child abuse, sexual assault, and domestic-partner battering.

As a tangible approach to this goal, President William J. Clinton's first legislative action was to sign the Family Medical Leave Act in 1993, which, in part, provided families with an easier means to care for their elder relatives. His administration also expanded Medicare benefits to help older Americans and cracked down on fraud. More recently, in 1998, the NCEA received a $1 million grant designed to expand the agency and its services. In 2003, this agency commissioned the National Research Council Panel to Review Risk and Prevalence of Elder Abuse and Neglect, indicating that other leaders will be as supportive of elder care. Indeed, astute elected officials will take this position not only for humanitarian reasons but for electoral reasons as well: as the country ages and today's adult baby boomers become tomorrow's senior citizens, candidates will need elders' support for election.

THE AGING POPULATION

Despite improvements in elder care during the past 20 years, health care providers can expect to see more cases of elder abuse and mistreatment in the coming decades simply because the American population is aging. Better and more accessible health care, advanced technology, less invasive procedures, and pharmacologic advances are keeping older Americans alive and in many cases healthier than ever before. The introduction of Medicare in the mid-1960s was a major step toward this goal. The emphasis on primary care introduced in the 1980s and its role in disease prevention, risk reduction, cancer screening, and promotion of healthier lifestyles for both young and old has undoubtedly contributed to the "graying of America" (2,18).

Population statistics and projections are indeed staggering. Life expectancy has increased dramatically in this century alone. The U.S. Census Bureau projects the life expectancy of an American child born in 1990 to be more than 75 years, compared with an average life span of 47 years for a child born in 1900 (20). A person who reached age 65 in 1990 could expect to live for an additional 17.2 years (20). These data represent a marked increase over the 12 additional years expected in 1900 and even a significant increase over the 15.2 additional years anticipated by a 65-year-old in 1970 (2,20). The fastest growing segment of the elderly population is the "old old," that is, over age 75. Often this age-group is further divided into the "very old," between ages 75 and 84, and the "oldest old," age 85 and over. This growth is demonstrated by recent population statistics, which reported a 38% increase in the number of Americans aged 85 or older from 1980 to 1990. Similarly, the number of centenarians doubled in these 10 years (2,20).

Elderly persons represent an ever-increasing percentage of all Americans. In 1980, there were 25.5 million people older than 65 in the United States, representing 11.3% of the population (21). In comparison, the 2000 census documented 35 million people in this age-group, constituting 12.4% of the total US population (22). Over 12 million of these senior citizens were in the very old age-group, and an additional 4.2 million were aged 85 or older when they welcomed the new millennium (22). These oldest demonstrated the most rapid relative population growth. By the year 2020, more than 52 million Americans will be 65 or older (23).

This "elder boom" will bring even more interactions between the elderly and the health care system. It should come as no surprise that elderly people utilize health care resources more often and with disproportionate frequency than the population at large. This applies for both routine care and emergency services. Recent statistics from a 1994 report generated by the American Association of Retired Persons (AARP) showed that patients aged 65 and older accounted for 35% of all hospital stays and 46% of all inpatient care days (24). The seniors' outpatient visits also outnumber those of the general population by nearly 2:1 (2). There will be particular stress placed on emergency physicians and emergency service providers (25). Several studies have demonstrated, as one might expect, that elderly people use emergency services more frequently than the general population (21,26–29). This amounted to an estimated 13.6 million visits to emergency departments (EDs) nationally in 1990 (21). The elderly also are more likely to require a comprehensive level of emergency care. They are more frequently admitted, and they need an intensive care unit more often than younger patients (21). These trends imply what another group of authors conclude on the basis of actual data: elder use of emergency services is in fact more efficient than that of young people (29). Perhaps cases of elder abuse and mistreatment will increase in proportion to the projected population growth. Perhaps its incidence and prevalence will drop as elders, their caregivers, and their health care providers become better educated and more cognizant of available resources. Those involved in the care of elders hope for the latter.

DEFINITIONS AND TERMINOLOGY

Definitions of what constitutes elder abuse and mistreatment vary substantially. This variance has been a major barrier to understanding the true prevalence of abused or mistreated elders. Indeed, the terms "abuse" and "mistreatment" may be used synonymously or synchronously with one another depending on which authors are read. The different types of maltreatment are also subject to different definitions. Extensive literature reviews performed for this book and by other authors (17,30) have found no generally accepted meanings for these expressions. Furthermore, what constitutes abuse, mistreatment, or any other act in the opinion of one clinician, social worker, or layperson may not for another. Many authorities, including the American Medical Association (AMA) (31), prefer the term *mistreatment* to include both abuse and neglect (13,18,32). *Inadequate care* has also been proposed as a more universal phrase (33). In addition, clinical or common sense criteria for abuse may not be consistent with specific legal definitions. There is discrepancy even with regard to who is considered an elder. Most writers use the age of 65 as the accepted cutoff, but a few studies have included patients as young as 60 (1,11,34,35). One can become very confused. It is best to keep in perspective that the ultimate goal is the safety and welfare of the elderly. Rather than add a new author's interpretation into the mix, the reader should consider the relevant terminology and some of their existing definitions. The following practical definitions have already been published.

A broad definition of elder abuse or mistreatment is any adverse act of omission or commission against an elderly person (36). There is no consideration for intent in this most basic meaning. Other researchers restrict abuse to acts of commission with the intent to cause harm or injury (2). A Connecticut-based group that has compiled significant data since 1982 includes intent in its working definition of abuse: the willful infliction of physical pain, injury, or mental anguish, or the willful deprivation by a caretaker of services necessary to maintain physical and mental health (37). The US Congress in 1985 introduced the Elder Abuse Prevention, Identification and Treatment Act, which sought in part to clarify terminology (Table 10-1) (38). Its definition of abuse is similar to that of the aforementioned group. In 1992, the AMA published a comprehensive and sensible set of terms and classifications (31) This listing (Table 10-2) was an improvement and foreshadowed what will likely become the gold

TABLE 10-1

U.S. CONGRESS DEFINITIONS

Abuse	Willful infliction of injury, unreasonable confinement, intimidation, or cruel punishment with resulting physical harm, pain, or mental anguish; or the willful deprivation by a caretaker of goods or services that are necessary to avoid physical harm, mental anguish, or mental illness
Physical harm	Bodily pain, injury, impairment, or disease
Exploitation	Illegal or improper act of a caretaker using the resources of an elder for monetary or personal benefit, profit, or gain
Neglect	Failure of a caretaker to provide the goods or services that are necessary to avoid physical harm, mental anguish, or mental illness

Adapted from Jones J, Dougherty J, Schelble D, et al. Emergency department protocol for the diagnosis and evaluation of geriatric abuse. *Ann Emerg Med* 1988;17:1006–1015.

standard for all those involved in the care of the elderly: the National Elder Abuse Incidence Study (NEAIS) of 1996 (39). This project, undertaken by the NCEA through the U.S. Department of Health and Human Services Administration on Aging, empowered a panel of experts to define terms prior to the study of domestic elder abuse. After a pilot testing period of definitions, the final versions were selected and utilized (Table 10-3).

Neglect is a term that is even more nebulous than *abuse*. Some authors consider neglect less serious than abuse with regard to intent (40). Others pointedly remark that neglect, although conceptually different, should not be deemed a lesser form of abuse and can be just as harmful (41). The Connecticut researchers define neglect as the failure of a designated or responsible caregiver to meet a dependent elder's needs, or the inability of an elderly person without a caregiver to provide himself or herself with the means to maintain physical and mental health (37,42). Some experts specifically designate this latter situation as self-neglect (41). Interestingly, neither the congressional nor the AMA framework addresses the concept of self-neglect. Abandonment is defined as the desertion of an elderly person by an individual or group responsible for providing care or by an individual with the physical custody of an elderly person (39).

This jargon can confuse even an experienced provider. The clinician should learn these terms and become familiar with the working definitions so as to recognize examples of elder mistreatment and to communicate effectively with the appropriate authorities. Although various medical organizations, legislative bodies, and government agencies may all adopt seemingly crisp definitions, an individual form of elder mistreatment or abuse does not occur in a vacuum; a victim of one type of mistreatment too often suffers multiple abuses (18). The bottom line for the emergency provider is still to recognize when

TABLE 10-2

AMERICAN MEDICAL ASSOCIATION DEFINITIONS

Physical abuse	Acts of violence that may result in pain, injury, impairment, or disease
Physical neglect	Failure of the caregiver to provide the goods or services that are necessary for optimal functioning; avoidance of the older adult
Psychological abuse	Conduct that causes mental anguish in an older person
Psychological neglect	Failure to provide a dependent elderly individual with social stimulation
Financial or material abuse	Misuse of the elderly person's income or resources for the financial or personal gain of a caretaker or advisor
Financial or material neglect	Failure to use available funds and resources necessary to sustain or restore the health and well-being of the older adult
Violation of personal rights	Caretakers or providers ignoring the older person's rights and capability to make decisions for himself or herself

Adapted from Aravanis SC, Adelman RD, Breckman R, et al. *Diagnostic and treatment guidelines on elder abuse.* Chicago: American Medical Association, 1992.

TABLE 10-3

NATIONAL ELDER ABUSE INCIDENCE STUDY (NEAIS) DEFINITIONS

Physical abuse	The use of physical force that may result in bodily injury, physical pain, or impairment
Sexual abuse	Nonconsensual sexual contact of any kind with an elderly person
Emotional or psychological abuse	The infliction of anguish, emotional pain, or distress through verbal or nonverbal acts
Neglect	The refusal or failure to fulfill any part of a person's obligations or duties to an elder
Abandonment	The desertion of an elderly person by an individual who has assumed responsibility for providing care or by a person with physical custody of an elder
Financial or material exploitation	The illegal or improper use of an elder's funds, property, or assets
Self-neglect	The behaviors of an elderly person that threaten his or her own health or safety

Adapted from U.S. Department of Health and Human Services Administration on Aging and the Administration for Children and Families. *The national elder abuse incidence study*. Washington, DC: NCEA, 1998.

an elderly patient has suffered adverse physical or emotional health consequences as a result of abuse or neglect.

TYPES OF ABUSE/MALTREATMENT

Initial studies in different countries classified elder abuse into three or four categories: abuse, split often into physical and emotional/psychological; financial exploitation; and neglect (11,37,42,43). Tatara's report for NARCEA in 1990 further expanded the scope of abuse and mistreatment to include three additional types: self-neglect, sexual abuse, and miscellaneous (44). The miscellaneous category was designated for "all other types" of abuse, such as abandonment (perhaps the extreme form of neglect) and violations of a citizen's rights. Furthermore, certain abuses and most incidences of neglect could be either active (committed willfully) or passive (committed without intent) (41).

Physical abuse involves willful infliction of force that results in bodily harm, injury, impairment, or pain. Examples include hitting, slapping, striking with an object, pinching, kicking, pushing, shaking, burning, and rough handling (45,46). The most common instrument used by an abuser to inflict damage, pain, force, or punishment is his or her own hand. A less commonly recognized type of physical abuse is force-feeding. Other abusive behaviors include improper and perhaps unindicated use of physical restraints, intentional withholding of medication, or overmedicating, such as with an anxiolytic or other mood-altering drug.

Physical neglect involves physical harm brought to an elder as a result of a caregiver's failure to provide the means for well-being. Examples may include inadequate feeding or hydration, not enough physical

exercise or therapy, unsanitary living conditions, and poor personal hygiene care. Other neglectful behaviors include failing to provide or maintain basic assistive devices, such as eyeglasses, hearing aids, dentures, commodes, canes, walkers, and wheelchairs. The absence or inadequacy of safety precautions, such as bathroom handrails or bed side rails, also qualifies as physical neglect. Some authors specify that neglect is unintentional by definition (45), whereas others subdivide neglect into active and passive forms with regard to intent (41). An example of passive neglect would be an overburdened caregiver simply not having the time or resources to provide the level of care needed by an elder. If that same caregiver intentionally withheld basic items for that elder's quality of life, the neglect would be active.

Intent to cause harm is difficult to evaluate and even more difficult to prove. It is probably beyond the scope of the clinician to delve deeply into the issue of intent. The health care provider should be most concerned with damage control and safe disposition. An even more complex dilemma may arise in the area of self-neglect. Although the term is self-explanatory, self-neglect raises ethical issues and requires value judgments. An elderly person with moderate dementia, for example, who lives alone and cannot provide self-care, and who has signs of physical neglect, represents a case of passive self-neglect. A patient like this is probably incompetent and needs to be cared for, if necessary, against his or her will. Conversely, active self-neglect might involve a homeless adult who chooses not to utilize available community resources for the indigent and chooses a standard of living and personal hygiene below the socially expected norms (41). Other authors dismiss the notion of active self-neglect and specifically exclude this type of conscious and voluntary situation from elder abuse (39).

Psychological abuse is the infliction of mental or emotional anguish by threat, humiliation, or other nonverbal abusive conduct. It may be willful (45). Examples include verbal harassment, yelling, intimidation, and berating. Threatening an elder with punishment, physical abuse, or deprivation of basic needs also constitutes psychological abuse. Infantilization of a competent senior citizen is perhaps the most brazen of emotional abuses. A frustrated caregiver may be unaware of hurtful words hurled at a needy elder in moments of stress. Such negative remarks contribute to feelings of low self-esteem in any age-group, particularly in the elderly who may already harbor feelings of uselessness (47). Clinical depression is already highly prevalent among senior citizens (48); one's interactions at home should not fuel the fire.

Psychological neglect involves unintentional conduct that deprives an elder of good mental health. Examples include inadequate social stimulation caused by ignoring the victim, lack of companionship, or leaving the elder alone for inappropriately long periods of time (18). For instance, a caregiver might provide a dependent elder with adequate food, medical care, and housing but may not interact with that elder much at all. Such a caregiver may be supervising several seniors or may have other responsibilities that preclude him or her from providing even minimal social activity for an individual elder (47). Even facilitating a brief visit from a friend or giving assistance with a phone call to a relative might seem like undue effort for a harried provider.

Financial or material mistreatment may be abusive or neglectful. Directly exploitative behaviors include theft of an elder's money or property, or coercing an elder to change a will, make purchases, or sign any agreement against his or her will. Many elderly people have their checks cashed by others without proper authority. Likewise, elders can fall victim to slick confidence scams perpetrated by professional con men. Many instances of financial abuse involve senior citizens who possess substantial assets. However, even small incomes from government checks can become an incentive for an abusive caregiver to exploit an elder, especially when that money may be a household's only regular source of income (47). An exploiter with some official control over an elder's decisions, such as a chosen or appointed guardian, conservator, or someone with power of attorney, may abuse this authority. Financial or material neglect occurs when the elder or the caregiver fails to utilize available funds or resources immediately to meet the elder's needs.

Sexual abuse of an elder involves any nonconsensual sexual conduct or contact between an elder and an abuser. Examples include unwanted touching, fondling, and rape. Other kinds of sexual abuse may be less direct but just as unseemly: coerced nudity, explicit photography, indecent exposure, and lewd talk. Some people mistakenly believe that any sexual activity involving the elderly, even between consenting adults, is somehow inappropriate. This notion is clearly outdated and wrong. There is no reason for an elderly person to stop exploring sexuality on the sole basis of his or her age. Discouraging, restricting, or prohibiting consensual sexual relations between competent persons may be considered abusive. However, some elders may be incapable of consenting to sexual activity. One must be particularly cognizant not to dismiss the possibility that a senior citizen could be sexually assaulted or harassed. This subject is rarely addressed in studies of elder maltreatment, and there is not much data on the sexual abuse of elders. On a positive note, perhaps a contributing factor for the absence of data is infrequency of sexual abuse of elderly persons. One study reports that sexual abuse accounts for less than 1% of all elder mistreatment (49). This study notes that sexual abuse is particularly uncommon in a domestic environment; its usual setting is institutional.

The deprivation of an elder's rights represents a miscellaneous form of mistreatment. These rights may include an elder's right to privacy and his or her right to make decisions. These decisions for a competent elderly person may include medical, financial, or personal choices. Forcing an elder from a private residence without due process or placement of a competent elder in a nursing home against his or her will also fits this category. Medical professionals may unknowingly participate in elder rights violations with regard to reimbursements for certain hospitalizations. It has been suggested that the funding of hospital care based on diagnosis-related groups (DRGs) discriminates against the elderly by potentially denying them the longer hospital course that is often necessary to achieve recovery than for younger patients with similar diagnoses (50). DRG coding, with its emphasis on standardization of naturally varied and heterogeneous disease processes, does not account for age and its contribution to morbidity. There is no appreciation of the unique needs and characteristics of the elderly, such as slower recovery, comorbid illness, and possible inferior baseline function. That is not to suggest that all elders require longer hospital stays. Rather, assessment of any patient's level of functioning and the provision for reimbursement, at least in part, on the basis of function-related groups might eliminate this under-recognized iatrogenic mistreatment.

Besides grouping mistreatments by specific types of actions or inactions, elder abuse may also be classified by its setting. Abuse or neglect may occur at the elder's home or at the home of a caregiver. The caregiver would have some special relationship with the elder, such as spouse, sibling, child, other relative, or friend. This is referred to as domestic mistreatment (34,39). Institutional mistreatment takes place outside a private dwelling, as in a nursing home, assisted-living facility, group home, or in elder foster care. The perpetrators of this type of maltreatment have some professional or contractual obligation to care for the elder. Abusers and neglecters can include nurses, aides, and licensed private elder care providers. In addition, administrators of facilities can exploit elders with regard to financial or material abuses without ever meeting that elder face to face.

EPIDEMIOLOGIC FACTORS

The true incidence or true prevalence of elder abuse can only be estimated, but these approximations are frighteningly high for an enlightened and productive modern society. One must remember that the only cases of elder abuse that can be studied directly are those that have been reported. Thousands of cases go unreported each year, so data are skewed at best. Many studies that have attempted to enumerate these statistics have design flaws. There have been considerable discrepancies with regard to term definition, research methodology, data acquisition, sample size, and study goals. This situation makes any meta-analysis at this time impossible. Some studies attempt to extrapolate information using general population statistics to estimate national rates, whereas others confine the conclusions they draw to their data only. In addition, certain research groups have reported only on domestic elder mistreatment. Some other papers fail to include neglect as maltreatment. Sources of information also vary widely. Some focus on a small geographic area, whereas other studies compile data from nationally representative sites. Some studies directly sample cohorts of elderly patients in a community; some rely on previously collected information by protective service agencies; others retrospectively review hospital charts of elders, looking for evidence for or documented suspicion of mistreatment. The following text will review some of the more pertinent epidemiologic studies to date.

One of the earliest surveys, by Block and Sinnott in 1979, utilized both primary sources (actual community elders) and secondary sources (medical and elder care professionals) to acquire prevalence data. They found that 4.1% of elders who replied as primary respondents reported at least one incident of abuse (1). The U.S. House of Representatives Select Committee on Aging in 1981 reported a similar prevalence of 4% on the basis of secondary data obtained from state agencies. This prevalence translates into an estimated 1 million abused seniors yearly (39). Other studies estimate the prevalence to be as high as 2.5 million (51).

The first somewhat large-scale survey was conducted in Boston in the mid-1980s by Pillemer and Finkelhor, who interviewed more than 2,000 elders and reported a prevalence of 3.2% (17). This study was one of the first to use clearly defined parameters for the mistreatments sought: physical abuse, psychological abuse, and neglect. These authors modified a previously validated scale popular in the family violence literature called the *Conflict Tactics Scale* to the specifics of elder abuse. This instrument consists of a brief series of questions designed to elicit evidence and frequency of actions or verbal assaults that might have occurred during a conflict with a relative, friend, or caretaker. Just one reported case of physical violence was sufficient for a positive response to physical abuse. The guidelines for psychological abuse were different. This maltreatment was limited to verbal forms of abuses, and at least ten instances in a person's life after age 65 were required for a positive case of psychological elder abuse. The damaging effects of verbal emotional abuse appear to lie in the chronic nature of repeated infliction, not just once or twice, which explains why fewer instances of verbal assaults were not considered abusive. The assessment of neglect used a different sociological instrument called the *Older Americans Resources and Services (OARS)* test, which evaluated ten activities of daily living to ascertain whether or not any aid was withheld. Once again, ten aspects of neglect were needed for a positive result. At these rates, the national estimate of abused elder Americans ranged from just over 700,000 to nearly 1.1 million. Because of the narrowly defined terms, this study may have actually underestimated this problem's prevalence (51). In addition, an elder who reported fewer than ten separate incidents of verbal attacks or neglectful occurrences would have been excluded from the victim groups. European surveys of similar sample sizes reported comparable rates of abuse in the early 1990s, demonstrating that elder abuse is a global problem (11). These studies inquired additionally about financial or material exploitation as a type of mistreatment. Prevalence data are summarized in Table 10-4 (11,17,35,52).

In 1996, the NCEA conducted the most comprehensive study on elder abuse to date, the NEAIS. The U.S. Department of Health and Human Services published its results in 1998 (39). The study's fundamental goal was to determine the incidence of domestic elder abuse and neglect in the United States. Its design was quite elegant and its

TABLE 10-4

PREVALENCE OF ELDER MISTREATMENT (%)

Mistreatment	Lau/Kosberg (1978) (35)	Pillemer/Finkelhor (1988) (17)	Ogg/Bennett (1992) (11)	Comijs et al. (1998) (52)
All types	9.6	3.2	8.8	5.6
Physical violence	7.1	2.0	1.7	1.2
Psychological	5.0	1.1	5.6	3.2
Neglect	N/A	0.4	N/A	0.2
Financial/material	5.2	N/A	1.5	1.4

conclusions well supported. The NEAIS estimated approximately 450,000 (range 211,000–689,000) cases of domestic elder abuse and/or neglect during the study year. This figure does not include incidents of self-neglect and rises to approximately 551,000 (range 315,000–787,000) when all cases are totaled. Alarmingly, adult protective services (APS) could have expected notification on a mere 20% of these cases. The NEAIS concluded that nearly 450,000 elders suffered domestic abuse or neglect in 1996. Of this, only 16% of cases were reported to APS offices. That leaves 84% of victims below the tip of the iceberg and unidentified by APS. In other words, more than five times as many new instances of elder abuse and neglect occur in domestic settings as those about which APS already knows. The figures improve slightly when self-neglect cases are included in the calculations, but they are still dismal. Seventy-nine percent of elder sufferers of all mistreatments, including self-neglect, remain unknown to an APS agency. It is worthwhile to examine this study in depth. For a thorough review of the NEAIS, refer to the appendix at the end of this chapter.

VICTIM AND PERPETRATOR CHARACTERISTICS

The NEAIS and other data collectors have compiled demographic information about the victims of abuse and the perpetrators to better characterize both groups of people. Drawing definite conclusions is difficult because of the many differences in study design, but some patterns emerge upon examination of the literature. The available data suggest that victims of domestic elder abuse and neglect are more typically older than 75 or 80 years, depressed, and to some degree unable to provide self-care. Perpetrators in general are more likely male and closely related to the victim. Abusers also have a high rate of alcoholism and substance abuse.

Age has been shown as a risk factor for mistreatment. NEAIS results show that seniors in the over-80 group are abused or neglected two to three times beyond their proportion in the general population (39). APS agencies reported that this group held wide majorities in all categories of maltreatment except abandonment. Earlier studies have also suggested this on the basis that the most elderly may have the most overall heath problems and be the most dependent and susceptible to maltreatment (2,12,17,36). Although some recent studies have not found a direct link between frailty or dependence and the likelihood of abuse (13,43,53), it seems reasonable that an elder's overall physical infirmity and dependence may increase susceptibility to mistreatment (42). With regard to gender, the NEAIS data strongly demonstrated a female majority among victims in proportional excess to population differences (39). Figure 10.1 demonstrates a 2:1 female predominance in published data for the successive years 1990 through 1996. Whether gender is truly a risk factor is still in question. Some studies demonstrate statistical significance of a female majority (53), whereas others simply reflect a trend (13,43) toward this predominance. Others reveal the opposite: more men suffer reported mistreatments than women (17).

For some time, geriatrics authorities have felt that the mental health of an elder was an important risk factor for maltreatment (36). NEAIS researchers compiled data for both depression and dementia in abused elders. Both disorders were significantly prevalent among victims. Approximately 45% of NEAIS entrants were judged to be moderately or severely depressed, whereas more than 50% of them were at least "sometimes confused," if not "very confused" or completely disoriented (39). These numbers greatly exceed the prevalence of these mental illnesses in the general population (54,55).

It may surprise some people to learn that the most common perpetrator of mistreatment against elders is a very close relative, either the victim's own child (2,36,39) or spouse (17,53). Table 10-5 summarizes NEAIS data with regard to the perpetrators.

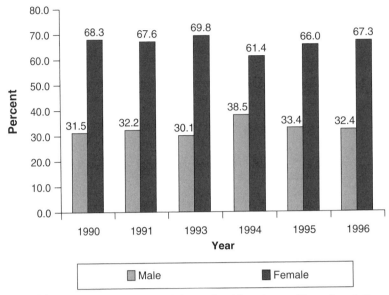

FIG. 10.1 Gender of victims of domestic elder abuse. (Reproduced from National Center on Elder Abuse. *Trends in elder abuse in domestic settings. Elder abuse information series no. 2.* Washington, DC: National Center on Elder Abuse, 1997).

Figure 10.2 demonstrates the predominance of an adult child as the abuser in all calendar years that the NCEA has published to date (1990 through 1996). A poor premorbid relationship between the elder victim and the younger perpetrator or a history of violence directed toward the child may contribute to future mistreatment (12). One characteristic that particularly stands out among abusers is substance abuse (42). Some experts assert that a history of substance abuse, most commonly alcoholism, in a care provider is the single most reliable predictor of elder abuse and neglect (36). Such a care provider would have impaired ability to

make care decisions, may be unable to control his or her behavior, and might be motivated to exploit an elder's material resources to support the addiction. A history of psychiatric illness in the perpetrator also predisposes that caregiver to abuse an elder. One study documented that 35% of abusers have an addiction problem or psychiatric ailment (56). Although sources differ, an additional circumstance that may characterize a person responsible for abuse involves how much the perpetrator depends on the victim (42). There often exists a significant degree of dependence with regard to money, housing, or even emotional issues that can predispose a relationship toward abuse or neglect.

While some authors focus on victim assessment and others on perpetrator evaluation to elucidate a handy chart of risk factors for elder abuse, one must bear in mind two important points. First, the care-giving relationship comprises very complex emotional and physical interactions between the elder and the provider. Many so-called risk factors that affect one person also invariably affect the other. For instance, some authors identify external stressors on a relationship as influential factors for mistreatment. Such stress may involve financial woes, bereavement, and illness that may afflict any family member. Second, there is enough controversy in the literature to make any conclusions drawn speculative at best. Unlike coronary artery disease, whose reliable risk factors have been well studied among many thousands of patients, elder abuse may

TABLE 10-5

NATIONAL ELDER ABUSE INCIDENCE STUDY (NEAIS) DATA: PERPETRATORS OF ELDER MISTREATMENT (%)

Perpetrator	APS Data	Sentinel Data
Adult child	47.3	30.8
Spouse	19.3	30.3
Friend/neighbor	6.2	5.7
Grandchild	8.6	4.2
Service provider	4.2	4.2
Other family member	8.8	24.0

APS, adult protective services.

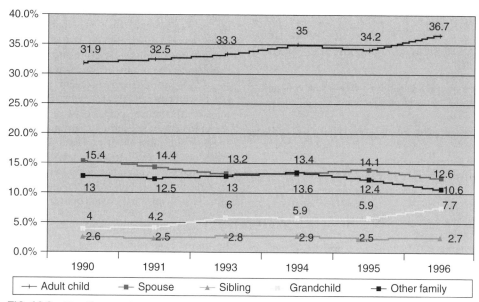

FIG. 10.2 Family members as perpetrators of domestic abuse. (Reproduced from National Center on Elder Abuse. *Trends in elder abuse in domestic settings. Elder abuse information series no. 2.* Washington, DC: National Center on Elder Abuse, 1997).

occur with few or no identifiable risk factors. The practitioner must approach every senior citizen who may be a victim of domestic violence with the same level of suspicion regardless of age, background, or comorbidity.

ASSESSMENT/SIGNS AND SYMPTOMS

Elders who have been neglected or abused may present daunting diagnostic challenges to the clinician. Some mistreated elders might display obvious physical findings that will arouse a provider's suspicion. Others' presentations will be subtle and may indeed be indistinguishable from or confused with sequelae of normal aging (57), disease processes, or accidental injury patterns. The vigilant clinician should always entertain the possibility of abuse or mistreatment in any elder who presents for care. Equal attention must be paid to institutionalized seniors. Asking a few additional questions in an inoffensive and caring manner regarding an elder's welfare as part of a routine history may elicit a discovery that would warrant additional inquiry. Knowledge of the risk factors for elder abuse and neglect as discussed in the preceding text should help direct the practitioner's approach to an elderly patient. Home health care providers are in a unique position to assess an elder's condition in the very setting where the mistreatment may be occurring.

An appropriate assessment requires time commitment. Although a busy emergency clinician may not

be the person performing the entire assessment, this provider should have enough knowledge to perform adequate screening to determine which patients may benefit from additional evaluation. The thought of an additional responsibility should not be discouraging. It is not the role of the emergency provider to do the complete appraisal. As a parallel, think of a patient who arrives with chest pain and a clinical presentation suggestive of unstable angina. The emergency physician treats the patient and in so doing accumulates enough data to reach a decision of whether additional evaluation (i.e., telemetry or cardiac care unit admission or cardiology consult) is indicated. Then an inpatient provider takes over. Similarly, resources for elder assessment should be available. Every practitioner needs to be familiar with the resources accessible at his or her site. Emergency departments EDs should develop and enact written protocols or clinical pathways for elder abuse, as many have done other forms of domestic violence. Unfortunately, few have.

Taking a medical history from a senior citizen in general is a complex and elaborate process. Adding the burden of evaluating for elder abuse can make this task even more difficult. As a starting point, the AMA has proposed a series of screening questions that can be employed by any health care provider (Table 10-6). Although this guide has yet to be validated as formally effective, it may be employed in an initial attempt to uncover mistreatment. Some authors recommend screening all elderly hospital patients, with particular urgent attention afforded to

TABLE 10-6

AMERICAN MEDICAL ASSOCIATION SCREENING QUESTIONS

1. Has anyone ever touched you without your consent?
2. Has anyone ever made you do things you did not want to do?
3. Has anyone taken anything that was yours without asking?
4. Has anyone ever hurt you?
5. Has anyone ever scolded or threatened you?
6. Have you ever signed any documents you did not understand?
7. Are you afraid of anyone at home?
8. Are you alone a lot?
9. Has anyone ever failed to help you take care of yourself when you needed help?

Adapted from Aravanis SC, Adelman RD, Breckman R, et al. *Diagnostic and treatment guidelines on elder abuse.* Chicago: American Medical Association, 1992.

those with cognitive or functional impairment (18). Indeed, it has been noted that such diminished capacity will not necessarily discredit an elderly victim's ability to report or describe abuse or neglect (7,31). The AMA encourages the questioning of all senior citizens regarding domestic violence regardless of whether signs and symptoms of mistreatment are present (31).

Certain points illustrating interviewing technique should be employed when screening an elder. First, it is important to interview any potential victim alone. The salient descriptions of maltreatment should be documented in the victim's own words. Specific and direct inquiries with regard to the frequency, type, and severity of maltreatment must be asked. Afterward, interviewing the caregiver (if available) separately may expose important discrepancies that might suggest a problem. All experts recommend that the elder be questioned and examined before interviewing the caregiver or suspected perpetrator. If nothing else, this method may, in some small way, reassure the elder that his or her story, in his or her own words, told in confidence, is of utmost importance to the clinician. The tone of the encounter should be nonjudgmental to elicit the most useful information. Although one's initial natural reaction to any abusive situation might be disgust and contempt, the health care provider must temper this reaction and approach the case in a nonconfrontational manner. Such a measured and calm approach has been shown to yield more data (2). The examiner should incorporate screening and other direct questioning in such a

way as to make these seem like a routine part of the assessment. This may help a patient feel more secure. Focusing on the elder as a whole patient, not simply as a victim, and approaching the problem as one of unmet patient needs may provide for a less intimidating interview process. Indeed, the first encounter by an emergency care provider may be the most spontaneous and useful source for information if conducted properly. It may pave the way for subsequent revelations during a social work or APS evaluation, especially because such formal consultations may seem very threatening to an elderly victim (18). General guidelines for the clinician during a patient encounter are presented in Table 10-7 (58).

General observations that are suggestive but by no means diagnostic of elder mistreatment include delays in getting medical attention, missed appointments, doctor or ED "hopping," and any physical abnormality that is inconsistent with the explanation provided by either the elder or the caregiver. There may be suspicious inconsistencies between two given histories. Also, noting how an elder interacts with the caregiver may prove invaluable. Inappropriate or abusive behavior may be observed directly. An absent caregiver may suggest neglect or abandonment. The elder may appear afraid of the care provider or act very docile and obedient. Spontaneous and inappropriate crying may occur. More examples of historical revelations and physical findings are detailed in Table 10-8. This list is by no means all-inclusive and may not help at all in many cases. Some studies demonstrate that typical physical signs of elder abuse correlated poorly with reports (12). Nevertheless, the emergency care provider must

TABLE 10-7

GUIDELINES FOR THE ENCOUNTER

1. Express concern
2. Validate patient concerns
3. Assess and treat medical problems
4. Assess cognitive and functional status
5. Document findings and preserve evidence and chain of custody
6. Assess psychosocial needs and safety
7. Involve appropriate consultants
8. Ensure safe disposition
9. File report

Adapted from Ramsey-Klawsnik H. Assessing physical and sexual abuse in health care settings. In: Baumhover LA, Beall SC, eds. *Abuse, neglect and exploitation of older persons: strategies for assessment and intervention.* Baltimore, MD: Health Professions Press, 1996:67–87.

TABLE 10-8

PERTINENT FINDINGS ON HISTORY AND PHYSICAL EXAMINATION

Physical Abuse and Neglect

Patterned injuries: slap marks, fingertip pressure bruises, rope or ligature marks on wrists/ankles, bite marks

Bruises: especially on areas of the body not over bony prominences, multiple ages

Wounds: laceration, abrasion, puncture, especially if untreated or in various stages of healing, decubiti

Head injury: traumatic alopecia, scalp swelling

Burns: cigarette marks, scald burns with an immersion line, absent satellite splash burns

Fractures: spiral/oblique orientation without a given twisting mechanism, multiple fractures of different ages, mechanism not consistent with history

Subdural hematoma: from violent shaking with cerebral atrophy and direct blow

Nutrition: dehydration, cachexia, weight loss, electrolyte abnormalities, fecal impaction

Drug levels: subtherapeutic or toxic, or presence of a drug not prescribed

Disease patterns: untreated chronic disorders, excessive exacerbations of chronic disease

Poor hygiene: filth, soiled with excrement, infestation, dental caries

Personal effects: inadequate clothing, shoes, glasses, hearing aid, dentures

Living conditions: fire hazard; infestation; inadequate heating, air conditioning, or plumbing

Psychological Abuse and Neglect

Communication: ambivalence, withdrawal, poor eye contact, cowering, noncommunication

Mood/affect: agitation, depression, passivity, anxiety, hopelessness

Behavior: fear, apprehensiveness, shame, paranoia, infantile behavior

Motor: involuntary movement, rocking, sucking, trembling

Psychosomatic: poor appetite, disturbed sleep patterns, post-traumatic stress disorder (may result from physical abuse as well)

Interactions: caregiver insists on remaining with the patient at all times, elder fearful of the caregiver

Sexual Abuse

Wounds: located over breasts or genitalia

Infection: new sexually transmitted disease without reported sexual activity

Bleeding: unexplained vaginal or anal bleeding

Pain/tenderness: on pelvic or rectal examination

Abandonment

Institutional desertion: leaving an elder at a hospital without means of return

Public desertion: leaving an elder at a public location to be picked up by police or emergency medical service

Homelessness

Self-Neglect

Many of the above

maintain a high index of suspicion and take appropriate steps to ensure the safety and well-being of the elder. Such measures may be extremely varied to meet the individual needs of each patient relative to the resources available to the provider. Communication with a reliable primary care physician to convey possible concerns and ensure follow-up may suffice in some cases. Hospital admission is always an option to guarantee what should be a safe environment and adequate care. The involvement of a geriatrics consult team, if available, may be appropriate, as may consultation with a hospital social worker or direct referral to an APS agency.

The physical examination and diagnostic workup in the ED likewise must be tailored to meet the individual patient's needs. A guideline with regard to elder care in general is to err on the side of conservative practice. If a test or procedure is being considered in the first place, then it should be ordered. The so-called cost-effective strategies and evidence-based medicine are often not in the best interests of the elderly. All practitioners should become patient advocates when treating the aged, especially when the possibility of abuse or neglect arises. The evaluation of the elderly involves, at a minimum, head-to-toe physical examination in a hospital gown, on a stretcher or a bed. Trying to examine a frail senior citizen with a physical or mental handicap who is fully or partially clothed and seated in a wheelchair will only do the patient a disservice. It may seem time consuming or inconvenient to perform this simple task, but only a meticulous examination will uncover occult findings that may be consistent with maltreatment. Ancillary data may include baseline laboratory tests, such as complete blood count, basic chemistry profile (CHEM-7, albumin), coagulation panel, urinalysis, and toxicology screen with drug levels if indicated. These tests may provide clues to aid in the evaluation of bruises, altered mental status, dehydration, and malnutrition. Radiographic evaluation of the elderly should also be utilized liberally. Unlike the abused pediatric population, no constellation or types of fracture patterns have been elucidated for abused elders (59). However, senior citizens are more likely to sustain fractures on the basis of bone demineralization, osteoporosis, or metastatic disease. Any significant bony tenderness or unexplained soft-tissue swelling should be considered a fracture until proved otherwise. Similarly, age-related cerebral atrophy and vein fragility contribute to the development of a subdural hematoma from even relatively mild head trauma (60). For this reason, a computed tomography scan of the brain should be an important part of the diagnostic workup in cases of suspected or possible elder abuse. Any history or evidence of sexual assault should be fully assessed by a trained forensic examiner specializing in this field by colposcopy, evidence collection, and venereal culturing. The neurologic evaluation should include an assessment of cognitive status. This can be administered through tools such as Folstein's Mini Mental State Examination (61) or the Short Portable Mental Status Questionnaire (62).

Even experienced providers can be fooled by findings that may mimic abuse. Skin bruises, for instance, may represent senile purpura (Fig. 10.3) or may develop secondary to thrombocytopenia or coagulopathy. Fractures that appear traumatic may actually be pathologic as a result of underlying disease. A senior with poor visual acuity may not be able to maintain good hygiene. Cachexia or weight loss can result from underlying malignancy. Certain cultural practices, such as spooning, coining, or moxibustion, endured willingly, leave wounds that mimic physical abuse (63).

Even if suspicious or questionable findings are present, the diagnosis of elder abuse or neglect may require more time than is practical for an emergency care provider. The primary goals of this provider are (a) to treat any active medical issues and (b) secure a safe environment for the elder until all issues can be addressed. If this safe environment is an acute care hospital bed at 10 p.m. on a Friday because no family is present or reliable or because the hospital's resources are unavailable, then this must

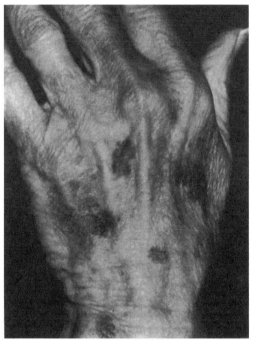

FIG. 10.3 Senile purpura. (Reprinted with permission from: Habif TP. Light-related diseases and disorders of pigmentation. In: Habif TP, ed. *Clinical dermatology: a color guide to diagnosis and therapy*, 3rd ed. St. Louis: Mosby-Year Book, 1996:601).

be the disposition. The emergency care provider must stand firm and act as the patient's advocate in this scenario, which may be met with resistance from administrators or gatekeepers.

Comprehensive evaluation includes the following:

- Patient demographics: name, age, social security number, address, phone number
- Physical health: medical history, medications, advance directive
- Functional status: limitations, normal activities of daily living
- Cognitive status: confusion, dementia
- Mental health: psychosis, depression
- Personal hygiene: cleanliness, appropriateness of clothing, continence
- Support system: family/friends with contact numbers
- Current care providers: names, relationship, and contact numbers
- Financial resources: income amount and sources
- Social situation: type of dwelling, living alone, isolated
- History of violence: domestic violence, in the past or current
- Physical examination
- Ancillary tests: radiography, laboratory studies

- Documentation of injuries/lesions: sketch and photographs
- Legal contacts: next of kin, power of attorney, conservator, and guarantor
- Safety in current living arrangement

Naturally, this information must be documented accurately. A descriptive narrative should be supplemented with sketches or diagrams of physical lesions. Photographs provide an excellent means of documentation. These must be labeled properly and should have some reference to scale in view and the means to positively identify the subject, such as an initial picture showing the victim from the waist up.

REASONS FOR ABUSE

The reasons for elder maltreatment are as varied as the individual elders themselves. They encapsulate a broad and complex range of physical, sociological, psychological, and cultural factors. Certainly, no single or simple explanation can account for such a complicated process. Many purported causes focus on sociological theories, which are of lesser importance to the practicing clinician, especially an emergency care provider. A thorough understanding is not necessary for the clinician to recognize, diagnose, treat, and refer cases of elder abuse or mistreatment; however, an overview is helpful. Many authors have examined the issue of why people mistreat their elders; no consensus has been reached.

Some theories focus on the impairment and dependence of the elder. Such a person would become more vulnerable to mistreatment by another. The perpetrator may be able to take advantage of the elder with less risk of being caught. Furthermore, a dependent elder may not report or corroborate an abusive situation because he or she might lose the caregiver. Some abusive family members report that a lack of gratitude in return for care given to an impaired victim has led to maltreatment (64). Perhaps more common is the following situation: an elderly person's impairments worsen over time, and eventually that person's needs exceed the caregiver's capacity to provide adequate care. The caregiver may simply ignore or neglect the situation or directly lash out at the elder. Another study found the opposite: that abused victims were not more likely to be functionally impaired than nonabused controls (65). Conversely, the more important aspect of the abuser–victim relationship was the perpetrator's dependence on the victim. In many cases, a caregiver may be financially or emotionally dependent on the elder. This could precipitate a dangerous situation in which a caregiver materially exploits an elder or attempts to assert authority over the victim to preserve a sense of power or dominance.

Some authors offer evidence to dispute the notion that abused elders are frailer than their nonabused counterparts (12,45,65–67).

Other characteristics of the abuser have led to psychoanalytic theory of abuse and neglect. Some authorities propose that the psychopathology of a perpetrator alone may be enough to precipitate mistreatment, particularly physical abuse (18). When the perpetrator is a child of the elder, an additional factor may be an unresolved filial crisis. This theory proposes that the child's relationship with his or her parent never advanced beyond the parent–child discord of adolescence. A mature relationship between adults was never cultivated as the child aged, and unresolved conflict that should have been settled as the adolescent developed contributes to later abuses (67). Additional theories focus on transgenerational family violence. These hypotheses pose that violence toward family members is a learned phenomenon that becomes a normative behavioral pattern among children who are exposed to it repeatedly while growing up. Some perpetrators actually report overt retaliation for past victimization as reasons to abuse or neglect elderly parents (8).

Another theory focuses on generalized discrimination against the elderly, known as *ageism*. Common myths held by many people that fuel ageism include senior citizens being unproductive and resistant to change. Often abusers and mistreaters correlate age with functional impairment and assume that all elderly individuals suffer from or will succumb to Alzheimer's disease. Nothing could be further from the truth. Although the cause of this debilitating form of dementia has yet to be fully elucidated, it is clear that age is only one of many factors (2). Unfortunately, many laypersons are not enlightened to the potential contributions and value of senior citizens and discriminate against them, either willfully or unknowingly.

The typical studies that attempt to understand "why" are small series of relatively few patients. Although interesting to behavioral scientists or sociological theorists, such conceptual models do not translate well into practical terms. It is easy for the clinician to become lost in a sea of social or behavioral hypotheses when attempting to understand elder abuse and neglect. Perhaps this is because elder mistreatment should not have a solid foundation in explanations, reasons, or causes. Too much explaining may lead to rationalization of these despicable acts, for which society should, under no circumstances, accept any justification.

REPORTING

The reporting of elder abuse and neglect is the cornerstone to intervention, treatment, and prevention. Most states have statutes that cover mandatory reporting of suspected elder abuse. Naturally, laws vary from state to state. Some states specifically name which professionals, such as health care providers, clergy, financial personnel, or long-term care employees must, by statute, report. Some states do not mandate the reporting of elder abuse by a health care provider specifically. Some states broadly sweep this statutory requirement upon anyone by stating that "any person" has a duty to report. Notably, a few states specifically do not mandate reporting as a statutory requirement for anyone, including a health care provider (68).

The Eldercare Locator, a national hotline, can be reached at 1-800-677-1116. Trained operators refer callers to the appropriate local agency. Table 10-9 lists by state the contact phone numbers for reporting suspected elder mistreatment. Reporting will aid in the understanding of this problem by providing additional databases for analysis. The source of any report to authorities may be the elder person; however, more commonly it is another person. That person could be someone with frequent and close contact, such as a family member or friend, or a professional with an episodic connection to the victim, such as a home health care provider, social worker, financial manager, nurse, or physician. The last group represents persons particularly accessible to improving the ability to detect elder mistreatment through awareness and education efforts. Unfortunately, physicians report elder abuse infrequently (51,69), despite the standpoint taken by

TABLE 10-9
STATE REPORTING CONTACTS

State	Domestic Elder Abuse	Institutional Elder Abuse
Alabama	800-458-7214	800-458-7214
Alaska	800-478-9996	800-730-6393
	907-269-3666	907-334-4483
Arizona	877-767-2385	877-767-2385
Arkansas	800-482-8049	800-582-4887
California	888-436-3600	800-231-4024
Colorado	303-866-2800	303-866-2800
	800-773-1366	800-773-1366
Connecticut	888-385-4225	860-424-5241
Delaware	800-223-9074	800-223-9074
District of Columbia	202-541-3950	202-434-2140
Florida	800-962-2873	800-962-2873
Georgia	404-657-5250	404-657-5728
	888-774-0152	888-878-6442
Hawaii, Oahu	808-832-5115	808-832-5115
Hawaii, Maui	808-243-5151	808-243-5151
Hawaii, Kauai	808-241-3432	808-241-3432
Hawaii, East Hawaii	808-933-8820	808-933-8820
Hawaii, West Hawaii	808-327-6280	808-327-6280
Idaho	208-334-3833	208-334-1899
Illinois	800-252-8966	800-252-4343
Indiana	800-992-6978	800-992-6978
Iowa	800-362-2178	515-281-4115
Kansas	800-922-5330	800-842-0078
	785-296-0044	
Kentucky	800-752-6200	800-752-6200
		800-372-2991
Louisiana	800-259-4990	800-259-4990
Maine	800-624-8404	800-624-8404
Maryland	800-917-7383	800-917-7383
Massachusetts	800-922-2275	800-462-5540

(continued)

TABLE 10-9

(Continued)

Michigan	800-996-6228	800-882-6006
Minnesota	800-333-2433	800-333-2433
	651-296-5563	651-296-0382
Mississippi	800-222-8000	800-227-7308
Missouri	800-392-0210	800-392-0210
Montana	800-551-3191	406-444-4077
	800-332-2272	
Nebraska	800-652-1999	800-652-1999
		402-595-1324
Nevada	800-992-5757	800-992-5757
New Hampshire	800-351-1888	800-442-5640
	603-271-4386	603-271-4396
New Jersey	800-792-8820	800-792-8820
New Mexico	800-797-3260	800-797-3260
	505-841-6100	505-841-6100
New York	800-342-3009	By region:
		Buffalo: 800-425-0314
		Hudson Valley: 800-425-0320
		Long Island: 800-425-0323
		NYC: 800-425-0316
		N. E. State: 800-220-7184
		Rochester: 800-837-9018
		Syracuse: 800-425-0319
North Carolina	800-662-7030	800-662-7030
North Dakota	800-451-8693	800-451-8693
Ohio	866-886-3537	800-282-1206
Oklahoma	800-522-3511	800-522-3511
Oregon	800-232-3020	800-232-3020
Pennsylvania	800-490-8505	800-254-5164
	717-783-6207	717-783-6207
Puerto Rico	787-725-9788	
	787-721-8225	
Rhode Island	401-462-0050	401-785-3340
South Carolina	800-868-7318	800-898-2850
South Dakota	605-773-3656	605-773-3656
Tennessee	888-277-8366	888-277-8366
Texas	512-834-3784	512-438-2633
	800-252-5400	800-458-9858
Utah	801-264-7669	801-264-7669
	800-371-7897	800-371-7897
Vermont	800-564-1612	800-564-1612
Virginia	888-832-3858	888-832-3858
	804-371-0896	804-371-0896
Washington	866-363-4276	800-562-6078
West Virginia	800-352-6513	800-352-6513
Wisconsin	608-266-2536	800-815-0015
		608-246-7013
Wyoming	307-777-6137	307-777-7123
		307-322-5553

Adapted from U.S. Department of Health and Human Services Administration on Aging and the Administration for Children and Families. *The national elder abuse incidence study,* Washington, DC: NCEA, 1998, and the National Center on Elder Abuse State Elder Abuse Hotlines, 2005.

the AMA that they "are in an ideal position to recognize, manage, and prevent elder mistreatment" (31). One facet of elder mistreatment that this mandate overlooks is provider awareness. Physicians are indeed in an ideal position to intervene, but only by first becoming better educated about this problem. The AMA's first step, recognition, can be achieved through better physician education. Studies suggest that the latter steps, improved management and prevention, should naturally follow when clinicians have an appropriate knowledge base (70). Unfortunately, formal training appears inadequate, with only 25% of residency-trained emergency physicians receiving any education in this area during their residencies.

Fortunately, overall reporting has increased. NCEA data indicate that in 1986 a total of 117,000 reports of elder mistreatment were received by state APS agencies. Each year thereafter for the next decade, the number of reports rose steadily (71), such that by 1996, the year of the NEAIS, this sum had grown to 293,000 nationwide (39). This remarkable increase of 150% may be attributed in part to increased awareness and dedication of resources and to mandatory reporting laws. Of note, over this period, the total elder population increased by only 10% (39). NEAIS data with regard to reporting of elder mistreatment are presented in Tables 10-10 and 10-11. Notable are the different distributions of reporters of self-neglect compared with those who report non–self-inflicted domestic abuse and neglect. The population projection estimates calculated by NCEA researchers concluded that more than five times as many events of mistreatment were unreported as were reported to authorities. Previously published data indicated that anywhere from 1 in 5 to as few as 1 in 14 cases were reported to APS agencies (7,31,69).

TABLE 10-10

NATIONAL ELDER ABUSE INCIDENCE STUDY (NEAIS) DATA: REPORTERS OF ELDER ABUSE AND NEGLECT (%)

Family	20
Hospitals	17.3
Law enforcement	11.3
In-home service providers	9.6
Friend/neighbor	9.1
Physician/nurse/medical clinic	8.4
Out-of-home service providers	5.2
Bank official	0.4
Public health officials	0.1
Victim	8.8
Others	5.1

TABLE 10-11

NATIONAL ELDER ABUSE INCIDENCE STUDY (NEAIS) DATA: REPORTERS OF SELF-NEGLECT (%)

Hospitals	19.8
Friend/neighbor	19.1
In-home service providers	12.3
Law enforcement	11.7
Physician/nurse/medical clinic	11.5
Out-of-home service providers	7.8
Family	6.5
Bank official	0.4
Public health officials	0.0
Victim	1.4
Others	26.5

The NEAIS did not differentiate among specific health care providers in its "hospitals" category. Therefore, these data cannot provide insight into physician reporting. Other statewide studies addressed this question specifically, with embarrassing results. A Michigan group sought to characterize reporting patterns among physicians by examining all reported cases of suspected elder abuse in Michigan from 1989 to 1993. In this state, more than 17,000 total cases were reported, with physicians supplying only 2% of the reports. Nonphysician health care providers performed more admirably, accounting for 26% of the total, and 25% of reports originated from social workers or mental health workers. Interestingly, the largest overall reporting body was the community at large (41%) (69). This may suggest that cases of elder mistreatment that went unreported in the community may be the most difficult to detect, even for physicians. The authors acknowledge that some extraneous factors may contribute to physicians' low representation, such as the delegation of reporting duties to other staff or electing not to report suspected cases. However, common sense dictates that major barriers exist in physician reporting of suspected elder abuse and neglect.

Elderly victims do not report abusive situations for a myriad of reasons. Traditionally, there have been considerable obstacles to the detection and reporting of elder mistreatment. This situation is not dissimilar to other forms of domestic violence, which until recently have been considered private matters exempt from public or government inquiry (2). Often victims do not come forward to keep the mistreatment a private affair. It is hoped that these ingrained beliefs will break down as society recognizes with increasing fervor its role in acknowledging elder abuse as a form of domestic violence. Some seniors, having been victims of ageism in the past, do not believe they will be considered trustworthy and honest historians when reporting abuse or mistreatment. Some, because of physical or emotional handicap, may have great difficulty communicating about this sensitive topic. Others hope that it will simply go away by itself. Some even learn to tolerate abuse or neglect as part of their lives, perhaps becoming convinced by a perpetrator that it is deserved. An elderly person may feel ashamed at reporting maltreatment, especially if he or she was duped, or if the perpetrator is a friend or family member. The victim may fear repercussions such as further or worsening abuse by a perpetrator if a report is made. He or she may fear separation from family or the loss of individual freedoms if the abuse is revealed. Alternatively, a victim may try to protect an abuser if the abuser is a friend or relative or the victim's only caregiver. Perhaps the most frightening prospect is the acceptance of maltreatment simply because a pattern of victimization has been established. This has been proposed to relate to elder abuse in a similar way to its application in the understanding of battered women, that is, some adult battered women show a pattern of repeated sexual assault as children. It is possible that this model extends into old age and contributes to abuse (2).

Differences in the perception of abusive situations among the elderly of various ethnic groups have recently been examined by two professors of social work using a sample of 90 elderly women (72). This approach is a novel and important one for gaining insight into the victims of elder mistreatment. All previous authorities from the diverse backgrounds of professionals who participate in elder care (medicine, nursing, social work, psychology) have focused on their skilled perceptions of what constitutes abuse of the elderly. Naturally, their definitions and classifications are based on formal education and training. Despite their good intentions, few of these authorities are senior citizens themselves, so a "grassroots" perspective is lacking. This survey examined lay seniors' views and acknowledged that these perceptions may not be entirely consistent with practitioners' judgments. Furthermore, certain significant cultural patterns of what would be defined as abuse and what would trigger help-seeking behavior were found among the three ethnic groups queried. Analysis of such behaviors and further studies should help professionals develop new and effective operational definitions and practical strategies for intervention.

For obvious reasons of protecting one's own interests, perpetrators do not report mistreatment. However, studies of abusers show that they tend to rationalize their actions and minimize or deny the

harm inflicted. Often perpetrators believe their actions to be justified because the victim was deserving of the consequences. They may feel provoked by an elderly person's behavior or demeanor to mistreat that person and not recognize that mistreatment is indeed occurring. Mentally ill or substance-abusing care providers may use their illness as an excuse for abusive or neglectful behavior, or their impairment may truly prevent them from knowing what they are doing. Even if an abuser expresses remorse after an incident, one study shows that this remorse is transient and the victim is eventually subjected to more and worsening abuses (2,73).

Barriers to reporting also exist within the medical community. Confusion over what constitutes abuse or neglect and over their varying definitions contributes. Other commonly cited reasons for poor physician reporting include fear of legal entanglements, unfamiliarity or ignorance of reporting statutes and procedures, fear of making a situation worse, and confidentiality issues and preserving the relationship with the patient (18,69,74,75). A national survey of more than 700 practicing emergency physicians performed in 1996 sought to gain insight into physician awareness and perceptions of this problem (76). This study revealed some startling results. Nearly one third of respondents characterized elder maltreatment as a rare occurrence, and more than 80% of physicians reported that they rarely asked elderly patients in the ED direct questions about mistreatment. These data correlate with an earlier survey of Alabama ED personnel, done in 1988. In Alabama, more than 22% of ED physicians believed that "very few" senior citizens were victims of abuse (77). A Connecticut-based research group found similar results when they reviewed more than 500 ED charts (78). These collectors used local APS data to compile a list of substantiated cases of community-based elder abuse. They then researched these elders' visits to local EDs in the 5 years prior to their initial identification by an APS agency as an abuse victim. Their trained reviewers retrospectively found that more than 37% of these visits were related with high probability to abuse, on the basis of the findings reported in the ED chart. Yet only 9% of these encounters resulted in an APS referral. Alarmingly, even in those cases of an obvious injury, physicians inquired about family violence less than 14% of the time. Table 10-12 lists the most commonly reported reasons for failure to report suspected elder mistreatment. This list reflects inadequacies in the system that must be addressed on local, state, and national levels by government agencies, private organizations, and professional societies to provide for the welfare of the abused and neglected elderly. To compound matters, the Policy Statement on the Management of Elder Abuse

TABLE 10-12
REASONS ELDER MISTREATMENT IS NOT REPORTED

Reasons	%
Minor injuries or subtle signs only	41
Victim denial	27
Unfamiliarity with reporting procedure	26
Unclear about definitions	19
Failure to recognize the mistreatment	19
Ignorance of reporting laws	18
Inadequate community resources to respond	17
Patient confidentiality concerns	4
Incident already reported	4
Patient was admitted	4
Fear of legal involvement	2
Liability risks	2
Belief that it is the victim's responsibility to report	2

Adapted from Jones JS, Veenstra TR, Seamon JP, et al. Elder mistreatment: national survey of emergency physicians. *Ann Emerg Med* 1997;30:473–479.

and Neglect, published in 1997 and reaffirmed in 2001 by the American College of Emergency Physicians (ACEP), places the emergency physician in direct conflict with the mandatory reporting laws that exist in most states in America (79). In this statement, ACEP opposes mandatory reporting of elder abuse and neglect when a patient is mentally competent. This mandate recognizes the "autonomy of the competent elder and the confidentiality of the relationship" with the patient. It does encourage the recognition and management of this problem and reporting events "when appropriate," in accordance with the patient's wishes. Certainly, many clinicians will encounter this ethical and legal dilemma as they become more familiar with elder abuse and treat its victims.

An important question to consider with a competent elder is how much weight should be given to that victim's assessment of the situation and what he or she desires as a plan of action (72). What may seem to a practitioner as a clear-cut case in which an elder would benefit from involvement of social services and/or law enforcement may not be perceived as such by the victim, perhaps with good reason. The clinician must not practice in a vacuum; one must be aware of hospital resources, local agencies, and state laws. There must be an open dialogue between the clinician and the elder, which involves family members or caregivers, if appropriate. The provider must listen to the patient and understand any hesitation to seek help, but the provider must also take the time to

explain his or her point of view. A sincere approach with free exchange may convince a reluctant patient that filing a report is the right thing to do. This way, both provider and patient are in agreement on the course of action. The physician should aggressively utilize institutional resources such as social workers and case managers, who are assuming a larger role and a more recognizable presence in EDs throughout the country. These providers may possess the training, insight, and skills to reach a reluctant elder. The quick solution would be to fall back on a mandatory reporting statute and to state there is no choice in the matter. However, this could impose another unwelcome circumstance on an already victimized senior citizen and prove to be counterproductive. It is advisable to sit down (literally) and try earnestly to persuade a competent elderly victim that help is available. Above all, any practitioner must act according to what he or she believes is in the best interests of the patient. Remember, the old man or old woman underneath the bedsheet is somebody's grandparent, just as the doctor or nurse behind the starched white coat is somebody's grandchild.

The genuine value of mandatory reporting was demonstrated by a study of the events reported in California in 1984, shortly after mandatory reporting was instituted in this state. The total number of reports increased dramatically in that year. Nearly 85% of victims willingly accepted help that was offered as a result of the report (80). Presumably, many of these elders would have declined to file a report on a voluntary basis, thereby being cast adrift until the next abusive or neglectful experience. The profound implications of this finding are difficult to dispute. More recently, a compilation of data from all states found that statutory requirements for mandatory reporting correlated positively with an increase in the absolute number of filed reports and with an increase in the number of investigations that were subsequently undertaken (81). Clearly, mandatory reporting serves to capture a group of vulnerable senior citizens and administer to them the service and care to which they are entitled. Providers must also be aware that, in jurisdictions in which mandatory reporting applies, failure to report an incident could subject that provider to sanctions, which can include criminal prosecution, punishment by a fine or a jail sentence, and civil liability (68).

The reporting of elder abuse or neglect naturally goes hand in hand with its detection. The training of medical providers in the recognition of elder mistreatment will serve the senior population when a victim interacts with the medical community. In 1999, the NCEA spearheaded a major initiative to improve the detection of maltreatment in the community at large and uncover the so-called hidden victims of abuse. This program, Community Sentinels for Elder Abuse Prevention, utilized average citizens who, through their jobs or volunteerism, naturally came into contact with a number of elderly persons on a regular basis. These laypersons were specifically trained to detect potential victims. The APS agencies in the communities where this program was launched all reported an increase in the number of referrals. By partnering with such community resources that are mobilized, health care providers can achieve even loftier goals. Overall awareness will be raised in 2006: June 15 of this year has been designated World Elder Abuse Awareness Day. Many national and global organizations are contributing to this event, which should serve to enlighten both the medical and the lay communities.

INSTITUTIONAL ABUSE

The expected growth of the elderly population will contribute to a dramatic rise in the number of senior citizens living in nursing homes or other institutions that provide all types and levels of care. The 2000 Census documented over 1.5 million people older than 65 living in nursing homes (22). Federal and state governments oversee and monitor almost all such facilities in this country. Their agencies estimate that 3.5 million elderly will occupy such institutions nationwide by the year 2030 (82). This will expose millions of elders to the possibility of institutional mistreatment. The types of abuse that occur in a residential or nursing facility are not particularly different from what has already been described with regard to domestic elder abuse and neglect. All of the previously mentioned forms of maltreatment can occur in an institutionalized setting. The perpetrator may be a staff member, as is most commonly the case, or the abuser may be a fellow resident/patient or an intruder. One form of mistreatment that is unique to a nursing facility is failure to establish and follow a long-term plan of care or rehabilitation for a patient (7,51). This can result in profound physical and emotional distress for an isolated and infirm senior citizen. Experienced practitioners who evaluate and treat nursing home patients on emergency or chronic bases need only remember the multitude of patients whose problem lists include the diagnosis "failure to thrive" to understand the potential scope of this problem. In addition, many disorders common to institutionalized patients, such as pressure sores, dehydration, and urinary tract infections, could likely be avoided with more attentive care.

Institutionalized elders are placed at risk by their vulnerable physical and cognitive states as well as by the inexperience and inadequate training of staff (7,31). The most likely staff perpetrators of this form of mistreatment are nurses' aides (2,83). These persons have the most contact with the patients but have the least training and the lowest educational status among professional care providers. Many nursing homes suffer from understaffing, insufficient funding, and high employee turnover (7,31). Often their employees receive no specific instruction in the care of the elderly and perform their duties without proper supervision. With these inadequacies, the results of a large survey of nursing facility care providers ($n = 577$) may not be terribly shocking: more than 20% of those interviewed reported having witnessed physical abuse committed by another staff member, and a full 70% reported having witnessed psychological abuse (14). Furthermore, 10% confessed that they themselves had committed an act of physical abuse, and 40% admitted guilt with regard to the infliction of psychological abuse (14). Naturally, such a survey would likely underreport the true number of abusive situations based on reporter bias, which makes these data even more striking. Of note, more than 60% of these employees were nursing aides, and fewer than 50% of the total had any training beyond high school.

The vast range in levels of care at different types of facilities contributes to the difficulty in monitoring for abuses. Facilities that provide skilled nursing services or some level of medical care are required to uphold certain standards of care. Such sites are typically more actively regulated than a boarding facility for the elderly with mild cognitive impairments who do not need nursing supervision (31). Since the 1990s, there has been tremendous political effort to settle on a "Patient's Bill of Rights" for all Americans. Nursing home residents have been fortunate to have this agenda legislated since 1987 as the Nursing Home Reform Act. This law set national standards of care for nursing facilities and provided specific rights to which each resident is entitled. Such rights protect patients from all forms of abuse, inappropriate use of restraints, and Medicaid discrimination. This law guarantees access to advocates such as a personal physician and an ombudsman. Although the mere existence of such a law does not necessarily mean that it is being obeyed, it provides for investigation and supervision by the federal Office of the Inspector General and stiff penalties for violations. It is an important step toward ensuring proper care for institutionalized senior citizens. The NCEA recently conducted a review of the literature on preventing abuse in nursing homes and other such institutions (84). Useful strategies that were identified included strict enforcement of mandatory reporting, improving employees' working conditions, creating and supporting resident councils, and comprehensive screening and background checks during hiring.

THE PHYSICIAN, THE LAW, AND ETHICS

It is of paramount importance that clinicians familiarize themselves with the laws regarding elder abuse in the state(s) in which they practice. The federal OAA, while providing definitions and funding research and training in elder mistreatment, is much more limited in its scope than current federal laws covering child abuse and domestic violence. Therefore, individual state's laws are even more pertinent to everyday practical management of this problem. The first statutes appeared in 1977, and as of mid-1999 all 50 states plus the District of Columbia had specific statutes that address elder abuse and neglect. In general, each jurisdiction has statutes that cover three categories of elder care: APS, institutional abuse, and a long-term care ombudsman program (LTCOP) (85).

It is not possible or practical in this chapter to detail each state's specific codes. Rather, the clinician should be aware that wide variation exists with regard to each individual state's requirements and specifications. For instance, many states have no separate law for institutionalized elders. Those that do define "institution" or "long-term care facility" differently. Furthermore, some states include mental health sites under the umbrella of "institutional," whereas others specifically do not. In general, all state laws will define abuse, provide social services for victims, delineate eligibility for services, and institute a means for reporting and investigation. Here again one encounters the problem of jurisdictional variability. Definitions and terminology differ from state to state, as do the ages and circumstances around which a victim may receive help from APS. Some states include both acts of commission and acts of omission as prohibited conduct, whereas others do not. In many states, it is not enough merely to be a mistreated or neglected senior citizen; there must also exist some defined statutory disability or impairment to apply a state APS law. Specific types of abuse, such as sexual assault, may be separately categorized. Most states require reporting of suspected elder abuse or neglect to appropriate authorities. However, some jurisdictions allow reporting on a voluntary basis.

The LTCOP exists specifically to provide an advocate for residents of a long-term care facility. The role and authority of the ombudsman vary from state to state, but in general this person acts to ensure that residents' rights under federal laws are being protected and not violated. He or she interacts with law enforcement and local or state APS as appropriate if an inquiry leads to suspected abuse or criminal activity. Certainly much of what is considered elder maltreatment is criminal. A perpetrator may be prosecuted under criminal laws that pertain to the nature of the abuse, such as assault, theft, and rape. Some states have enacted specific criminal laws that address crimes against the elderly, often with stiffer penalties (85). These jurisdictions may classify forms of elder mistreatment as felonies, misdemeanors, or either, depending on legal specifications. Some states specifically reclassify a crime to a higher offense when the victim is a senior citizen (86). Often the age of a victim is used as an aggravating factor at a sentencing proceeding. Although this subject is very daunting, the busy practitioner need not be an expert in the law to manage these victims. He or she must have an overall familiarity with the laws that pertain in his or her jurisdiction. More importantly, the clinician must acknowledge this lack of expertise and utilize appropriate services and agencies to provide optimal care in an unfortunate situation.

Mandatory reporting clauses have triggered a volatile debate among providers. Currently, all but nine states have legislated mandatory reporting of suspected elder mistreatment. The so-called voluntary states are Colorado, Kentucky, Illinois, New Jersey, New York, North Dakota, Pennsylvania, South Dakota, and Wisconsin (68,86). Even within this narrow sphere of reference, jurisdictional variability persists: each state has designated different professionals as mandatory reporters. In general, persons such as physicians, nurses, and mental health or social workers are almost always included among those required by statute to report. Some states specifically include others, such as attorneys, dentists, clergy members, and even ambulance personnel (86). As previously discussed, such laws may place a practitioner at odds with a patient's wishes and with ACEP's policy statement. With regard to the latter, a closer examination of this policy reveals that it opposes mandatory reporting specifically to the criminal justice system. Notably absent is a mention of reporting to a social services agency or to a hospital social worker. Depending on individual state laws, a report made to APS may or may not automatically trigger notification of law enforcement. Most practicing clinicians will not know this unless they are intimately familiar with their state's provisions. Furthermore, even if a report is made, some statutes specifically enable the elder to refuse an investigation. If the mental competency of an elder is in question, ACEP's policy implies no opposition to mandatory reporting. Certainly, clinicians would agree with this on all levels. It is the situation of a competent elderly person refusing intervention that presents a legal and ethical dilemma. The legal predicament is fairly concrete: a law may mandate the practitioner to act specifically against a patient's wishes. If push comes to shove, the provider has a statutory requirement to report suspected elder abuse in those jurisdictions. Most states with such laws include provisions for reporter immunity from any liability associated with compliance.

The ethical predicament of filing an unwelcome report, either for legal reasons or because the clinician truly believes that doing so is in the patient's best interests, may be more disturbing to practitioners. Such a quandary deserves a forum for dialogue and discussion. There is a paucity of information available in the medical literature that addresses this ethical issue, yet this is the concern that may place the greatest emotional burden on both the elder and the clinician. Our enlightened society champions the potential contributions of senior citizens and encourages them to act as independently thinking, productive members. However, a case of elder mistreatment may force a practitioner to usurp a person's most basic societal liberty: the freedom to choose how to manage his or her life. A provider, naturally, should always strive for what is in a patient's best interests. It is highly likely that reporting a case of elder abuse to an appropriate APS agency or a hospital social work department would benefit an elder. The likelihood that harm will be done is low. Even an uncooperative victim of abuse or neglect at the very least becomes known to APS. This way, periodic checks can be made and the elder becomes aware of available services. These small steps toward making initial contact may avert a disastrous future event.

Opponents of mandatory reporting clauses commonly cite four distinct reasons. First is the violation of the elder's right to self-determination. Elderly people are presumed competent, unless examination suggests otherwise, and critics maintain that taking this decision away from them perpetuates ageism. Second, detractors allude to patient–physician confidentiality and the need for the clinician to establish a relationship based on trust. Another potential shortcoming is that mandatory reporting may discourage self-reporting and may deter an elder from seeking help on his or her own. Lastly, some opponents fear that mandatory reporting will overwhelm already overburdened social services with reports that lack validity. These concerns should be considered. Likewise, strong arguments exist for mandatory reporting. The most important considerations and the central themes that the clinician must always revisit are the safety and welfare of the elder. This may supersede confidentiality or self-determination interests. Legally, the inclusion of immunity clauses for mandatory reporters legislates that the duty to disclose and report indeed outweighs other factors such as confidentiality. Some language goes as far as specifically waiving patient–physician privilege (87). Furthermore, a senior citizen may already feel deterred from self-reporting and may not have the

benefit of adequate support to choose freely whether or not to file a report. Another consideration is that there may be a public good served by reporting elder abuse. If the maltreatment constitutes criminal activity, then the public at large, in addition to the victim, stands to benefit from reporting and prosecution.

A practitioner who is subject to mandatory reporting may be held criminally or civilly liable for failing to comply with a statutory requirement. Most statutes designate that a willful act of noncompliance is a criminal offense. Fortunately for practicing clinicians, the enforcement of such clauses is very rare (86). Of more concern to practitioners should be civil liability. The civil courts have traditionally been used to hold medical providers accountable, and this circumstance does not change with regard to elder abuse. Most laws stipulate that a reporter need have only a reasonable level of suspicion that maltreatment exists to initiate a report. A provider is expected to uphold this standard and can be held liable if failure to report results in damages to a victim.

A new twist on civil liability recently emerged. In 1997, a California physician was sued in civil court for both malpractice and elder abuse for allegedly undertreating a hospice patient for pain (88). The use of elder abuse statutory violations in this case placed the defendant at greater risk. There are no restrictions placed on pain and suffering awards based on elder abuse claims, whereas damages claimed in traditional malpractice cases in California are limited to $250,000 under that state's Medical Injury Compensation Reform Act (MICRA). A jury awarded the family of the deceased the sum of $1.5 million. The judge reduced the amount of the award to the traditional limit of $250,000, which was upheld at appeal. Despite the judicial restraint imposed on the verdict, the jury's decision reflects the public's willingness to sympathize with suffering patients and the claimant's attorneys' ingenuity to discover novel ways to circumvent tort reform and financial caps on malpractice awards. Indeed, a website that gives guidelines and background on "using state elder abuse laws in pain treatment cases" has been posted (89). Two more recent California court decisions upheld efforts to evade MICRA restrictions and allowed claimants to bring suits against physicians under elder abuse statutes. This type of threat may be used as leverage against health care providers and organizations to force a monetary settlement before a jury trial ensues.

Other legal issues that clinicians encounter frequently when treating elderly patients involve decision-making power. A competent elder is presumed capable of making decisions. Furthermore, such a competent person may revoke or change any previous agreement that was entered into voluntarily. All states have laws that enable a senior citizen to grant someone else the power of attorney. Statutes vary, but essentially such an agreement must be entered into voluntarily and while the granter is competent. The term "durable" refers to a clause that specifically permits the power of attorney to continue after the granter becomes incompetent and therefore incapable of revoking this power. It should be noted that not all power-of-attorney agreements contain a durable clause. Typically, such power is classified into two separate areas: health care/medical decision-making and financial matters. The specifics of different agreements vary: one person may hold joint power of attorney in both areas, or different people may hold power in each area. Likewise, an elder may appoint a financial manager but not specifically a medical attorney. Sometimes state courts will appoint a person to have power of attorney when an elder is unable to perform this duty. This appointee is called a guardian or conservator.

More recently, additional efforts at the federal level have been ongoing to champion the cause of elder Americans. The Elder Justice Act was first introduced into Congress in its 2003 session and is scheduled for reintroduction. If this bill is passed, several landmark developments would be legislated. Administratively, this act would establish an Office for Elder Justice in both the U.S. Department of Health and Human Services and the U.S. Department of Justice. A provision also exists for the creation of an office of APS within the U.S. Department of Health and Human Services. These offices would coordinate, at the federal level, national efforts to prevent elder abuse and neglect and enhance law enforcement. Another important mandate included in this proposal is to require by law an FBI criminal background check for nursing aides employed by long-term care institutions (90). One advocacy group, the National Association of State Units on Aging (NASUA), exists to advance policies that promote elder and dependent adult health and welfare. This group submitted a comprehensive proposal for reform of the OAA when that act comes before Congress for reauthorization. The NASUA drafted specific statutory language to change certain elements of the OAA. These changes are designed to increase federal funding to programs designated under the OAA, broaden the federal government's role, add programs specifically to meet special needs of older persons with dementia, and establish funds to begin evidence-based research into elder health (91). These initiatives are intended to promote independence, health, and safety among the diverse and growing elder population.

Practitioners should be familiar with the terminology that applies in their jurisdiction to meet the needs of the elderly patient. One must also be wary that guardians, conservators, and attorneys are not exempt from perpetrating abuse against those whose interests they have agreed to serve. Prudent clinicians should also become familiar with applicable legal trends and decisions in their states of practice.

CONCLUSION

Unfortunately, the specter of elder abuse is alarmingly prevalent among senior citizens today. It is a difficult problem to understand and study, with a multitude of causative factors. Therefore, a simple solution is lacking. Fortunately, however, elder mistreatment has become more visible through interdisciplinary recognition of patterns of abuse and neglect, resource availability, and legislative action. As shocked as medical professionals and members of the community at large should be at such transgressions, we must not stand still with mouths agape. Medical professionals especially should hail the opportunity to affect the life of an elderly person so profoundly. We are familiar with helping the elderly through many trying times: an acute disease process, new limitations set by a debilitating condition, and the illness or death of a spouse or loved one, to name a few. All clinicians have taken specific action toward the healing of the bodies and the minds of elders stricken with many conditions: heart failure, stroke, Parkinson's disease, dementia, and others. We must add elder mistreatment to the list of common diseases of the elderly and always be on guard to diagnose, treat, and intervene on behalf of a victim. A critical point for the emergency care provider is that any suspected case of elder mistreatment should be reported. It is not necessary for the provider to be the accuser, the judge, or the jury. Indeed, the provider must shun these roles and remain an objective observer, all the while being an advocate for the patient without being judgmental. The provider must simply recognize that a situation deleterious to the patient may be occurring. In many cases, such a situation will be neglect because a caretaker is overwhelmed or uneducated about proper care for the elder in his or her charge. Often a caregiver welcomes outside involvement that assists in providing better overall physical and emotional care for an elderly individual.

A proactive approach can help: hospitals and communities need to provide adequate resources that are easily accessible to clinicians and potential victims. Legislative bodies must allocate more funds for research, treatment, and intervention. The elderly must be sought out, reminded of their rights, and informed that people and resources are willing and able to help them. Hospital protocols should be developed in advance and all personnel well versed in their application. To do any less, or to ignore a potential abusive or neglectful situation, can result in more harm to a potential victim. Clinicians universally are instructed to "do no harm," yet many may not realize the damaging consequences of passive acquiescence. Through such vigilance, the physical, emotional, and financial welfare of our senior citizens can be preserved, protected, and cultivated as we await their next contribution to our lives.

APPENDIX: THE NATIONAL ELDER ABUSE INCIDENCE STUDY

The NEAIS primarily sought to answer one question: what is the incidence of domestic elder abuse and neglect in the United States? The study employed rigorous definitions and methodology to collect and interpret data. Its figures were utilized to calculate an estimate of national elder abuse incidence within a 95% confidence interval. NEAIS was designed to limit its scope to cases of domestic, not institutional, elder mistreatment because of legislative directive. Specifically, the Family Violence Prevention and Services Act of 1996 (PL 102–295) mandated that the abuse, neglect, and exploitation of elderly Americans be studied so as to prevent family violence in the domestic setting. Therefore, elderly residents of nursing homes, group homes, assisted-living facilities, acute or subacute care hospitals, or any institution were not included. If the incidence data presented in this chapter seem lower than expected, consider that many thousands of cases of elder abuse do occur in such establishments (14). Cases of self-neglect were reported separately. The congressional legislation provided for funding of this study through the Administration for Children and Families and the Administration on Aging, both under the auspices of the U.S. Department of Health and Human Services. The NCEA performed the research through both the American Public Welfare Association and a private survey research company with experience in domestic violence survey techniques. Data were collected from a nationally representative sample of 20 counties in 15 states over 8-week-long blocks of time in 1996. The study periods in different counties were staggered throughout 1996 to account for seasonal variation.

Researchers classified elder mistreatment into the seven types of maltreatment listed in Table 10-3. They defined their terms explicitly, and one instance of any kind of mistreatment was sufficient to include an elder as a victim. Standardized definitions were drafted for NEAIS by a panel of experts after an analysis of states' nomenclature, local discussions, and consensus meetings. NEAIS used two sets of sources in each selected county to acquire data: social services agencies and designated community sentinels. Local APS or Area Agency on Aging (AAA) organizations contributed the reports that came to the database during the study weeks. These reports may or may not have been substantiated by that agency, and only substantiated reports were considered positive. Details with regard to the nature of the abuse, the characteristics of both the victim and the perpetrator, and the original informant were also collected.

Sampling local APS offices is a useful means of gaining insight into elder abuse. However, one of the inherent flaws is that for a case of elder abuse or neglect to be recorded, it must be recognized and reported to that agency. As with all types of domestic violence, many incidents go unreported. This reality has been described as the "iceberg theory" (Fig. 10.4). Only a small portion of an iceberg is visible above the water line. The larger submerged segment cannot be seen and its true dimensions remain unknown. Similarly, the unreported elder mistreatment cases lurk below the tip of the iceberg and somewhere beyond any APS agency's outreach program.

To capture elder abuse cases not initially reported, a sentinel approach was also used. This approach had already been developed as an alternative to general population studies. It has been used in large national incidence studies of child abuse (92). The sentinels were people in the community who had frequent contact with the elderly but were not APS case workers. More than 1,100 law enforcement officers, hospital workers, elder care providers, home nurses, bank employees, and other citizens of the study areas were independently selected to perform this duty. They received specialized training to recognize the signs and symptoms of all forms of elder mistreatment. Because sentinels directly observed cases of elder abuse, neglect, or self-neglect, these cases were presumed substantiated. Sentinels reported any instances directly to NEAIS; some also reported their cases to the appropriate APS agency. Investigators accounted for this circumstance by eliminating any duplication of a reported case from the database. Likewise, a single elder was included only once in the study, even if he or she was the victim of more than one episode of maltreatment during the study period. In this manner, incidence, not prevalence, could be determined.

APS sources contributed 1,466 cases of elder abuse, neglect, and self-neglect to NEAIS prior to their substantiation. Sentinels contributed 140 cases, bringing the total number of unduplicated cases for study to 1,606. NEAIS investigators incorporated a sophisticated system of weighting and adjustment to their data and used population statistics to calculate an estimated national number of case reports of domestic elder mistreatment. By the APS figures,

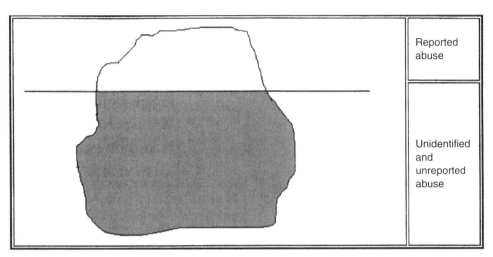

FIG. 10.4   Iceberg theory of elder abuse. (Reproduced from The National Elder Abuse Incidence Study. Prepared by *The national center on elder abuse at The American Public Health Services Association* in collaboration with Westat, Inc., September 1998).

this study estimated that in 1996 there were more than 236,000 unduplicated reports of domestic elder maltreatment (abuse, neglect, or self-neglect) filed in the United States. This estimated number is comparable to the actual total number of case reports received by all state APS agencies that year, 290,314. The gap between these numbers would close when one considers that the latter figure does not account for duplication of cases or repeatedly victimized elders. Indeed, before NEAIS statisticians adjusted for duplication, the estimated number of national APS reports was more than 286,000. The difference between this unadjusted estimate and the actual total is less than 1.5%, demonstrating the accuracy of the NEAIS estimate. Of these reports, nearly half are substantiated. This percentage figure actually underestimated the number of truly abusive or neglectful circumstances because nonsubstantiation of a report does not guarantee that such a situation is absent. Rather, an unsubstantiated report of elder mistreatment might mean that levels of proof or other statutory requirements were not met but a dangerous condition might still exist. Also, some cases still remained under active investigation when researchers compiled data. Other investigations were terminated because the alleged victim declined to cooperate, died, moved, or otherwise was lost to follow-up. Surely some of these reported events would have achieved substantiation. Figure 10.5 depicts the outcomes of APS investigations.

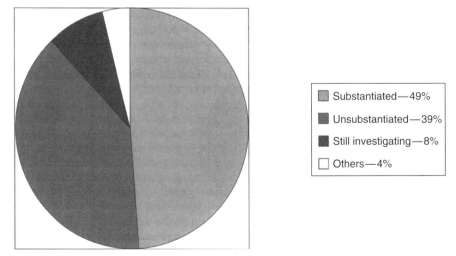

FIG. 10.5   NEAIS data: outcomes of APS investigations.

It is unclear why NEAIS researchers selected age greater than 60 years for their definition of elderly; most previous studies on elder abuse and elder utilization of services chose age greater than 65 years (13,17,21,25,26,37,43,52,53,78,93). A limitation of the sentinel method involves an inherent underestimation of abused or neglected elders. The sole basis for the use of sentinels is that they will have contact with the elderly in the community. However, unlike child abuse where school represents a universal community institution where all children must congregate, no such place exists for the elderly. Therefore, the most isolated seniors, who may be at the greatest risk, rarely leave home to interact with a community member. Additionally, the NEAIS investigators acknowledge that many of their data have wide confidence intervals because of a small sample size. More resources dedicated to expanding the sample size and lengthening the study time could limit the confidence intervals and provide more accurate and precise statistical estimates. One additional criticism not identified by the authors concerns reporting by the sentinels. The presumption of NEAIS is that victims reported to the study by sentinels would have gone unnoted by APS. This is not necessarily true. Perhaps the sentinel, even without specific training for the purposes of this study, would have recognized a possible case of abuse, neglect, or exploitation and reported it to APS or other authorities. After all, the sentinel did by definition have contact with the elder. Many were trained observers, such as police officers, nurses, and physicians, whose skills may have enabled them to detect a suspicious situation prior to NEAIS training. Despite its flaws, this study represents the most comprehensive effort to date and shall serve as a foundation for continued research and awareness well into the 21st century.

NEAIS indicated that the most common form of domestic maltreatment involved neglect. Self-neglect was the most common type overall, uncovered in 38% of all substantiated APS and sentinel reports. When self-neglect cases were excluded, neglect still represented the most common mistreatment of the remaining incidents, nearly 50%. Table 10-13 lists the percentage of types of maltreatment discovered in all the substantiated cases. This analysis is consistent with an earlier NARCEA survey that found that more than half of all cases of domestic maltreatment reported to APS agencies in 1990 and 1991 involved self-neglect (18). The distribution of harm types for the remaining cases demonstrated that the most prevalent form of non–self-perpetrated mistreatment was still neglect. Table 10-14 summarizes this information. Self-neglect and neglect were also the most common

TABLE 10-13

NATIONAL ELDER ABUSE INCIDENCE STUDY (NEAIS) DATA: ANALYSIS OF SUBSTANTIATED CASES WITH DISTRIBUTION OF HARM TYPES (%)

Physical	25.6
Psychological	35.4
Financial/material	30.2
Neglect	48.7
Abandonment	3.6
Sexual	0.3
Others	1.4

aberrant behaviors among a cohort of elders living in New Haven, Connecticut, who were longitudinally studied for more than 10 years (93). Other researchers with more narrow inclusion criteria for neglect have published prevalence data showing neglect to be much less common than other forms (Table 10-4). Neglect may be the most difficult type of harm to prove. This is suggested by the substantiation rates found in NEAIS, which are shown in Table 10-14. Only about half of all cases reported to APS in 1996 met validation requirements. As one might expect, physical abuse was the type of maltreatment most frequently verified. APS workers in the individual New Haven area were able to substantiate all forms of neglect with greater frequency than the rate reported by NEAIS's national compilation of agencies (93). Their data show verification rates of 78% for self-neglect, 71% for neglect, and 75% for abuses. Variance from state to state would be expected because of differences in individual statutes and availability of resources. In any case, all types of abuse and neglect are sufficiently prevalent to warrant concern among health care providers.

TABLE 10-14

NATIONAL ELDER ABUSE INCIDENCE STUDY (NEAIS) DATA: SUBSTANTIATION RATES FOR ADULT PROTECTIVE SERVICES (APS) REPORTS (%)

All case types	48.7
Physical	61.9
Psychological	54.1
Financial/material	44.5
Neglect	41.0
Abandonment	56.0
Sexual	N/A

REFERENCES

1. Davidson JL. Elder abuse. In: Block MR, Sinnott JD, eds. *The battered elder syndrome: an exploratory study.* College Park: University of Maryland, 1979:49–66.
2. Quinn MJ, Tomita SK. *Elder abuse and neglect,* 2nd ed. New York: Springer-Verlag, 1997:9–10.
3. Stearns PN. Old age conflict: the perspective of the past. In: Wolf R, Pillemer K, eds. *Elder abuse: conflict in the family.* Dover: Auburn House, 1986:3–29.
4. Attorney General's Task Force on Family Violence. *Final report.* Washington, DC: US Government Printing Office, 1984.
5. Burston GR. Granny-battering. *Br Med J* 1975;3:592.
6. Baker AA. Granny battering. *Mod Geriatr* 1975;5:20–24.
7. Aravanis SC, Adelman RD, Breckman R, et al. Diagnostic and treatment guidelines on elder abuse and neglect. *Arch Fam Med* 1993;2:371–381.
8. Wolf RS. Elder abuse: ten years later. *J Am Geriatr Soc* 1988;36:758–762.
9. Kurrle SE, Sadler PM, Cameron ID. Elder abuse: an Australian case series. *Med J Aust* 1991;155:150–153.
10. Kurrle S. Abuse of the elderly: a hidden problem. *Aust Fam Physician* 1992;21:1742–1748.
11. Ogg J, Bennett G. Elder abuse in Britain. *Br Med J* 1992; 305:998–999.
12. Homer AC, Gilleard C. Abuse of elderly people by their caregivers. *Br Med J* 1990;301:1359–1362.
13. Lachs MS, Berkman L, Fulmer T, et al. A prospective community-based pilot study of risk factors for the investigation of elder mistreatment. *J Am Geriatr Soc* 1994;42:169–173.
14. Pillemer K, Moore DW. Abuse of patients in nursing homes: findings from a survey of staff. *Gerontologist* 1989; 29:314–320.
15. Coyne AC, Reichman WE, Berbig LJ. The relationship between dementia and elder abuse. *Am J Psychiatry* 1993;150:643–646.
16. Reis M, Nahmiash D. Validation of the Indicators of Abuse (IOA) screen. *Gerontologist* 1998;38:471–480.
17. Pillemer K, Finkelhor D. The prevalence of elder abuse: a random sample survey. *Gerontologist* 1988;29:51–57.
18. Rosenblatt DE. Elder mistreatment. *Crit Care Nurs Clin North Am* 1997;9:183–192.
19. Kosberg JI. Preventing elder abuse: identification of high risk factors prior to placement decisions. *Gerontologist* 1988; 28:43–50.
20. U.S. Bureau of the Census. *Sixty-five plus in America.* Curr Popul Rep (Special Studies), Series 1023-178, 1992.
21. Strange GR, Chen EH, Sanders AB. Use of emergency departments by elderly patients: projections from a multi-center data base. *Ann Emerg Med* 1992;21:819–824.
22. U.S. Census Bureau. *The 65 years and over population: 2000.* Census 2000 Brief. 2001.
23. Schneider EL, Guralnik JM. The aging of America: impact on health care costs. *JAMA* 1990;263:2335–2340.
24. American Association of Retired Persons. *A profile of older Americans.* Washington, DC, 1994.
25. McNamara RM, Rousseau E, Sanders AB. Geriatric emergency medicine: a survey of practicing emergency physicians. *Ann Emerg Med* 1992;21:796–801.
26. Lowenstein SR, Crescenzi CA, Kern DC, et al. Care of the elderly in the emergency department. *Ann Emerg Med* 1986;15:529–535.
27. Baum SA, Rubenstein LZ. Old people in the emergency room: age-related differences in emergency department use and care. *J Am Geriatr Soc* 1987;35:398–404.
28. Gerson LW, Skvarch L. Emergency medical service utilization by the elderly. *Ann Emerg Med* 1982;11:610–612.
29. Spaite DW, Cris EA, Valenzuela TD, et al. Geriatric injury: an analysis of prehospital demographics, mechanisms, and patterns. *Ann Emerg Med* 1990;19:1418–1421.
30. Tatara T. *Elder abuse in the United States: an issue paper.* Washington, DC: NARCEA, 1990.
31. Aravanis SC, Adelman RD, Breckman R, et al. *Diagnostic and treatment guidelines on elder abuse.* Chicago: American Medical Association, 1992.
32. Hudson MF. Elder mistreatment: its relevance to older women. *J Am Med Women's Assoc* 1997;52:142–146.
33. Fulmer TT, O'Malley TA. *Inadequate care of the elderly: a health perspective on abuse and neglect.* New York: Springer-Verlag, 1987.
34. Tatara T. *NARCEA's suggested state guidelines for gathering and reporting domestic elder abuse statistics for compiling national data.* Washington, DC: NARCEA, 1990.
35. Lau EE, Kosberg JI. Abuse of the elderly by informal care providers. *Proceedings of the annual meeting of the Gerontological Society,* Dallas, TX, 1978:10–15.
36. Kosberg JI, Nahmiash D. Characteristics of victims and perpetrators and milieus of abuse and neglect. In: Baumhover LA, Beall SC, eds. *Abuse, neglect, and exploitation of older persons: strategies for assessment and intervention.* Baltimore, MD: Health Professions Press, 1996:31–49.
37. Lachs MS, Williams MA, O'Brien S, et al. The mortality of elder mistreatment. *JAMA* 1998;280:428–432.
38. Jones J, Dougherty J, Schelble D, et al. Emergency department protocol for the diagnosis and evaluation of geriatric abuse. *Ann Emerg Med* 1988;17:1006–1015.
39. U.S. Department of Health and Human Services Administration on Aging and the Administration for Children and Families. *The national elder abuse incidence study.* Washington, DC: NCEA, 1998.
40. Johnson T. Critical issues in the definition of elder mistreatment. In: Pillemer K, Wolf R, eds. *Elder abuse: conflict in the family.* Dover: Auburn House, 1986:167–196.
41. Fulmer TT, Gould ES. Assessing neglect. In: Baumhover LA, Beall SC, eds. *Abuse, neglect, and exploitation of older persons: strategies for assessment and intervention.* Baltimore, MD: Health Professions Press, 1996:89–103.
42. Lachs MS, Pillemer K. Abuse and neglect of elderly persons. *N Engl J Med* 1995;332:437–443.
43. Lachs MS, Williams C, O'Brien S, et al. Risk factors for reported elder abuse and neglect: a nine-year observational cohort study. *Gerontologist* 1997;37:469–474.
44. Tatara T. *Suggested state guidelines for gathering and reporting domestic elder abuse statistics for compiling national data.* Washington, DC: National Aging Resource Center on Elder Abuse, 1990.
45. McCreadie C. Introduction: the issues, practice and policy. In: Eastman M, ed. *Old age abuse: a new perspective.* London: Chapman & Hall, 1994:3–22.
46. O'Malley TA, O'Malley HC, Everitt DE, et al. Categories of family mediated abuse and neglect of elderly persons. *J Am Geriatr Soc* 1984;32:362–369.
47. Sengstock MC, Steiner SC. Assessing nonphysical abuse. In: Baumhover LA, Beall SC, eds. *Abuse, neglect, and exploitation of older persons: strategies for assessment and intervention.* Baltimore, MD: Health Professions Press, 1996:105–122.
48. Blazer DG. The epidemiology of psychiatric disorders in late life. In: Busse EU, Blazer DG, eds. *Geriatric psychiatry.* Washington, DC: American Psychiatric Press, 1989:235–262.
49. Tatara T. Understanding the nature and scope of domestic elder abuse with the use of state aggregate data: summaries of

the key findings of a national survey of state APS and aging agencies. *J Elder Abuse Negl* 1993;5:35–57.

50. Wilkinson TJ, Sainsbury R. Diagnosis related groups based funding and medical care of the elderly: a form of elder abuse? *NZ Med J* 1995;108:63–65.

51. Kleinschmidt KC. Elder abuse: a review. *Ann Emerg Med* 1997;30:463–472.

52. Comijs HC, Pot AM, Smit JH, et al. Elder abuse in the community: prevalence and consequences. *J Am Geriatr Soc* 1998;46:885–888.

53. Paveza GJ, Cohen D, Eisdorfer C, et al. Severe family violence and Alzheimer's disease: prevalence and risk factors. *Gerontologist* 1992;32:493–497.

54. German PS, Shapiro S, Skinner EA, et al. Detection and management of mental health problems of older patients by primary care providers. *JAMA* 1987;257:489–493.

55. Jolley S, Jolley D. Psychiatry. In: Pathy MSJ, ed. *Principles and practice of geriatric medicine*, 3rd ed. London: John Wiley and Sons, 1998:1031–1053.

56. Steiner RP, Vansickle K, Lippmann SB. Domestic violence: do you know when and how to intervene? *Domestic Violence* 1996;100:103–116.

57. O'Brien JG. Screening: a primary care clinician's perspective. In: Baumhover LA, Beall SC, eds. *Abuse, neglect, and exploitation of older persons: strategies for assessment and intervention*. Baltimore, MD: Health Professions Press, 1996:51–64.

58. Ramsey-Klawsnik H. Assessing physical and sexual abuse in health care settings. In: Baumhover LA, Beall SC, eds. *Abuse, neglect, and exploitation of older persons: strategies for assessment and intervention*. Baltimore, MD: Health Professions Press, 1996:67–87.

59. Lachs MS, Fulmer T. Recognizing elder abuse and neglect. *Geriatr Emerg Care* 1993;9:665–681.

60. Levy DB, Hanlon DP, Townsend RN. Geriatric trauma. *Geriatr Emerg Care* 1993;9:601–620.

61. Folstein MF, Folstein SE, McHugh PR. Mini-mental state: a practical method of grading the cognitive state of residents for the clinician. *J Psychiatr Res* 1975;2:189–198.

62. Pfeiffer E. A short portable mental status questionnaire for the assessment of organic brain deficit in elderly patients. *J Am Geriatr Soc* 1975;23:433–441.

63. Look KM, Look RM. Skin scraping, cupping, and moxibustion that may mimic physical abuse. *J Forensic Sci* 1997;42:103–105.

64. Ansello E. Causes and theories. In: Baumhover LA, Beall SC, eds. *Abuse, neglect, and exploitation of older persons: strategies for assessment and intervention*. Baltimore, MD: Health Professions Press, 1996:9–29.

65. Pillemer KA. Risk factors in elder abuse: results from a case control study. In: Pillemer KA, Wolf RS, eds. *Elder abuse: conflict in the family*. Dover: Auburn House, 1986:239–263.

66. Korbin JE, Anetzberger G, Thomasson R, et al. Abused elders who seek legal recourse against their adult offspring. *J Elder Abuse Negl* 1991;3:1–18.

67. O'Connor F. "Granny-bashing": abuse of the elderly. In: Hutchins N, ed. *The violent family: victimization of women, children and elders*. New York: Human Sciences Press, 1988:104–114.

68. American Bar Association. *Facts about law and the elderly*. 1998. Available at http://www.abanet.org/media/factbooks/eldtoc.html. Accessed on August 17, 2005.

69. Rosenblatt DE, Cho K, Durance PW. Reporting mistreatment of older adults: the role of physicians. *J Am Geriatr Soc* 1996;44:65–70.

70. Tilden VP, Schmidt TA, Limandri BJ, et al. Factors that influence clinicians' assessment and management of family violence. *Am J Public Health* 1994;84:628–633.

71. Tatara T, Kuzmeskus L. *Types of elder abuse in domestic settings*. Washington, DC: NCEA, 1998.

72. Moon A, Williams O. Perceptions of elder abuse and help-seeking patterns among African-American, Caucasian American, and Korean-American elderly women. *Gerontologist* 1993;33:386–395.

73. Sonkin DJ, Durphy M. *Learning to live without violence*. San Francisco: Volcano Press, 1982.

74. Brewer RA, Jones JS. Reporting elder abuse: limitations of statutes. *Ann Emerg Med* 1989;18:1217–1221.

75. Jones JS. Elder abuse and neglect: responding to a national problem. *Ann Emerg Med* 1994;23:845–848.

76. Jones JS, Veenstra TR, Seamon JP, et al. Elder mistreatment: national survey of emergency physicians. *Ann Emerg Med* 1997;30:473–479.

77. Clark-Daniels CL, Daniels RS, Baumhover LA. Abuse and neglect of the elderly: are emergency department personnel aware of mandatory reporting laws? *Ann Emerg Med* 1990;19:970–977.

78. Lachs MS, Williams CS, O'Brien S, et al. ED use by older victims of family violence. *Ann Emerg Med* 1997;30:448–454.

79. American College of Emergency Physicians. Policy statement: management of elder abuse and neglect. *Ann Emerg Med* 1998;31:149–150.

80. Garfield AS. Elder abuse and the states' adult protective services response: time for a change in California. *Hastings Law J* 1991;42:809–932.

81. Jogerst GJ, Daly JM, Brinig MF, et al. Domestic elder abuse and the law. *Am J Public Health* 2003;93:2131–2136.

82. Kusserow RP. *Resident abuse in nursing homes*. Washington, DC: US Government Printing Office, 1990.

83. Payne B, Cikovic R. An empirical examination of the characteristics, consequences, and causes of elder abuse in nursing homes. *J Elder Abuse Negl* 1996;7:61–74.

84. Teaster PB. *A response to the abuse of vulnerable adults: the 2000 survey of state adult protective services*. Washington, DC: National Center on Elder Abuse, 2006.Available at http://www.elderabusecenter.org/pdf/research/apsreport030703.pdf. Accessed on January 5, 2006.

85. Goldstein MZ. Elder neglect, abuse, and exploitation. In: Dickstein LJ, Nadelson CC, eds. *Family violence: emerging issues of a national crisis*. Washington, DC: American Psychiatric Press, 1989:101–124.

86. Moskowitz S. Saving granny from the wolf: elder abuse and neglect—the legal framework. *Conn Law Rev* 1998; 31:77–204.

87. Velick MD. Mandatory reporting statutes: a necessary yet underutilized response to elder abuse. *Elder Law J* 1995;3:165–190.

88. Foubister V. Doctor faces charges for allegedly undertreating pain. *Am Med News* 2000;43:11.

89. Bazelon Center for Mental Health Law. *Using state elder abuse laws in pain treatment cases*. 2001. Available at. http://www.painlaw.org/elderabuse.html. Accessed on August 16, 2005.

90. National Center on Elder Abuse. *Laws and legislation: elder justice act of 2003*. 2003. Available at http://www.elderabusecenter.org/default.cfm?p=elderjustice.cfm. Accessed on January 5, 2006.

91. National Association of State Units on Aging. *2003 survey of state unit on aging elder rights system development activities: progress in elder rights*. Washington, DC, 2004.

92. Sedlak AJ, Broadhurst DD. *The third national incidence study of child abuse and neglect (NIS-3)*. Washington, DC: United States Department of Health and Human Services, 1996.

93. Lachs MS, Williams C, O'Brien S, et al. Older adults: an 11-year longitudinal study of adult protective service use. *Arch Intern Med* 1996;156:449–453.

11

TREATING SURVIVORS OF INTIMATE PARTNER ABUSE: FORENSIC IDENTIFICATION AND DOCUMENTATION

■ DANIEL J. SHERIDAN

I ntimate partner abuse has profound physical and psychological health effects on millions of Americans and is now a crime in every state. The objectives of this chapter are to (a) give an overview of the dynamics of domestic abuse, (b) provide a brief legal overview, (c) describe clinical forensic assessments and documentation, (d) identify common domestic violence injuries, and (e) review the principles of forensic photography.

Estimates vary, but each year in the United States at least 4 million women experience ongoing physical, psychological, sexual, and financial abuse from a male intimate partner (1). The number of men abused by female intimates is estimated in the tens of thousands (1), and there is growing recognition of abuse occurring in gay and lesbian intimate relationships (2–4).

Although there is overlap in assessment and intervention techniques between these varying types of intimate partner abuse, this chapter will focus primarily on women victimized by male intimates.

ABUSE OF WOMEN

The battered-women's movement originally conceptualized domestic violence as a social, public policy, and criminal justice concern (5–9)—a view still strongly supported by many (10,11). However, early in the battered-women's movement, a few visionaries recognized abuse of women as a major health issue (12–16).

During the past 20 years, as the number of clinical and research articles on the health consequences of abused women has swelled, domestic violence has come to be viewed as a major public health concern. Nevertheless, only a handful of health professionals have examined the health link between abuse, domestic homicide, and the role of clinical forensics, despite growing documentation of the seriousness of physical, psychological, and sexual domestic violence (17–27).

Sequelae from physical abuse of women by male intimates are relatively easy to assess. There are physical findings: bruises, lacerations, sharp injuries, fractures, old and new scars, patterned injuries, pain, and bleeding. Physical injuries from domestic violence can be lavaged, debrided, sutured, x-rayed, scanned, and photographed. However, physical abuse is almost never the first form of abuse experienced by battered women. The first form of domestic violence is a combination of verbal and emotional abuse. These include name-calling, public embarrassment, veiled and explicit threats of harm, harassment, lies, "mind games," and other psychological manipulations. Sexual assault of women by current or former male intimates is a common yet under-recognized problem (28–30). Assessing and intervening in situations of domestic financial abuse is seldom viewed as being in the purview of medical treatment; however, this form of abuse is a common power and control tactic and a major barrier to women leaving abusive relationships (31,32).

For many women, the forms of abuse change and escalate when they attempt to leave the abusive relationship. For thousands of battered women, leaving the abusive relationship is marked by increased harassment and danger. Tragically, for more than 2,000 women every year, leaving an abusive relationship results in their death and sometimes in the deaths of their children at the hands of their abusive male partners (20,33,34). Data from three domestic homicide studies (33) demonstrated that estrangement from the abusive relationship disproportionately explained the risk of homicide in women, especially between 2 months and a year following separation. These data support the assertion that the first year out of an abusive relationship is the most deadly for battered women. Wilson and Daly (33) concluded that physically leaving an intimate relationship was a risk factor for homicide and that beginning the process of leaving was "an important risk factor in uxoricide" (33). They also stated that countless more women are subjected to near-lethal and increased violence, jealousy, coercion, threats, and other control tactics during the process of leaving relationships.

"If I Can't Have You, No One Can"

Wilson and Daly (33) prefaced their paper with a quotation from a man who killed his wife after being separated for a month, saying that if he could not have her, no one could. That same threat has been echoed in hundreds of the domestic violence histories given to this author in clinical practice. Campbell (20) titled her discussion of power and control in homicides of female partners "If I Can't Have You, No One Can." Homicide data from police files in Dayton, Ohio, from the 1980s, demonstrate that more than 64% of the 28 women killed by an intimate or formerly intimate male partner had a history of being physically abused. In the same percentage of cases, the police reports indicated that male jealousy was a primary motive (19). This finding supports arguments that male jealousy connotes male control and ownership (20).

Campbell (20) also reviewed domestic homicides against women who had either left the relationship or had expressed an intention to leave. Thirteen (46%) of Campbell's sample of murdered women had actually left the relationship ($n = 11$) or had threatened to leave ($n = 2$). All four of the male victims of homicide in Campbell's study used violence against their estranged wives just before the wives' use of homicide. The police records reported that the murdered men had expressed jealousy toward the women having a new male intimate and were trying to get back together at the time of the deaths. Campbell cited one case in which a man

"constantly harassed his ex-wife and returned many times to the house to violently accost her for months after the divorce" (20). On one such occasion, the ex-husband was let into the home by one of his children. The woman locked herself in her bedroom, and then shot and killed her ex-husband when he kicked down the bedroom door and came toward her. Despite what appeared to be a case of self-defense, the woman was convicted of voluntary manslaughter and sentenced to 20 years in prison (20).

THE PROCESS OF LEAVING AN ABUSIVE RELATIONSHIP: REASONS FOR STAYING VERSUS BARRIERS TO LEAVING

It is common for health care providers who treat severely abused women to wonder why a woman would stay in an abusive relationship. Why would she return time and time again? Why does she stay? When one questions why a woman stays in an abusive relationship, in essence, the health care provider is holding the battered woman accountable for her abuser's behavioral choices. Unfortunately, health care providers rarely say to the abusive male, "Why do you abuse?" Instead of questioning why she stays, it is better to reframe the question as, "What are her barriers to leaving?"

Psychological Barriers to Leaving

Several psychological explanations for why women stay in abusive relationships have been developed. They include brainwashing (35), mind control and active recapture techniques (36), the Stockholm syndrome (37,38), and traumatic bonding (39,40).

Sonkin (35) and many others (41–44) have compared psychological abuse in domestic violence with brainwashing of war and political prisoners, for example, Biderman's chart of coercion, which depicts eight brainwashing techniques used on prisoners of war and political prisoners—isolation, monopolization of perception, induced debility and exhaustion, threats, occasional indulgences, degradation, demonstrating omnipotence, and enforcing trivial demands (45).

On the basis of decades of clinical counseling experience, Boulette and Andersen (36) believe that cult members and battered women experience similar forms of brainwashing and mind control and share many common characteristics. Using parallels from cultic mind control and brainwashing techniques, they hypothesized that women often become trapped in abusive relationships. They describe cultic systems as exerting totalistic and demanding degrees of extreme control over an individual's freedom through various degrees of psychologically coercive and deceptive behaviors, including social isolation, confusion and guilt, threats of harm, love with strings attached, lying, and distortions of reality.

Battering that includes mind control, according to Boulette and Andersen (36), includes early verbal and/or physical dominance that can begin during or shortly after the courtship phase. Gradually, the batterer emotionally and geographically isolates and sometimes literally imprisons the woman, cutting her off from family and friends. During this process, the batterer weakens the woman's access to a support network, minimizes her escape options, and fosters the development of his partner into a more docile and behaviorally malleable person. To enforce this process, the abuser uses fear arousal and maintenance techniques that include actual and verbal threats of physical harm, direct threats with weapons, humiliation, public embarrassment, and intimidation by fear (36).

So often are the women blamed for causing the violent and coercive behaviors by their male abusers that the women begin to self-blame. This induction of guilt by the battering male toward the woman is occasionally softened by his contingent expressions of love. If she does not adequately acknowledge his love for her, he continues to degrade, devalue, and malign her until she capitulates (36). The abusive male is often jealous, accusing the woman of infidelity even while blatantly flaunting his own promiscuity. The problems within these violent relationships and dysfunctional families are expected to be kept secret at all costs. Breaking the family secret has been accompanied by the male abusers' threats of increased or lethal harm (36). To compensate for the cognitive dissonance resulting from experiencing the above behaviors, many battered women develop an enforced loyalty to the abusive male partners, exaggerating the socially acceptable behaviors and verbalizing a need to change and rescue the men from their violent actions (38). Women have described this behavioral pattern as cyclic, noting that it leads to feelings of powerlessness and helplessness (9,36), alternating with a sense of hopefulness when the abuser exhibits some positive behaviors. The abusers temporarily modify their behavior so that the women believe there is hope that the violence, threats, manipulations, and isolation will eventually end (36).

The brainwashing of battered women, whether conceptualized as being similar to that of a prisoner of war or a cult member, often occurs insidiously and over an extended period. This gradual process provides a partial explanation for the difficulty some battered women have in objectively assessing the severe levels of abuse and danger and in questioning their capacity to leave their abusers.

However, these techniques are less explanatory for battered women who begin experiencing severe physical, sexual, and psychological abuse early in the intimate relationship before brainwashing occurs. A frequently asked question is, "Why don't these women just leave?" Two highly related models have been used to explain this phenomenon: the Stockholm syndrome (38) and traumatic bonding (39,40).

The Stockholm Syndrome: Bonding with Your Captor

The Stockholm syndrome represents an attempt to explain the seemingly paradoxical response of some hostages to their captors. First attributed to a hostage situation in a bank in Stockholm, and subsequently identified in multiple hostage and kidnapping situations, hostages sometimes develop a significant fondness and attraction to their captors. The Stockholm syndrome (38) is characterized by four conditions:

1. The captor threatens and has the capacity to kill the captive.
2. The captive cannot safely escape; therefore, he or she is totally dependent on the captor.
3. The captive is isolated from others outside the hostage situation and is dependent on the captor.
4. The captor is perceived as showing some degree of kindness or benevolence toward the captive.

When the Stockholm syndrome is applied to battered women, the captive (battered woman) accurately identifies that the aggressor (the abuser) has the power of life and death and actively identifies with the aggressor through pathologic transference and traumatic psychological infantilism (38). Women in ongoing abusive relationships with male intimates experience varying levels of physical abuse interspersed with transient periods of kindness and benevolence from their abusers. Battered women are sometimes literally held hostage by their abuser at knifepoint or gunpoint. Many home hostage situations that result in police intervention and media coverage involve domestic violence. When battered women say, as they often do, that they feel as if they are prisoners in their own homes, they may be struggling with the dynamics of brainwashing, mind control, and the transference effects of the Stockholm syndrome.

Traumatic Bonding: Intermittent Good–Bad Behavior

Women in abusive relationships frequently minimize the seriousness of the abuse and tend to justify and defend the severe abusive behaviors of their abuser. This seemingly illogical connectedness with the aggressor, especially after severe trauma, has been explained by a model of traumatic bonding (39,40), which was developed to explain powerful emotional attachments in abusive relationships created by intermittent abuse and power imbalances. Traumatic bonding can quickly solidify as the subjugated person develops a continual lowering of self-esteem and decreased ability to live independently. At the same time, the abusive person develops an inflated sense of power. The stronger person becomes increasingly dependent on the weaker to maintain the feeling of power, a feeling the abuser does not want to relinquish.

The unpredictability of this intermittent abuse, coupled with periods of reconciliation, feigned (or partially sincere) contrition, and isolation from the reality checks of family and friends, is a catalyst that accelerates traumatic bonding and the battered women's fantasies of loving partners (40). Traumatic bonding can occur early in a relationship (39,40); in fact, it appears to occur for some women during the dating relationship (46). Intermittent abuse, in which women separate the "good-man image" from the "bad-man image," was identified (46) in a sample of 90 college students, 43% of whom reported a history that experts interpreted to be psychologically abusive.

Active Recapture Measures

From their extensive clinical practices, Boulette and Andersen (36) recognized that many battered women struggle to shed the traumatic bonds that make them feel like prisoners in their own homes. This can be a difficult and, at times, immobilizing process that requires overcoming multiple barriers to leaving, including active recapture techniques such as cocky disbelief, confused searching, bargaining, pleading, threatening, and revenge (36).

Initially, an abusive man is shocked that his wife or girlfriend would dare to leave him. He is convinced that she cannot exist without him, and sometimes he has so thoroughly convinced her that she cannot make it without him that she does return to him, begging his forgiveness (36).

If she does not reenter the relationship, he begins a period of anxious and/or panicked searching (36). When he discovers where she is staying, he sends bargaining messages that include promises of changed behavior, highlighting future love, fidelity, and kindness (36). Most women, from this researcher's clinical experience, do not want the relationship to end. They want to return to an ideal relationship full of love, fidelity, and kindness. Promises of change can be an effective recapture technique (9,36).

Over time and after multiple broken promises of change by the abuser, the battered woman stops being swayed by his bargaining tactics. The abuser then often activates the recapture technique of pleading, during which time he pleads and begs for another chance, frequently shedding tears and exhibiting physiologic signs of remorse (36). The woman may interpret tears and sobbing as signs of love. She feels sorrow and pity for the man and guilt for precipitating his tears. Men who are successful with the recapture technique of pleading often have brief periods of improved behavior (36), which Walker (9) described as the honeymoon phase. However, when pleading fails to recapture the abused woman, the abusive man can quickly escalate to the recapture techniques of threats and revenge (36). Threats of physical, sexual, and financial harm to her, the children, and family escalate. He may threaten to kidnap the children or have her institutionalized. Interspersed in the threats are instances of physical abuse and destruction of property and/or pets (36). If she persists in her efforts to stay out of the abusive relationship, the batterer plans revenge tactics that could culminate in the woman being severely injured or killed. Johnson (47) described severe threats and serious abuse as patriarchal terroristic control intended to control women and keep them from leaving the abusive relationship. These recapture and patriarchal terroristic methods help perpetuate the woman's sense of being a prisoner in her home and help facilitate the processes of mind control, brainwashing, and traumatic bonding (36,38,40,47).

From Fear to Fatigue: Clinically Identified Barriers to Leaving Abusive Relationships

From extensive clinical experience, this author has compiled a practical list of terms that help the health care provider to better understand a battered woman's barriers to leaving. They are discussed in the following sections.

Fear

A battered woman stays in an abusive relationship because of fear of being further abused and/or fear of failure. Her abuser may say to her, "If you try to leave me, I'll kill you. I'll hurt the kids." He may say, "I know you can hide from me, but I know where your mother lives, where your sister lives. I dare you to leave. If you hide from me, you'll read about your family in the papers." Or maybe he has convinced her she cannot live without him. She is afraid of failure. She is afraid that if she leaves him she will not be able to provide food and shelter for her children.

Finances

A battered woman stays in an abusive relationship because she cannot afford to leave. Ending a relationship, even a nonabusive one, is expensive and usually results in financial loss for both parties. In many abusive relationships, the abuser has so controlled the finances that the woman has little or no access to money.

Father

A battered woman stays in an abusive relationship because she wants her children to be with their father. She does not want to be a single mother. As long as the man is relatively good to the children, she will stay and endure his abusive behavior toward her. One of the prime motivators for women to begin the process of leaving is when the abuser begins to threaten and/or hurt the children. Another motivator is when the children begin to mimic his abusive language or his abusive physical behavior.

Faith

A battered woman stays in an abusive relationship because her religion has taught her that marriage is for life, through good times and bad times, until death. Until very recently, religious leaders in the community had little or no training in domestic violence awareness and interventions. It is not uncommon for a battered women, on seeking religious counseling, to hear from the clergy, "Be a better wife. Pray harder. Offer it up. Cook better meals." Some untrained clergy may try to do couples counseling, which is contraindicated in most ongoing abusive relationships.

Forgiveness

A battered woman stays in an abusive relationship because she forgives her abuser when he says he is sorry for hurting her. Most battered women do not want the relationship to end. They want the abuse to end. Most abusive relationships do not begin on the first date. If on her first date with a man, he called a woman a fat pig, broke her nose, and then forced her to have sex with him, undoubtedly, the chances for a second date would be slim. However, in most abusive relationships, the woman has seen a side of the man that can be good and caring, tender, and loving. She has seen a man who can be quite wonderful and has the ability to shower her with love, attention, and affection. When he tells her he is sorry for hurting her, often with tears in his eyes, she wants to believe he will change. She wants to believe it was extenuating stressors that made him hurt her. She wants to believe it was the stress from his job, the stress from the children, or the stress from his first wife that made him hurt her. She wants to believe he will change back to the man with whom she fell in love. And she believes she can help change him.

Fantasy/Fix

A battered woman stays in an abusive relationship because she has a fantasy that she can fix her abuser. She believes if she loves him a little harder, does everything he asks of her, limits her activities outside the home, and keeps the children from increasing his stress, then the relationship will improve. She does not understand that she cannot fix him because *he* does not believe anything is wrong with him. He blames her for all their problems. She does not understand that only he can change his own behaviors and attitudes.

Family

A battered woman stays in an abusive relationship for extended-family reasons. Either her family does not yet know that she is in an abusive relationship or her family has become somewhat estranged from her because she keeps returning to the abusive relationship. She may not have easy access to her family support system if she and her abuser have moved a great distance away.

Friends

A battered woman stays in an abusive relationship because she has not been able to maintain many friendships and lacks a social support network. Social isolation is common among abused women of all ages. The more emotionally and/or geographically isolated one is from a support and safety network, the more difficult it is to leave.

Familiarity

A battered woman stays in an abusive relationship because she was brought up in an abusive home and accepts that being beaten by a man is a necessary part of being a woman. She may have witnessed her grandmother being beaten or maybe her mother was beaten. She knows her older sister is being beaten. This author has had many battered women say to him, "Don't you beat your wife? Don't all men beat women?"

Full

A battered woman stays in an abusive relationship because she has tried to leave but discovered that the emergency women's shelter was full and all the beds were occupied. Or perhaps there was space for her, but the shelter has a policy of not allowing teenage boys into the home. She stays because she does not want to leave her teenaged son at home without her to protect him.

Find

A battered woman stays in an abusive relationship because she knows, from prior attempts at leaving, that her abuser will search for her until he finds her, even if it means searching state by state.

Fatigue

A battered woman stays in an abusive relationship because she has become too physically and emotionally exhausted to leave. She is so fatigued that she cannot muster the energy needed to develop and implement a safety plan.

LEGAL OVERVIEW

Physical abuse within intimate relationships is now a crime in every state. As such, medical documentation of domestic violence has potential forensic (pertaining to the law) implications. What the provider writes or does not write in the medical record may be crucial in court. Unfortunately, health care providers tend to underdocument domestic violence histories, examinations, and findings (17, 25,27,48). Health care providers need to know whether reporting domestic violence cases to police is mandatory in their community or state. For example, in California the health care provider not only needs to make a telephone report to the police in a timely manner but must also give the police a written summary of the battered patient's history. This must be done, even if the patient instructs the provider to keep the information confidential. In Illinois, although the police are routinely called to the medical treatment area when any suspected crime victim or perpetrator presents for treatment, the provider is not obligated to divulge to the police any information gathered during the history or examination. The decision to talk or not talk with the police is entirely up to the victim.

In many communities, the address where the abuse reportedly occurred determines the police agency that needs to be notified of the domestic violence crime. If the victim was abused in one community or county and travels to a health facility in another city or county, the local police may not want to get involved. It is not uncommon for the health care provider to find herself or himself in the middle of police jurisdiction turf battles. To avoid some of these conflicts, it is helpful for the health care agency to develop, *a priori*, networking relationships with all regional law enforcement agencies. In some states, police notification depends on the severity of the patient's injuries or, if the injury was penetrating, whether it was caused by a knife or a firearm.

Health care providers who work at institutions at or near state borders often need to become familiar with reporting requirements of the two states and two sets of legal terminology. For example, in the State of Oregon, if one person inflicts an injury on another, it is the crime of assault, with assaults ranging from misdemeanors to felonies. In the State of Washington, the identical act is called a *battery*, with the level of battery ranging from misdemeanor to felony.

If legal advocacy is provided to battered patients, the provider must have a working knowledge of the definitions of various violence-related crimes. What level of abuse is most probably a misdemeanor? What level is a felony? For what types of violent crimes do the police send only a patrol officer, as opposed to cases in which the police may dispatch a detective and/or an evidence specialist? In rural settings, the level and timeliness of police response may vary significantly from that provided in an urban setting.

Health care providers need to know whether there is mandatory arrest or proarrest in their state. It is not uncommon for an abuser to bring his wife or girlfriend to the health care setting for treatment of the injuries he just inflicted. Often he will wait in the waiting room or hover around the woman in the examination/treatment area. With mandatory arrest of domestic violence perpetrators, the odds go up that the reported abuser will be arrested (on site) if the police come to the medical facility. In situations in which the police are governed by domestic violence proarrest statutes, the responding officer(s) have much more discretionary power to decide whether to arrest the abuser.

All states have implemented some form of domestic violence civil court remedies in the form of either specialized restraining orders or orders of protection. Health care providers need to know what form of civil remedy is issued in their state. These protective orders can be quite helpful in several general areas and can be crafted to address unique issues of the victim. In general, restraining/protective orders can give the victim immediate, emergency, temporary custody of the children; make the reported abuser leave the home; and order the reported abuser to stay 500 ft away from the victim or not come to the victim's workplace or school. This author has often gone to the court and obtained restraining or protective orders on behalf of battered women who are going to be hospitalized for more than a couple of days. The appropriate legal forms were completed and signed by the victim and then notarized by a hospital representative (usually from the business office) at the patient's bedside. The author went to court as the victim's proxy. Some judges telephoned the hospital and spoke directly with the patient, whereas others accepted the paperwork without question. In all these cases, the orders were modified to include a clause that the reported abuser was not to come within 500 ft of the hospital, thereby giving the hospital, its staff, and other patients some additional safety and legal protection. Violations of many types of civil restraining/protective orders often result in criminal sanctions and can give local law enforcement the power to arrest simply because the civil order was violated.

ASSESSMENT AND IDENTIFICATION

During the 1990s, routine screening for domestic violence in all health care settings had been recommended as the norm (49,50). However, in 1996 and again in 2004, a U.S. Preventative Services Task Force found a lack of evidenced-based research for or against screening for intimate partner abuse (51). Despite the lack of case-controlled trial studies that show the efficacy of screening for intimate partner violence, routine screening by health providers is still being recommended.

For any screening to be effective, the health care provider needs to understand that the woman's privacy and safety are paramount. The health care provider will never elicit a history of abuse from a woman if her husband/boyfriend, any children older than 3 years, his mother, her mother, or other people who may be later "quizzed" by the abuser are in the examination room. Whether it is because of fear of further harm and/or embarrassment, a woman will not share her abuse history in front of an audience. It is best to establish a policy within every health care institution that all patients will be interviewed and/or examined alone for some period during their visits. This author has also found sitting at the same eye level as the patient, when culturally appropriate, to be an effective interviewing technique with women being assessed for battering.

Many types of routine abuse screens are used in health care settings. Among the most tested and used is a five-item Abuse Assessment Screen (AAS) developed by Helton (52) and modified by the Nursing Research Consortium on Violence and Abuse (Table 11-1) or a shortened three-item version of the AAS (53) (Fig. 11.1). The AAS is as effective at screening for abuse (53) as the 19-item Conflict Tactics Scale (CTS) (54) and the 30-item Index of Spouse Abuse (55). When the AAS was further tested on a large, ethnically stratified cohort of women, it was found to be an extremely effective domestic violence screening tool (56).

However, it is not acceptable to just routinely screen for the presence or absence of domestic violence. If, during a routine domestic violence screening process, a woman shares that she has been slapped and kicked during the past year and has been forced into sex by her husband/boyfriend when she did not want to participate, additional assessment is

TABLE 11-1

FIVE-ITEM ABUSE ASSESSMENT SCREEN

1. Are you ever afraid of your partner?
2. Do you feel your partner tries to control you?
3. Do you feel emotionally abused or hurt by your partner?
4. Has your partner ever hit, slapped, kicked, or otherwise physically hurt you?
5. Has your partner ever forced you into sex when you did not want to participate?

From Helton A. *Protocol of care for the battered women.* Houston: Houston Chapter of the March of Dimes, 1986.

required. If a patient told a health care provider that she was experiencing crushing chest pain, shortness of breath, sweating, and pain shooting down her left arm, it is doubtful the provider would move on to assess the patient's bunions. A reasonable provider would ask additional cardiac assessment questions while obtaining physical findings and tests. The symptoms could be nothing more than atypical indigestion or they could be symptomatic of a life-threatening cardiac crisis.

Battered women may be at just as much risk of lethal sequelae as the above fictitious patient. Therefore, if there is a positive history of recent abuse on routine assessment, the next logical clinical step for the prudent provider would be to administer the 23-item Harassment in Abusive Relationships: A Self-report Scale (HARASS) tool (57) (Fig. 11.2) coupled with the administration of the 20-item Danger Assessment (DA) instrument (58) (Fig. 11.3). Both tools are self-report scales and take a few minutes to complete.

The HARASS tool was developed for clinical use by women in the process of leaving abusive relationships (57). It was designed to be used in conjunction with Campbell's DA (58) to better identify battered women at risk for increased abuse and/or domestic homicide. The HARASS tool, which has a Cronbach's α of 0.93 for the OFTEN scale and 0.92 for the DISTRESS scale, has preliminary evidence (through factor analysis) for three subscale groupings. These groupings had logical support in the literature and were named as follows: (a) *stalking-like behaviors*, (b) *threatening behaviors*, and (c) *controlling-his-commodities behaviors*, which encompass children, property, and forced sex. All these behaviors have been linked to domestic homicide. The HARASS scale was positively and significantly correlated with the concurrent administration of the DA but was not redundant (57).

Campbell (58) developed the DA to attempt to predict the known link between intimate partner

Abuse Assessment Screen

1. **WITHIN THE LAST YEAR**, have you been hit, slapped, kicked, or
otherwise physically hurt by someone?   YES   NO

   If YES, by whom? _____

   Total number of times _____

2. **SINCE YOU'VE BEEN PREGNANT**, have you been hit, slapped,
kicked, or otherwise physically hurt by someone?   YES   NO

   If YES, by whom? _____

   Total number of times _____

MARK THE AREA OF INJURY ON THE BODY MAP. SCORE EACH INCIDENT
ACCORDING TO THE FOLLOWING SCALE: SCORE

1 = Threats of abuse including use of a weapon

2 = Slapping, pushing; no injuries; and/or lasting pain

3 = Punching, kicking, bruises, cuts, and/or continuing pain

4 = Beating up, severe contusions, burns, broken bones

5 = Head injury, internal injury, permanent injury

6 = Use of weapon; wound from weapon

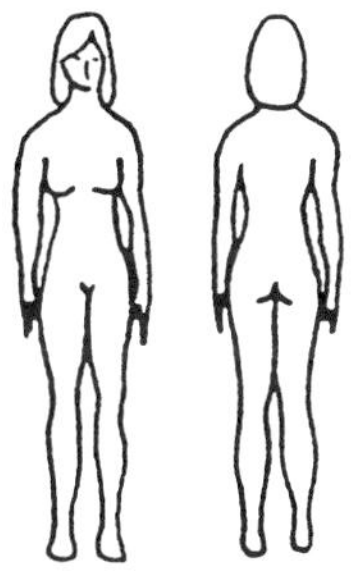

If any of the descriptions for the higher number apply, use the higher number.

3. **WITHIN THE LAST YEAR**, has anyone forced you to have
sexual activities?   YES   NO

   If YES, by whom? _____

   Total number of times _____

Developed by the Nursing Research Consortium on Violence and Abuse.
Readers are encouraged to reproduce and use this assessment tool.

FIG. 11.1   Three-Item Abuse Assessment Screen.

abuse and homicide. On the basis of her extensive clinical research experience and published lists of possible lethal danger signals in abusive intimate partner relationships (59,60), Campbell has incorporated behavioral warning signals that have been clinically associated with domestic homicide into the DA instrument. The DA is not a scale for initial domestic violence assessment; it has been designed for use in clinical and/or research settings for women who have already been identified as being abused. All items on the DA have been established as correlates of homicide, and as such, the DA is "best thought of as a statistical risk factor assessment rather than a (clinical) prediction instrument" (58). The DA and several questions from the HARASS tool were used in an 11-city study that sought to identify risk factors for femicide in abusive relationships (61).

Prediction of violent behavior in general, and life-threatening and potentially lethal violence in particular, has been fraught with inaccuracy (62). Campbell (58) and Sheridan (57) recommend that the DA and the HARASS tools be used with caution

H arassment in

A busive

R elationships:

A

S elf-report

S cale

Many women are harassed in relationships with their abusive partners, especially if the women are trying to end the relationships. You may be experiencing harassment. This instrument is designed to measure harassment of women who are in abusive relationships or are in the process of leaving abusive relationships. By completing this questionnaire, you may better understand harassment in your life. If you have any questions, please talk with the service provider who gave you this tool.

Harassment is defined as a persistent pattern of behavior by an intimate partner that is intended to bother, annoy, trap, emotionally wear down, threaten, frighten, terrify and/or coerce a woman with the overall intent to control her choices and behavior about leaving the abusive relationship.

There are no right or wrong answers. Do not put your name on the form. The instrument takes about 10 minutes to complete.

A

Copyright 1998, Daniel J. Sheridan, PhD, RN

For each item, circle the number that best describes how often the behavior occurred. Next, rate how distressing the behavior is to you. If the behavior has never occurred, circle 0 (NEVER) and go to the next question. If the question does not apply to you, circle NA (NOT APPLICABLE). If you are still in the relationship please circle below MY PARTNER. If you have left the relationship, please circle below MY FORMER PARTNER.

THE BEHAVIOR

HOW OFTEN DOES IT OCCUR?

0 = Never
1 = Rarely
2 = Occasionally
3 = Frequently
4 = Very frequently
NA = Not applicable

HOW DISTRESSING IS THIS BEHAVIOR TO YOU?

0 = Not at all distressing
1 = Slightly distressing
2 = Moderately distressing
3 = Very distressing
4 = Extremely distressing
NA = Not applicable

MY PARTNER/FORMER PARTNER (circle one)

	THE BEHAVIOR	HOW OFTEN DOES IT OCCUR?	HOW DISTRESSING IS THIS BEHAVIOR TO YOU?
1.	Frightens people close to me	0 1 2 3 4 NA	0 1 2 3 4 NA
2.	Pretends to be someone else in order to get to me	0 1 2 3 4 NA	0 1 2 3 4 NA
3.	Comes to my home when I don't want him there	0 1 2 3 4 NA	0 1 2 3 4 NA
4.	Threatens to kill me if I leave or stay away from him	0 1 2 3 4 NA	0 1 2 3 4 NA
5.	Threatens to harm the kids if I leave or stay away from him	0 1 2 3 4 NA	0 1 2 3 4 NA
6.	Takes things that belong to me so I have to see him to get them back	0 1 2 3 4 NA	0 1 2 3 4 NA
7.	Tries getting me fired from my job	0 1 2 3 4 NA	0 1 2 3 4 NA
8.	Ignores court orders to stay away from me	0 1 2 3 4 NA	0 1 2 3 4 NA
9.	Keeps showing up wherever I am	0 1 2 3 4 NA	0 1 2 3 4 NA
10.	Bothers me at work when I don't want to talk with him	0 1 2 3 4 NA	0 1 2 3 4 NA
11.	Uses the kids as pawns to get me physically close to him	0 1 2 3 4 NA	0 1 2 3 4 NA
12.	Shows up without warning	0 1 2 3 4 NA	0 1 2 3 4 NA

B

FIG. 11.2 Harassment in Abusive Relationships: A Self-report Scale (HARASS). (Permission to use the HARASS tool in clinical settings has been universally granted by its creator. Dr. Sheridan would appreciate notification if the HARASS tool is used in formal research studies.)

THE BEHAVIOR	HOW OFTEN DOES IT OCCUR? 0 = Never 1 = Rarely 2 = Occasionally 3 = Frequently 4 = Very frequently NA = Not applicable						HOW DISTRESSING IS THIS BEHAVIOR TO YOU? 0 = Not at all distressing 1 = Slightly distressing 2 = Moderately distressing 3 = Very distressing 4 = Extremely distressing NA = Not applicable					
13. Messes with my property (for example, sells my stuff, breaks my furniture, damages my car, steals my things)	0	1	2	3	4	NA	0	1	2	3	4	NA
14. Scares me with a weapon	0	1	2	3	4	NA	0	1	2	3	4	NA
15. Breaks into my home	0	1	2	3	4	NA	0	1	2	3	4	NA
16. Threatens to kill himself if I leave or stay away from him	0	1	2	3	4	NA	0	1	2	3	4	NA
17. Makes me feel like he can again force me into sex	0	1	2	3	4	NA	0	1	2	3	4	NA
18. Threatens to snatch or have the kids taken away from me	0	1	2	3	4	NA	0	1	2	3	4	NA
19. Sits in his car outside my home	0	1	2	3	4	NA	0	1	2	3	4	NA
20. Leaves me threatening messages (for example, puts scary notes on the car, sends me threatening letters, sends me threats through family and friends, leaves threatening messages on the telephone answering machine)	0	1	2	3	4	NA	0	1	2	3	4	NA
21. Threatens to harm our pet	0	1	2	3	4	NA	0	1	2	3	4	NA
22. Calls me on the telephone and hangs up	0	1	2	3	4	NA	0	1	2	3	4	NA
23. Reports me to the authorities for taking drugs when I don't	0	1	2	3	4	NA	0	1	2	3	4	NA

C

Optional:

List other harassing behaviors that you have experienced. Circle how often and how distressing the behaviors are to you.

THE BEHAVIOR	HOW OFTEN DOES IT OCCUR? 0 = Never 1 = Rarely 2 = Occasionally 3 = Frequently 4 = Very frequently					HOW DISTRESSING IS THIS BEHAVIOR TO YOU? 0 = Not at all distressing 1 = Slightly distressing 2 = Moderately distressing 3 = Very distressing 4 = Extremely distressing				
24. _____	0	1	2	3	4	0	1	2	3	4
25. _____	0	1	2	3	4	0	1	2	3	4
26. _____	0	1	2	3	4	0	1	2	3	4

Please answer a few additional questions:

_____ Your age in years

Check the statement that best describes you.

☐ Married, living with an abusive partner.
☐ Single, living with an abusive partner.
☐ Married, living apart from an abusive partner.
☐ Single, living apart from an abusive partner.

How long were you in the above relationship? _____

Are you still in the relationship? ☐ YES ☐ NO

If you have left the relationship, how long have you been out? _____

What is your approximate annual income? _____

How many years of school have you completed? _____

Check the statement that best describes you.

☐ Asian/Pacific Islander
☐ Black/African American
☐ Caucasian/White
☐ Hispanic
☐ Native American/American Indian
☐ Other_____

D

FIG. 11.2   (Continued).

DANGER ASSESSMENT

Jacquelyn C. Campbell, Ph.D., R.N.
Copyright, 2003

Several risk factors have been associated with increased risk of homicides (murders) of women and men in violent relationships. We cannot predict what will happen in your case, but we would like you to be aware of the danger of homicide in situations of abuse and for you to see how many of the risk factors apply to your situation.

Using the calendar, please mark the approximate dates during the past year when you were abused by your partner or ex-partner. Write on that date how bad the incident was according to the following scale:

1.   Slapping, pushing; no injuries, and/or lasting pain
2.   Punching, kicking; bruises, cuts, and/or continuing pain
3.   "Beating up"; severe contusions, burns, broken bones
4.   Threat to use weapon; head injury, internal injury, permanent injury
5.   Use of weapon; wounds from weapon

(If **any** of the descriptions for the higher number apply, use the higher number.)

Mark **Yes** or **No** for each of the following. ("He" refers to your husband, partner, ex-husband, ex-partner, or whoever is currently physically hurting you.)

_____ 1.   Has the physical violence increased in severity or frequency over the past year?
_____ 2.   Does he own a gun?
_____ 3.   Have you left him after living together during the past year?
            3a. (If you have *never* lived with him, check here___)
_____ 4.   Is he unemployed?
_____ 5.   Has he ever used a weapon against you or threatened you with a lethal weapon?
            (If yes, was the weapon a gun?____)
_____ 6.   Does he threaten to kill you?
_____ 7.   Has he avoided being arrested for domestic violence?
_____ 8.   Do you have a child that is not his?
_____ 9.   Has he ever forced you to have sex when you did not wish to do so?
_____ 10.   Does he ever try to choke you?
_____ 11.   Does he use illegal drugs? By drugs, I mean "uppers" or amphetamines, speed, angel dust, cocaine, "crack", street drugs or mixtures.
_____ 12.   Is he an alcoholic or problem drinker?
_____ 13.   Does he control most or all of your daily activities? For instance, does he tell you who you can be friends with, when you can see your family, how much money you can use, or when you can take the car? (If he tries, but you do not let him, check here: ____)
_____ 14.   Is he violently and constantly jealous of you? (For instance, does he say "If I can't have you, no one can.")
_____ 15.   Have you ever been beaten by him while you were pregnant? (If you have never been pregnant by him, check here: ____)
_____ 16.   Have you ever threatened or tried to commit suicide?
_____ 17.   Has he ever threatened or tried to commit suicide?
_____ 18.   Does he threaten to harm your children?
_____ 19.   Do you believe he is capable of killing you?
_____ 20.   Does he follow or spy on you, leave threatening notes or messages on an answering machine, destroy your property, or call you when you don't want him to?

_____   Total "Yes" Answers

Thank you. Please talk to your nurse, advocate, or counselor about what the Danger Assessment means in terms of your situation.

FIG. 11.3   Danger Assessment (DA) instrument. (Permission to use the DA tool in clinical settings has been universally granted by its creator. Dr. Campbell requests notification if the DA tool is used in formal research studies.)

and as part of clinical discussions with women involved in abusive relationships as an informal predictor of potential homicide. The data obtained from the additional assessment questions can help guide the health care provider and the patient to develop better safety plans. In the 11-city study of femicide in abusive relationships, Campbell et al. (61) noted the following to be exceptionally high preincident risk factors:

- The perpetrator's access to a firearm
- Previous threats with a weapon
- Perpetrator's stepchild living in the home
- Estrangement, especially from a controlling partner
- Stalking
- Forced sex
- Abuse during pregnancy
- Telling the abusive partner she is leaving him for another man

DOCUMENTATION OF DOMESTIC VIOLENCE

Historically, documentation of histories of abuse has been both sparse and forensically useless. It is common to read poorly written medical histories, such as:

> a 43-year-old female presenting with history of multiple facial trauma, struck by known assailant.

A much more forensically useful entry would be:

> a 43-year-old female presenting with history of multiple facial trauma states that she was struck four times on the right side of her face with a closed fist and kicked one time on the left ear by her husband, James Jones (DOB April 19, 1958), at 11:30 a.m yesterday at the corner of Fourth and Main Street, witnessed by her two children, David, 22, and Nicholas, 19.

Even when medical documentation is not sparse, it is often "sanitized." For example, an abused patient is rushed to the emergency department by paramedics immediately after being beaten. In an "unsanitized" progress/admission note, the provider documents not only the patient's presenting physical trauma but also that the patient is visibly upset and crying. The provider writes that the patient states her boyfriend, George Thomas Duffy, knocked her to ground, forced the barrel of handgun into her mouth, and said, "If you ever leave me, bitch, I'll blow your mother ?#%ing head off and drown your &%#ing kids." The "sanitized" entry may read, "Patient reports being knocked to ground by known assailant who then threatened her and her children." It should be evident that the first entry

is much more forensically useful than the second. Statements made by the victim in the unsanitized progress note may also be viewed as an "excited utterance," which is a statement made by a victim or witness immediately or shortly after experiencing some type of traumatic event. Excited utterances are presumed by the courts to be true statements. Courts often allow excited utterances to be introduced as evidence, as exceptions to the hearsay, because the presumption is that the victim was too excited and did not have time to fabricate a lie.

Histories of abuse in the patient record should always be detailed and unsanitized, even if the reported abuse occurred days, weeks, or years ago. When a medical care provider documents patient statements made in the routine course of health care delivery, the statements have been viewed by the courts as truthful and are allowed in court as evidence (*White v Illinois*, 1992). Statements made to and recorded by health professionals are often referred to as "medical exceptions to hearsay."

Realistic constraints on time management of busy health care providers make it almost impossible to chart, verbatim, the histories provided by abused patients. However, extensive fact-filled paraphrasing of the presenting history of abuse and a summary of past abuse events are invaluable in court. Verbatim documentation of select, poignant statements made by the abused patient is ideal. If the reported or suspected abuser is present, any statements and/or behaviors by him that are threatening, controlling, and/or in conflict with the patient's history should also be documented, especially if he directly (or indirectly) threatens the patient or staff.

TYPES OF INJURIES

Unfortunately, health care providers often misuse common forensic medical definitions. There is a taxonomic system of forensic terminology that should be used consistently in all medical documentation. The following sections are based in part on common preferred forensic definitions (17,48,63–65) and on the author's extensive clinical experiences.

Patterned Injuries

Patterned injuries are those in which the provider has reasonable certainty that the presenting injury was caused by an unknown object, a specific object, or a specific mechanism.

Pattern of Injuries

"Pattern of injuries" refers to injuries in various stages of healing, including old and new patterned injuries, fractures, and scars.

Abrasions

An abrasion is the scraping of the skin or mucous membrane, usually caused by friction against an object or surface. Most abrasions are superficial; however, the longer a person is dragged against a rough surface, and the rougher the surface, the more extensive the injury. Battered women are often dragged along the ground by the abuser. The ground surface helps determine the type of abrasion. Being dragged (supine) along a carpeted surface by one's feet usually results in "rug burn" abrasions to the woman's lower back and elbows. Being dragged (prone) on a carpet by one's feet may result in rug burns to the anterior chest, breasts, abdomen, and/or knees. Being pulled along a carpeted surface could result in rug burns to the posterior or anterior shoulder area, depending on how much twisting motion is being applied either by the abuser or by the woman as she tries to break free. Carpet fibers (trace evidence) may be present in or around the wound and should be documented, photographed, and preserved as evidence.

Being dragged along the pavement (concrete and/or asphalt) through the same mechanisms as in the preceding text will result in similar, but probably more severe, abrasion injuries that often contain trace evidence such as dirt, cinders, glass, and pebbles. Being dragged along a dirt or grass surface usually produces less severe abrasion injury but an abundance of trace evidence.

During strangulation assaults, the abuser may inflict fingernail scratch abrasions to the battered woman's neck (Figs. 11.4 through 11.6). While being strangled, the battered woman may try to pry the assailant's hands from her neck and in so doing scratch herself. The assailant may have fingernail scratch abrasions on his face, neck, and arms inflicted by the woman in self-defensive efforts.

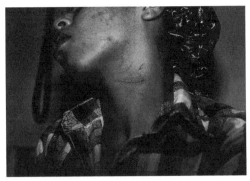

FIG. 11.5 Patterned, fingernail-like scratch abrasions to left lateral side of the neck caused by a strangulation mechanism of injury.

Being strangled with a rough rope or cord may produce ligature abrasions in a more circular pattern around the neck. Rope abrasions can also have a looped pattern (Fig. 11.7).

A variety of abrasions are caused by punch injuries inflicted by assailants wearing rings. Simple wedding bands seldom leave an abrasive imprint injury. However, raised rings, especially those with pointed corners, can cause significant abrasion injury or worse (laceration and/or partial or complete avulsion). Abrasion injuries from rings are usually linear or curvilinear and centered in the middle of a punchlike contusion (Figs. 11.6 and 11.8). The more angled the point of impact, the longer the abrasion. When punched straight on by an assailant wearing a ring with a stone, a victim may

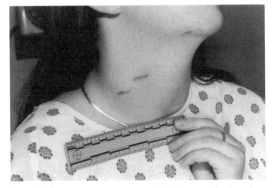

FIG. 11.4 Patterned, fingernail-like scratch abrasions to the right lateral side of the neck and chin caused by a strangulation mechanism of injury.

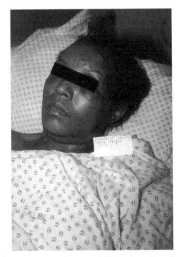

FIG. 11.6 Patterned, punchlike abrasion from a ring with a stone to the midforehead; sutured partial avulsion injury to the nose; punchlike contusion to the left eye involving the sclera; and strangulation-related abrasions to the neck.

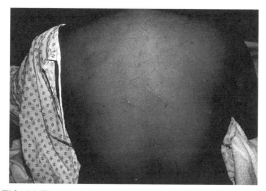

FIG. 11.7   Newer, patterned, looped, cordlike contusions to the right upper posterior shoulder and left lower posterior shoulder; patterned, looped, cordlike scar to the right-sided midlateral back; patterned, scabbed, cordlike abrasions to the midback; patterned, kick/stomp heel-like contusion to the left-sided midback; and patterned foot kick/stomplike, with heel imprint and sole imprint to upper left posterior, superior shoulder.

have a punchlike contusion with a circular, oval, semicircular, or horseshoe-shaped abrasion in the center of the injury. Whenever any form of ring-related abrasion is suspected, it would be prudent to secure the suspect's ring. Inside the ring may be trace evidence (skin and blood), or the ring pattern may be matched to the injury pattern.

Avulsion

An avulsion injury is the tearing away of a structure or part. Partial avulsions are more common and can result from blunt force trauma over bony surfaces. Punch injuries to a woman's face can result in

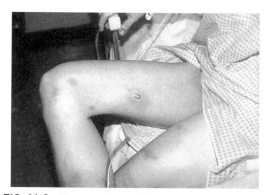

FIG. 11.8   Patterned, punchlike contusion to right medial thigh, with a patterned imprint abrasion from a ring with a stone; patterned, fingertip-like contusions to right medial knee and left anterior medial thigh from a reported marital rape.

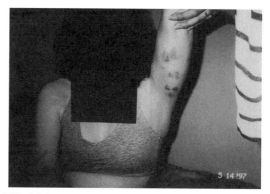

FIG. 11.9   Multiple, patterned, fingertip contusions to the left upper arm.

complete or partial avulsions to her nose, lips, chin, and forehead (Fig. 11.6). Being struck with a solid object with a jagged edge can avulse tissue anywhere on the body.

Bruise/Contusion

A bruise is the superficial discoloration in the skin or any other organ caused by hemorrhage due to broken blood vessels as a result of blunt force trauma. A bruise is also called a *contusion*. More specifically, in a contusion, there is usually swelling, pain, tenderness, and discoloration of the injured site. The causes of contusions in domestic violence injuries are almost endless. Any significant blunt force mechanism of injury will cause bruising. However, there are some classic patterned contusions that are frequently seen on battered women.

Blunt force injury caused by the assailant's fingertips often causes dime-sized or nickel-sized circular contusions, which are most often seen on the victim's arms, especially the medial surface of the upper arms (Fig. 11.9). The bruises are often in a close, somewhat triangular pattern of two or three (index, middle, and ring fingers), with a distinct, often slightly larger, circular thumb tip imprint bruise opposite the others. Other common locations for fingertip bruising are the neck (bruise is inflicted during strangulation) and the inner, medial knees and thighs (bruise is inflicted during forced sexual assault) (Fig.11.8).

Punchlike contusions are frequently seen on many areas of a battered woman's body (Fig. 11.6). These contusions are usually oval to circular, with clearly demarcated edges of bruised and nonbruised skin (new injuries). Abusers often punch women in the arm, especially the left arm (Fig. 11.10). Because most people are right handed, an abuser typically throws a right-handed punch during a face-to-face argument. The right-handed victim will turn away

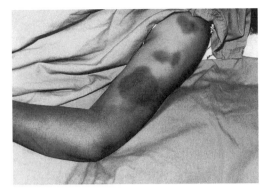

FIG. 11.10   Multiple, patterned, punchlike contusions to the left upper arm.

from the punch in a manner that "offers up" the left side to be struck. If the abuser lands a full punch, the contusion is usually well defined to her upper lateral arm.

If the victim raises her arm to block the punch, she will be bruised on the ulnar surface of the blocking arm (Figs. 11.11 and 11.12). These self-defense–like contusions to her forearms are usually less defined, and there can be linear lines of abrasion along with the contusions, which are caused by the assailant's arm sliding down her arm on impact. Midulnar bone contusions and fractures can result.

Many battered women report being abused in the car as they drive with their abusers. Usually the abuser is driving and the battered woman is in the passenger seat. In a full-sized vehicle, when he chooses to strike her, the abuser will punch or push with his right arm, making contact with her left arm and the left side of her face. This mechanism can also injure the victim's right side of the body, face, or head as she strikes the door and/or window. In a small vehicle, the abuser may start the episode by striking her with his right elbow, and as she cowers more to the right side of her seat, he may then begin

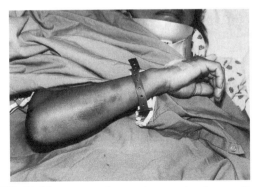

FIG. 11.11   Patterned contusions on the ulnar surface of the right arm, suggesting a defensive posture.

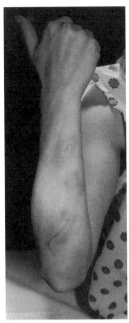

FIG. 11.12   Patterned contusions on the right lower arm, suggesting a defensive posture.

throwing full punches with his right arm. In this case, she may also have secondary right-sided injuries.

Many battered women examined by the author said that during abusive episodes in the car the abusers have tried to push them out of the moving car or that the women have tried to jump out of the moving car to escape the abuse. The women reported that they ended up dangling half in and half out of the car, dragging their hands and arms on the ground. This mechanism of injury usually results in severe "road-burn" abrasions in addition to the blunt force punch and/or elbow trauma. Battered women who totally exit a moving car usually present for emergency care with multisystem trauma with multiple types of injuries, external and internal.

Punchlike contusions to a battered woman's abdomen, chest, and back are common hidden injuries (Fig. 11.13). Although painful, these patterned contusions do not keep the woman from going out of the house because they cannot be seen in the normal course of her day. However, if the abuser wants to further isolate the woman, he will punch her in the face. Battered women with facial injuries often seclude themselves in their homes until the facial trauma injury has healed. When punched directly in the midface, battered women often develop bilateral, periorbital contusions; these contusions are also caused by certain nasal surgeries and as a sequela to basilar skull fractures (Fig. 11.14). Some health care professionals erroneously describe these injuries as bilateral periorbital ecchymoses.

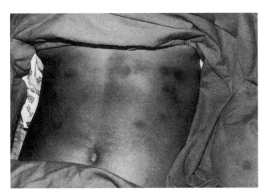

FIG. 11.13 Patterned, hidden, punchlike contusions to the upper abdomen, lower anterior chest.

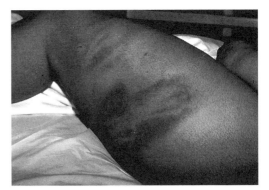

FIG. 11.15 Patterned, foot kick/stomplike contusion to the right, superior lateral thigh pushing blood outward from the point of impact, and patterned, foot kick/stomplike contusion to the right inferior lateral thigh.

Ecchymoses

Ecchymoses are not the same as contusions and bruises; these are hemorrhagic spots, larger than petechiae, that are nonelevated and usually painless. Contusions are caused by blunt force trauma and involve swelling and pain. Ecchymotic spots are caused by bleeding of a medical, hematologic nature, not trauma.

Battered women are frequently kicked or stomped by their abusers. This mechanism of injury can produce distinct patterns. When stomped by a foot with a heeled boot or shoe, a distinct pattern is seen (Figs. 11.7 and 11.15). A full-impact kick with heeled shoe or boot will leave the heel imprint and a bruise imprint from the sole of the shoe. A kick with a gym shoe may leave the distinct pattern from the sole. These types of patterned kick injuries are most visible on the back, buttocks, and thighs. Kick bruising to a woman's shins is most consistent with defensive posture injury. During the beating, the woman will curl up on the ground in a fetal-like position to protect her face, chest, and abdomen.

Lacerations

In addition to contusions, blunt force trauma can result in *lacerations*, which are wounds caused by the tearing of tissue, usually over bony prominences. Lacerations are not sharp injuries such as cuts or incisions. Unfortunately, many health care providers have developed an erroneous habit of calling any break in the skin from any cause a laceration. Lacerations are distinguished from sharp cutting injuries in a number of ways. Lacerations are usually jagged at the skin edges. When the wound is spread apart, lacerations do not have smooth edges, and they are of varying depths. Lacerations are often accompanied by bruising near the split area of skin.

Cuts/Incisions

Cuts or incisions produce openings in the skin that are usually straight. When spread apart, the tissue along the sides of sharp injuries is smooth and the depth is more consistent. If, on the basis of the examination or the patient's history, the health care provider cannot determine whether a break in the skin is a laceration or an incised, sharp injury, then its appearance should be documented and it should be referred to as a "wound."

Petechiae

With a strangulation mechanism of injury, the battered woman may develop facial petechiae, which are minute, pinpoint, nonraised, perfectly round, purplish–red spots caused by intradermal or submucosal hemorrhage. Petechiae can also be seen in the conjunctiva of the eye. Occasionally, facial and eye petechiae can be caused by nonabusive activities,

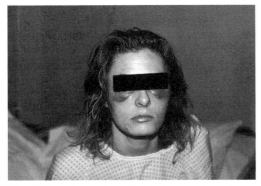

FIG. 11.14 Bilateral, periorbital contusions from a single punch to the midface/forehead (raccoon eyes).

such as childbirth, severe vomiting, or strenuous physical activity such as weight lifting.

Traumatic Alopecia

Battered women report that their abusers often pull them or drag them by the hair. Not only is this form of abuse acutely painful but it can also result in traumatic alopecia. Unless a segment of the scalp has literally been torn away in a scalping manner, traumatic alopecia can be difficult to photograph. To document traumatic alopecia, the author has carefully pulled a comb through the battered patient's hair and photographed the copious loose hairs removed by the comb.

Slap Injuries

Slap and punch injuries to the ears can produce enough force to rupture the ear drum(s). Unless there are other more severe injuries, the author has observed that battered women with ruptured traumatized membranes tend to delay seeking treatment. In general, any injured woman who has delayed seeking medical attention should be screened assertively for domestic violence. Slap injuries to flat areas of the body, such as the back, face, buttocks, or shoulders, can initially produce a patterned, erythemic outline of the hand. Within 24 hours, a slap injury could show sets of thin parallel linear bruises similar in width to the assailant's fingers. The blood vessels that are ruptured by the slap clear centrally to the edges of the points of impact (17).

Firearm Injuries

Battered women with firearm injuries are usually in need of emergency care. Evidence collection and preservation may be secondary to life-saving interventions. However, it is crucial that one member of the trauma/resuscitation team be delegated the task of evidence collection and preservation (see Chapter 4). All cut and removed clothing must be placed in separate paper bags, sealed, labeled, and secured in a locked, ventilated cabinet. Any trace evidence (e.g., soil, grass, glass) must be preserved and labeled accurately. All bullets and/or fragments must be wrapped in protective gauze, such as Telfa, and placed in a clean, dry, plastic container. Multiple bullets or bullet fragments should never be placed in the same container and allowed to bounce off each other. This motion destroys microscopic riflings and may prevent ballistics experts in the police crime lab from making a positive identification of the weapon. Health professionals, in most cases, are not adequately trained to determine which bullet hole is the exit or entrance wound. In fact, Randall found

health professionals to be accurate in determining bullet entrance and exit wounds only half of the time (66). Health professionals should never make any written opinions as to the caliber of the bullet used in the shooting.

Bite Marks

During domestic abuse, battered women are often subjected to biting, frequently in sexual areas. Vale and Noguchi found that women were bitten most frequently on the breasts, followed by the arms and legs (67). Bite injuries often result in unique patterned injuries that can be matched to the assailant's teeth (68). Protocols for the photographic documentation of bite injuries have been developed by the American Board of Forensic Odontology and include taking close-up photographs at both a 90-degree angle to the wound and at what appears to be the angle of the bite, if present (69). The photographs should also include shots with a right-angled ruler.

Sexual Assault

Sheridan (57) and Campbell (28) found that sexual abuse of women by intimate male partners occurred in nearly half of their cases, with forced sex often occurring after the women had left the abusive relationship. Therefore, every woman who has been identified as being battered needs to be assessed for the need for a forensic sexual assault examination. If the reported sexual assault occurred within the previous 120 hours, offering the victim a sexual assault examination has been considered standard. Most sexual assault examiners have been taught that after 120 hours there is no longer enough evidence in or on the victim to justify subjecting her to the trauma of a sexual assault examination. However, the 120-hour "rule" is not an absolute one, only a guideline. There may be numerous circumstances, based on victims' histories, to perform a forensic sexual assault examination after 120 hours. For example, consider doing an examination after 120 hours in case of victims who have not bathed or showered and/or are still wearing the same clothing worn during or immediately after an assault.

PHOTOGRAPHS AND BODY MAPS

Although detailed written histories of domestic abuse are essential components of thorough forensic examinations, taking photographs of all the injuries of battered women, new and old, is even more critical (see Chapter 17). Although taken for the medical documentation of observed and treated injuries, the photographs can be invaluable in criminal and/or civil court proceedings. The most important criterion for a "good picture" is that it be a true and accurate representation of what the health care provider examined and treated on the day of the examination. Most forensically trained abuse examiners prefer using 35-mm cameras with print film. However, prints from Polaroid and digital cameras are also effective in court. All photographic documentation systems have advantages and disadvantages.

Photographs should be taken after signed consent has been obtained. If the victim is unconscious, the photographs should be taken immediately and consent obtained when the patient's condition improves. Photographs of wounds should be taken before and after the wound is cleaned. Photographing the "dirty" wound may corroborate the victim's history as a result of the presence of trace evidence. All patterned injuries and patterns of injuries should be photographed. In fact, some patterned injuries become more apparent over time. Therefore, every abuse patient should be offered follow-up photography 1 and 2 days after initial treatment. Every series of photographs (no matter the camera style) should start with a full-frame identification picture of the victim. Then, for each wound on the victim, the patient should be photographed initially from several feet away, with each subsequent photo coming in closer and closer (Fig. 11.16). The final photo for each injury should be at the closest focal setting the camera can accommodate. Without special macro adapter lenses, most cameras cannot produce a focused picture when moved in closer than 2 ft.

If 35-mm print film is used, it is recommended that the photographer use 12-exposure film. In this author's experience, 12 exposures are usually enough to document the average patient's injuries. If 24- or 36-exposure film is used, there is a tendency to want to "not waste film" by photographing two or more patients on one roll. This is contraindicated. One patient per roll of film is the forensic standard. If a patient has multiple trauma, use multiple rolls of 12-exposure film. For each injury, there should be at least one photograph with a scale present and one photograph without the scale. Scales include rulers and coins. Quality camera shops sell ruler scales that have standardized gray or color reference scales. When using standardized scales, the film developer should be notified *a priori* so that appropriate adjustments can be made during film processing to produce colors true and accurate to those observed (48).

SAFETY PLANNING AND DISCHARGE OPTIONS

Every battered female patient should be asked whether she considers it safe to leave the treatment area or return home. For many of the reasons discussed earlier in this chapter, battered women often choose to return to the abusive relationship. This author has found it clinically useful to do safety planning with every battered patient around four issues. Anticipatory teaching is done for each woman.

The woman is asked what she would do if her husband/boyfriend began hitting her a week, a month, or a year from now. Most women reply that they would call 9-1-1 and seek police assistance. Although this behavior is strongly encouraged, the woman is instructed to state that she needs police help because she is being beaten and/or threatened by a man. The woman is instructed that it is not necessary to state that the assailant is her husband or boyfriend. Although police officers are more highly trained in domestic abuse responses than in years past, domestic calls are still viewed as a waste of time by some officers. The victim may get a quicker police response if the police think they are responding to an assault by a stranger.

A second safety planning technique is to ask the woman whether her abuser always carries a weapon (knife or gun). There are several reasons for this question. The health care provider needs to know whether the abuser is likely to be armed with a weapon, especially if he is sitting in the waiting room or shows up in the treatment area. Knowing this can help protect the health care provider, coworkers, and other patients. If the battered woman says her abuser is always or almost always armed with a weapon, she is instructed to share this information with the police anytime she makes an emergency call. This information may help keep law enforcement personnel safe and may result in a multiunit, faster response time.

A third safety plan includes teaching a battered woman to prepack an emergency "flight bag" with important materials that she or her children might need were they to flee the home in danger. First, she needs to be asked whether it is safe to have such a bag and where it can be safely hidden. Items to be included in the bag might be important documents (e.g., health, bank, court, birth, and citizenship records and emergency family/friend contact telephone numbers); spare money (including change for pay phones); a change of clothing, especially for the children; and small toys for small children.

A fourth safety plan taught to every battered woman consists of inviting her to use the 24-hour local emergency department as a short-term sanctuary for herself and her children. She is told that she can always return to the emergency department if she needs emergency safety. If necessary, she and her children can be assessed and treated. If no medical treatment is necessary, hospital and community social service and victim advocacy services can be obtained.

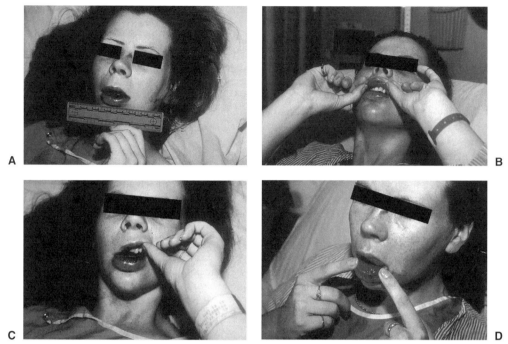

FIG. 11.16 The use of photographs to demonstrate mechanism of injuries. **A:** Victim has obvious facial trauma to her left eyelid, left lateral nose, and mouth. The left lateral nose contusion was caused by the nosepiece of her glasses being forcefully pushed into the nose from a punch injury to left eye. The patient's glasses absorbed much of the punch force and were broken (not pictured). Hence, the actual trauma to her left eye was limited to the upper eyelid. A second punch produced the mouth trauma. **B:** The force of the punch caused the upper teeth to leave patterned contusion, abrasion, and minor laceration trauma on the oral mucosa. **C:** A few of the victim's upper teeth are shown to demonstrate the source of the trauma in the fourth photo. **D:** The victim has a patterned puncture wound in the lower oral mucosa, corresponding to the teeth shown in (**C**).

ADULT MALTREATMENT SYNDROME

Every woman treated in a health care setting for an abuse-related condition must be assigned one or more adult maltreatment syndrome diagnoses in the ICD-9-CM diagnostic code book. The diagnoses are as follows:

995.80   Adult maltreatment, unspecified
995.81   Adult physical abuse
995.82   Adult emotional/psychological abuse
995.83   Adult sexual abuse
995.85   Adult abuse and neglect/other

The use of adult maltreatment syndrome diagnoses will be an asset during Joint Commission on Accreditation of Healthcare Organizations site visits if battered-women client charts are needed for review (17).

SUMMARY

The identification of domestic violence and the forensic documentation of histories and injuries by health care professionals are critical in preventing further abuse. The health care provider must have an understanding of the barriers that prevent women from leaving abusive relationships, as well as an understanding of the necessity for asking routine abuse screening questions and assessing the level of harassment and potentially lethal danger. Written and photographic documentation of abuse, safety planning, and community referrals to abuse services by health care professionals are now considered the minimal standard of care. Failure to meet these standards not only places the abused patient and her children at further risk of abuse but also places the provider at risk of a tort for not meeting the standard.

REFERENCES

1. Novella A. From the surgeon general, US Public Health Service. *JAMA* 1992;276(23):31–32.
2. Cruz JM, Firestone JM. Exploring violence and abuse in gay male relationships. *Violence Vict* 1998;13(2):159–173.
3. Renzetti CM. Violence in lesbian and gay relationships. In: O'Toole LL, Schiffman JR, eds. *Gender violence:*

interdisciplinary perspectives. New York: New York University Press, 1997:285–293.

4. Coleman VE. Lesbian battering: the relationship between personality and the perpetration of violence. *Violence Vict* 1994;9:139–152.

5. Loving N. *Responding to spouse abuse and wife beating: a guide for police*. Washington, DC: Police Executive Research Forum, 1980.

6. Pizzey E, Shapiro J. *Prone to violence*. Feltham, Middlesex, England: Hamlyn Publishing, 1982.

7. Roy M. A current survey of 150 cases. In: Roy M, ed. *Battered women: a psychosociological study of domestic violence*. New York: Van Nostrand Reinhold, 1977.

8. US Commission on Civil Rights. *Battered women: issues of public policy*. Washington, DC, 1978.

9. Walker LE. *The battered woman*. New York: Harper-Colophon Books, 1979.

10. Buzawa ES, Buzawa CG. *Domestic violence: the criminal justice response. Studies in crime and law*, Vol. 6. Thousand Oaks, CA: Sage Publications Inc., 1990.

11. Edwards SSM. *Policing "domestic" violence: women, the law, and the state*. Thousand Oaks, CA: Sage Publications Inc., 1989.

12. Drake VK. Battered women: a health care problem in disguise. *Image* 1982;14:40–47.

13. Lichenstein VR. The battered woman: guidelines for effective nursing intervention. *Issues Ment Health Nurs* 1981;3:237–250.

14. Lieberknecht K. Helping the battered wife. *Am J Nurs* 1978;78:654–656.

15. Parker B, Schumacher DM. The battered wife syndrome and violence in the nuclear family of origin: a controlled pilot study. *Am J Public Health* 1977;67:760–761.

16. Stark E, Flitcraft A, Frazier W. Medicine and patriarchal violence: the social construction of a private event. *Int J Health Serv* 1979;9(3):461–493.

17. Brockmeyer DM, Sheridan DJ. Domestic violence: a practical guide to the use of forensic evaluation in clinical examination and documentation of injuries. In: Campbell JC, ed. *Empowering survivors of abuse: health care for battered women and their children*. Thousand Oaks, CA: Sage Publications Inc., 1998:214–226.

18. Campbell JC. Misogyny and homicide of women. *Adv Nurs Sci* 1981;3(2):67–85.

19. Campbell JC. Nursing assessment for risk of homicide with battered women. *Adv Nurs Sci* 1986;8(4):36–51.

20. Campbell JC. "If I can't have you, no one can": power and control in homicide of female partners. In: Radford J, Russell DEH, eds. *Femicide: the politics of woman killing*. New York: Twayne Publishing, 1992:99–113.

21. Grant CA. Women who kill: the impact of abuse. *Issues Ment Health Nurs* 1995;16:315–326.

22. Lynch VA. Forensic nursing in the emergency department: a new role for the 1990's. *Crit Care Nurs Q* 1991;14(3):69–86.

23. Lynch VA. Forensic nursing: diversity in education and practice. *J Psychosoc Nurs* 1993;31(11):7–14.

24. Sheridan DJ, Belknap L, Engel B, et al. *Guidelines for the treatment of battered women victims in emergency room settings*. Chicago: Chicago Hospital Council, 1985.

25. Sheridan DJ. The role of the battered women specialist. *J Psychosoc Nurs* 1993;31(11):31–37.

26. Sheridan DJ. Family violence. In: Kitt S, Selfridge-Thomas J, Proehl JA et al., eds. *Emergency nursing: a physiologic and clinical perspective*, 2nd ed. Philadelphia, PA: WB Saunders, 1995:482–494.

27. Sheridan DJ. Forensic documentation of battered pregnant women. *J Nurse Midwifery* 1996;41(6):467–472.

28. Campbell JC. Women's responses to sexual abuse in intimate relationships. *Women's Health Care Int* 1989;8:335–347.

29. Eby KK, Campbell JC. Health effects of experiences of sexual violence for women with abusive partners. *Women's Health Care Int* 1995;14:563–576.

30. Campbell JC, Soeken K. Forced sex and intimate partner violence: effects on women's health. *Violence Against Women* 1999;5:1017–1035.

31. Pence E, Paymar M. *Power and control: tactics of men who batter*. Duluth, MN: Domestic Abuse Intervention Project, 1986.

32. Pence E, Paymar M. *Education groups for men who batter: the duluth model*. New York: Springer-Verlag, 1993.

33. Wilson M, Daly M. Spousal homicide risk and estrangement. *Violence Vict* 1993;8(1):3–16.

34. Wilson M, Daly M, Daniele A. Familicide: the killing of spouse and children. *Aggress Behav* 1995;21:275–291.

35. Sonkin DJ. *The counselor's guide to learning to live without violence*. Volcano, CA: Volcano Press, 1995.

36. Boulette TR, Andersen SM. "Mind control" and the battering of women. *Community Ment Health J* 1985;21(2):109–117.

37. Graham DLR, Rawlings EI. Bonding with abusive dating partners: dynamics of Stockholm syndrome. In: Levy B, ed. *Dating violence: young women in danger*. Seattle, WA: Seal Press, 1991:119–135.

38. Graham DLR, Rawlings EI, Rimini N. Survivors of terror: battered women, hostages, and the Stockholm syndrome. In: Yllo K, Bograd M, eds. *Feminist perspectives on wife abuse*. Thousand Oaks, CA: Sage Publications Inc., 1988:217–233.

39. Dutton DG, Painter SL. Traumatic bonding: the development of emotional attachments in battered women and other relationships of intermittent abuse. *Victimology: An Int J* 1981;1(4):139–155.

40. Dutton DG, Painter S. Emotional attachments in abusive relationships: a test of traumatic bonding theory. *Violence Vict* 1993;8(2):105–120.

41. Fortune MM, Horman D. *Family violence: a workshop manual for clergy and other service providers. Domestic violence monograph series*, Vol. 6. Rockville, MD: National Clearing House on Domestic Violence, 1981.

42. NiCarthy G. *Getting free: a handbook for women in abusive relationships*. Seattle, WA: Seal Press, 1986.

43. Tolman RM. The development of a measure of psychological maltreatment of women by their male partners. *Violence Against Women* 1989;3:159–177.

44. Walker LE. *The battered woman syndrome*, 2nd ed. New York: Springer-Verlag, 1999.

45. Biderman AD. Captivity lore and behavior in captivity. In: Grosser GH, Wechsler H, Greenblat M, eds. *The threat of impending disaster*. Cambridge, MA: MIT Press, 1964.

46. Raymond B, Bruschi IG. Psychological abuse among college women in dating relationships. *Percept Mot Skills* 1989;69:1283–1297.

47. Johnson MP. Patriarchal terrorism and common couple violence: two forms of violence against women. *J Marriage Fam* 1995;57:283–294.

48. Sheridan DJ. Forensic identification and documentation of patients experiencing intimate partner violence. *Clin Fam Pract* 2003;5(1):113–143.

49. American Medical Association. *Diagnostic and treatment guidelines on domestic violence*. Chicago, 1992.

50. Cole TB. Is domestic violence screening helpful? *JAMA* 2000;284(5):551–556.

51. U.S. Preventative Services Task Force. Screening for family and intimate partner violence: recommendation statement. *Ann Intern Med* 2004;140(5):382–386.

52. Helton A. *Protocol of care for the battered woman*. Houston: Houston Chapter of the March of Dimes, 1986.

53. McFarlane J, Parker B, Soeken K, et al. Assessing for abuse during pregnancy. *JAMA* 1992;267(3):3176–3178.

54. Straus MA. Measuring intra-family conflict and violence: the Conflict Tactics (CT) Scales. *J Marriage Fam* 1979;41:75–88.

55. Hudson WW, McIntosh SR. The assessment of spouse abuse: two quantifiable dimensions. *J Marriage Fam* 1981;43(4):873–885.

56. Soeken KL, McFarlane J, Parker B, et al. The abuse assessment screen: measuring frequency, severity, and perpetrator of abuse against women. In: Campbell JC, ed. *Empowering survivors of abuse: health care for battered women and their children.* Thousand Oaks, CA: Sage Publications Inc., 1998:195–203.

57. Sheridan DJ. *Measuring harassment of abused women: a nursing concern.* Unpublished doctoral dissertation, Portland, OR: Oregon Health Sciences University, 1998.

58. Campbell JC. Homicide of and by battered women. In: Campbell JC, ed. *Assessing dangerousness: violence by sexual offenders, batterers, and child abusers.* Thousand Oaks, CA: Sage Publications Inc., 1995:96–113.

59. Sonkin DJ, Martin D, Walker LE. *The male batterer: a treatment approach.* New York: Springer Publishers Inc., 1985.

60. Hart B. Beyond the "duty to warn": a therapist's "duty to protect" battered women and children. In: Yllo K, Bograd M, eds. *Feminist perspectives on wife abuse.* Thousand Oaks, CA: Sage Publications Inc., 1988:234–248.

61. Campbell JC, Webster D, Koziol-McLain J, et al. Risk factors for femicide in abusive relationships: results from a multi-site case controlled study. *Am J Public Health* 2003;93(7):1089–1097.

62. Limandri BJ, Sheridan DJ. Prediction of intentional interpersonal violence: an introduction. In: Campbell JC, ed. *Assessing dangerousness: violence by sexual offenders, batterers, and child abusers.* Thousand Oaks, CA: Sage Publications Inc., 1995:1–19.

63. DiMaio DJ, DiMaio VJM. *Forensic pathology.* New York: Elsevier Science, 1989.

64. Gordon I, Shapiro HA, Berson SD. *Forensic medicine*, 3rd ed. Edinburgh: Churchill Livingstone, 1988.

65. O'Toole M. *Miller-Keane encyclopedia and dictionary of medicine, nursing, and allied health*, 7th ed. Philadelphia, PA: WB Saunders, 2003.

66. Randall T. Clinician's forensic interpretations of fatal gunshot wounds often miss the mark. *JAMA* 1993;269(16):2058–2061.

67. Vale GL, Noguchi TT. Anatomical distribution of human bite marks in a series of 67 cases. *J Forensic Sci* 1983;28(1):61–69.

68. Gold MH, Roenigk HH Jr, Smith ES, et al. Evaluation and treatment of patients with human bite marks. *Am J Forensic Med Pathol* 1989;13(2):140–143.

69. American Board of Forensic Odontology. Guidelines for bite mark analysis. *J Am Dent Assoc* 1986;112(3):383–386.

NEW DRUGS OF ABUSE

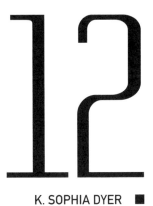

K. SOPHIA DYER ■

Alcohol still holds the lead as the most common drug of abuse and "social lubricant." However, many other drugs are used and abused by people from all strata of American society, and, unfortunately, these drugs remain in ready supply from local sources and through the Internet. Many of the substances of abuse discussed in this chapter are called "club drugs," a name based on the use of these substances as part of the culture of nightclubs, raves, and dance parties. But their use is not limited to the world of nightclubs. Many adults, teenagers, and children seek and use these drugs. Some are chronically addicted and others are occasional experimenters.

THE SPECTRUM OF NEW DRUGS OF ABUSE

Patterns of drug abuse differ by region. For example, methamphetamine might be seen commonly in one section of the country but unheard of in another. Some of these patterns are static; others reflect the gradual progression of the popularity of a substance. The types of drugs being abused in a community will likely be known to law enforcement agents. New drug patterns could first become apparent to emergency department physicians in a number of ways: a change in the number of intoxicated patients, an increase in the severity of their condition, or variation from the typical presentation of effect or overdose.

Laboratory examination of either the substance or biologic samples from patients can be helpful to public health officials and law enforcement officers. The detection of a contaminant or the introduction of a novel new drug can be vital information for both groups as they respond to community concerns about substance abuse. If the substance is the focus of a criminal investigation, the chain of custody must be preserved.

Variations imposed on chemical structures, which are not always intentional, can cause differences in clinical effect. For example, in an attempt to subvert existing regulations (the Controlled Substance Act), the amphetamine structure was modified and produced as 3,4-methylenedioxymethamphetamine (MDMA, Ecstasy). The Controlled Substance Act defined a substance as "controlled" only after the acceptance of its structure and effect—a retrospective approach that was changed by the Controlled Substance Analogue Enforcement Act of 1986. The 1986 act classifies chemical structures that are substantially similar to those of schedule I or II controlled substances. After this closing of the "loophole," a substance was considered illegal if it was used as a stimulant, depressant, or hallucinogen and designed for that purpose. These acts continue to be updated, as legal forces attempt to keep pace with those who distribute substances. In March 2000, γ-hydroxybutyrate (GHB) was added to the schedule I list (i.e., drugs with high abuse potential, such as heroin). GHB does not bear any structural similarity to the other schedule I or II drugs, but because of rising concerns about abuse, it was added to the list.

During the past 25 years, "designer drugs" have been implicated in mass poisoning and isolated instances of contamination. Both situations require public health and legal investigations. The early identification of extreme reactions to ingested drugs, atypical emergency department presentations of people who abuse the substances, and an increase in the number of people seeking emergency care after using the drug should be communicated to public health officials in an effort to avoid an epidemic of severe reactions and overdoses.

In 1991, New York City saw a rise in opioid overdoses in a heroin-abusing population. Investigation revealed a drug packaged as "Tango and Cash," which was found to contain a very potent form of fentanyl (1). A similar case involving heroin with a nonopioid contaminant occurred in several northeastern cities in the United States between 1995 and 1996. The heroin was contaminated with scopolamine, which caused a combined presentation of opiate and anticholinergic poisoning (2). In 1982, clandestine manufacturers intending to produce the meperidine analog MPPP (1-methyl-4-phenyl-4-propionoxypiperidine) actually made MPTP (1-methyl-4-phenyl-1,2,3,6-tetrahydropyridine), which destroyed users' substantia nigra, causing severe parkinsonism (3). Several comatose teenagers brought to an emergency department in Philadelphia had used the Internet to purchase the GHB they ingested at a party (4).

In addition to laboratory data, the history surrounding the presentation can be helpful to the emergency physician in the assessment and management of a patient suspected of being exposed to a drug of abuse. Suspicion or report of sexual assault should prompt an evaluation for sedative-hypnotics, hallucinogens, GHB or its analogs, benzodiazepines, or dissociative hallucinogens such as ketamine. The patient/victim might be able to identify the type of substance used (liquid, pill, injectable, inhalant) and the intended goal—hallucination, sedation, or stimulation. The report of pill or capsule ingestion suggests that a standard pharmaceutical might have been used. This possibility should be considered in the identification process for any "new" drug of abuse or "designer drug" presentation. The illegal procurement of pharmaceuticals has been reported and documented in relation to mass exposures. For example, in preparation for a dance party, teenagers stole baclofen from the doorstep of a neighbor who receives prescriptions by mail order. The results of distribution of the drug during the party were impressive: 14 children were evaluated at area hospitals, 9 of them requiring intubation (5). The intentional abuse of over-the-counter drugs remains an issue of concern. A poison control center evaluation of 2,214 intentional abuses among children aged between 6 and 14 showed that 38% involved nonprescription drug abuse, the most common being anticholinergics, caffeine, dextromethorphan (DXM), and ephedrine (6).

TESTING FOR DRUGS OF ABUSE

Emergency department physicians who request drug testing for a patient in their care should be aware of the strengths and limitations of the test methods available to them. Consultation with a clinical toxicologist, a clinical chemist, or a clinical pathologist can help identify the likely drug(s) in question. Important variables that should be considered in regard to the assessment of a patient for drug use are sample collection, the type of test to be performed, and the types of substances that could interfere with the accuracy of the results. The most common samples for drug testing are urine and blood; hair and meconium can also be used.

Before concluding that "the tox screen is negative," the physician must know the methodology used by the laboratory. Does it perform comprehensive screens for multiple substances or single tests for specific xenobiotics? In addition, the physician should be aware of the test's detection and confirmation limits, especially for new drug analogs. Some drugs (e.g., ketamine) are difficult to detect with standard screening methods; referral to a reference laboratory might be required. Other drugs of abuse, especially amphetamines, are often modified in clandestine "laboratories," so it is difficult for medical facilities to remain current with analytic techniques and precautions against cross-reactivity.

For some substances, testing can indicate use of the drug but not necessarily intoxication with it. In an analysis for the presence of cocaine, for example, the screen detects benzoylecgonine, a metabolite formed soon after ingestion; therefore, a negative test excludes intoxication, within the appropriate detection levels in testing, but a positive test within the detection interval does not allow a conclusion to be made about if and when the patient was intoxicated. Detection intervals vary with manufacturers, and they can be influenced by the nature of the abuse (chronic vs. occasional). For interpretation of drug test results, physicians are encouraged to consult a medical toxicologist, who is specifically trained to interpret the patient's presentation in relation to the results of the analysis.

Testing for drugs of abuse has applications in fields other than medicine; rapid testing is used by employers to screen potential and current employees for the presence of drugs. For jobs requiring a commercial driver's license, most companies test for the NIDA 5, the five substances for which the National Institute on Drug Abuse (NIDA) (www.nida.nih.gov) requires testing for federal employment: cannabinoids, cocaine (benzoylecgonine), amphetamines, opiates, and phencyclidine (PCP). Commercial testing is also available for barbiturates, benzodiazepine, methadone, propoxyphene (Darvon and Darvocet), MDMA, and inhalants such as toluene and xylene. The "NIDA 9" are amphetamine, opiates, cocaine, PCP, marijuana, barbiturates, benzodiazepine, propoxyphene, and methadone.

Testing for drugs of abuse as workplace screening is regulated by legislative influences and must consider workers' rights. It is common for laboratories to use one method of testing for initial screening and then confirm positive results with a different method. Laboratory testing is subject to governmental regulations. At the federal level, the Clinical Laboratory Improvement Amendments (CLIA) influence the testing of human specimens for medical purposes. Some point-of-care testing is exempt under CLIA, but most other testing is considered moderate to complex. Multiple requirements are listed under each degree of testing, ranging from written procedures to daily controls to on-site supervision. Further information on CLIA and its regulations can be found at www.cms.hhs.gov/clia.

Spectrochemical Tests

Many alcohol assays are based on spectrochemical analysis. This test method is based on chemical reactions that produce a light-absorbing product, typically using a specific wavelength of light. The quantity of a substance is determined by the amount of light (infrared or ultraviolet) absorbed. An example of spectrochemical testing is cooximetry used to determine the spectra of hemoglobins. Enzymes can be added to spectrochemical processes as catalysts for specific reactions.

Immunoassays

Immunoassays are one of the more common methods used to detect small concentrations of substances, typically in urine (other specimens can be used as well). The general principle of immunoassays is the use of selective and specific antibodies to recognize the composition of a drug. A limitation of immunoassays is their susceptibility to cross-reactivity. Examples of immunoassays are listed below:

- Enzyme-multiplied immunoassay technique (EMIT)
- Fluorescence polarization immunoassay (FPIA)
- Kinetic inhibition of microparticles in solution (KIMS)
- Cloned enzyme donor immunoassay (CEDIA)

- CEDIA and EMIT are commonly used as screens for drugs of abuse.

Thin-Layer Chromatography

Thin-layer chromatography (TLC) employs a thin silica gel designed to physically separate drugs and metabolites between its phases. After a solvent is allowed to migrate up the matrix, the gel is treated with reagents to analyze substances by color change. The addition of this identification step after separation made it possible for the technology to be used for drug screening. Some extraction techniques have the advantage of allowing measurement of the concentration of the substance being evaluated.

The advantage of TLC is that it can detect several substances. However, it is limited by a number of factors:

- Detection can be hampered if the quantity of substance present is low.
- TLC does not always allow the quantity to be determined.
- TLC is labor intensive if multiple extractions are required (but new commercial kits have reduced the labor requirement for urine screening).
- Detection limits vary with the test.
- Preparation for chromatography can require the introduction of organic solvents for extraction.

High-Performance Liquid Chromatography

High-performance liquid chromatography (HPLC) involves the application of high pressure to a stationary column. Drugs are identified by retention time in the column and ultraviolet spectroscopy—the amount of light absorbed is compared to a standard. The process has been automated to allow the processing of multiple columns with various solvents and light spectra. It has also been computerized to facilitate the comparison of retention times and spectra. The main disadvantage of high-performance liquid chromatography is its costly equipment.

Gas Chromatography/Mass Spectroscopy

Gas chromatography is available as a qualitative or quantitative method for volatile organic compounds. The compounds are separated by partitioning between the mobile gas phase and the stationary phase. Methanol, ethylene glycol, isopropanol, and basic drugs (sedatives, hypnotics, opioids) can be detected using this technique. The addition of mass spectroscopy can confirm, quantify, and identify larger groups of substances; libraries can be built to identify hundreds of drugs and their metabolites.

NEW DRUGS OF ABUSE

γ-Hydroxybutyrate and Related Compounds

GHB and the related compounds γ-butyrolactone (GBL) and 1,4-butanediol (BD) (Fig. 12.1) are used to induce recreational euphoria, for intentional attempts to intoxicate (as in date-rape cases), and as a purported bodybuilding agent. GHB is also used for the treatment of cataplexy, under the trade name Xyrem (Orphan Medical, Inc., Minnetonka, Minnesota). Varied effects are attributed to GHB and its relatives: improved mood, decreased anxiety, enhanced libido, amnesia, sleep, and muscular development. These compounds, under multiple names (Table 12-1), and the recipes for their manufacture can be found on the Internet. Liquid preparations that are manufactured may have dye additives in a variety of colors, so the reported color of the liquid might not be useful in identification. Hygroscopic-powder versions of the substances can be found packaged in capsules. The precursors of GHB (GBL and BD) are components of cleaners, paint removers, and other industrial chemicals. GHB and its related compounds are typically ingested orally, at times with alcohol or other sedative/hypnotic agents.

GHB has gained considerable attention as an agent used to facilitate sexual assault; the liquid form of the product can be concealed in drinks, although some people describe a salty, soapy, or chemical taste. The true scope of GHB-facilitated sexual assault is unknown. Underreporting, lack of confirmatory laboratory testing, and the relatively short period of time the drug can be detected in urine compound the difficulty in determining the actual incidence. Most hospital laboratories do not test for GHB.

Detection Methods

Laboratory analysis for the presence of GHB can be challenging because the compound occurs naturally in the body (in the brain, kidney, heart, and skeletal muscle (7,8)) and because ingested

TABLE 12-1

STREET AND CHEMICAL NAMES FOR γ-HYDROXYBUTYRATE AND RELATED COMPOUNDS

GHB	*Street names:* G, liquid ecstasy, Grievous Bodily Harm, gib, soap, scoop, Nitro *Chemical names:* γ-Hydroxybutyrate, Sodium oxybate
GBL	*Street names:* Blue Nitro, GH, Revitalizer, Gamma G, Renewtrient *Chemical names:* 2(3*H*)-furanone dihydro; butyrolactone; γ-butyrolactone; 4-butyrolactone; dihydro-2(3*H*)-furanone; 4-butanediol; 2(3*H*)-furanone, dihydro; tetrahydro-2-furanone; and butyrolactone γ
BD	*Street names:* Weight Belt Cleaner, Serenity, Thunder Nectar, Revitalize Plus, 1,4-B, BDO, Soma Solution, Dream On *Chemical name:* 1,4-butanediol
GVL	*Street names:* Tranquili-G, 4Sleep *Chemical names:* γ-valerolactone, dihydro-5-methyl-2(3*H*)-furanone, 4-hydroxypentanoicacid lactone, γ-methyl-γ-butrolactone, 4-methyl-γ-butyrolactone, 4-pentanolide

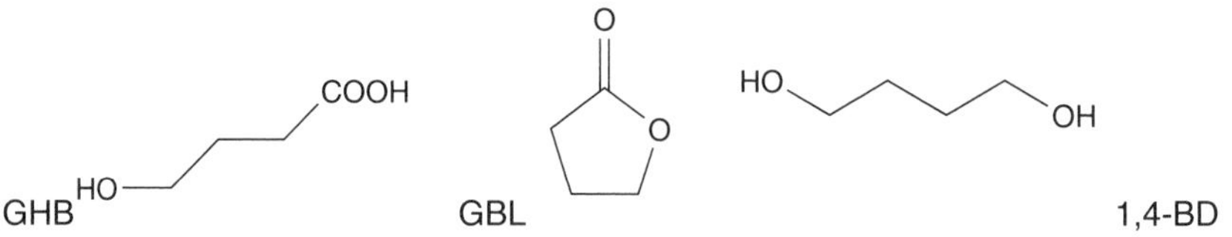

product is eliminated rapidly. GHB testing relies on the metabolism of BD and GBL *in vivo*. After analyzing samples from subjects presumed to be drug free, Elian (9) recommended cutoff values for endogenous levels of GHB of $1,000\ \mu$g per dL for urine and $500\ \mu$g per dL for blood. Chemists have also converted samples of GHB into GBL to facilitate analysis and have developed a method for direct analysis involving solid-phase and liquid–liquid extraction followed by gas chromatography/mass spectrometry (GC/MS) (10). Capillary electrophoresis has been reported as useful in the identification of GHB in both urine and serum (11). Availability of results depends on the capabilities of in-house or reference laboratories; many hospitals send specimens to reference laboratories.

It may be important for legal or forensic reasons to correctly identify the specific agent—GHB, GBL,

FIG. 12.1   Chemical structures of γ-hydroxybutyrate (GHB) and its precursors, γ-butyrolactone (GBL) and 1,4-butanediol (BD).

or BD—involved in a case. Some techniques for GHB identification can lead to shifts in chemical equilibrium between GHB and the lactone, GBL. But if the exact identification of GHB is needed, this should be communicated to the laboratory. Depending on the technique used, interference can come from urea or β-hydroxybutyric acid because of their similar spectral qualities but this can be controlled by laboratory techniques.

Other testing methods have been marketed to consumers concerned about the use of GHB and other substances for drug-facilitated sexual assault. An interesting drug-detection coaster is commercially available. The user is instructed to place a drop of a suspected drug-laced drink on the coaster. A color change indicates the presence of a "date-rape" drug. Analysis of this product showed that it does have some ability to detect GHB and ketamine, but its sensitivity is hampered by the need for high drug concentration, the matrix of the beverage, and the time requirement for the ketamine reaction (12).

Clinical Presentation

The clinical presentation of people intoxicated with GHB ranges from drowsiness to dose-related central nervous system depression, including respiratory depression. Alcohol can have an additive effect. Other reported effects include combative behavior and agitation. Symptoms can range from euphoria, amnesia, hypotonia, hypothermia, bradycardia, Cheyne-Stokes respiration, coma (maybe altering with agitation), seizures or seizure-like activity, salivation, myoclonic movements, severe respiratory depression, and death (13–16). A more bizarre presentation involved self-mutilation: a woman under the influence of GHB extracted many of her own teeth (17).

Most patients will recover in 6 hours. In general, supportive care is sufficient, but respiratory support might be required in severe poisoning. Severe GHB presentation can be confirmed with GHB levels, but quantitative serum levels do not correlate with the degree of coma or time to awakening (18). Coingestions should be considered. In a study of blood specimens of 149 suspected GHB cases, 54 specimens confirmed GHB; other substances found were ethanol, MDMA, marijuana, methamphetamine, cocaine, and citalopram (19). Another interpretation of these findings is that many patients who present with GHB as the suspected cause of their symptoms are not confirmed by positive GHB test results. A withdrawal syndrome is recognized as a consequence of chronic dosing and dependence on GHB. Its manifestations can include anxiety, insomnia, psychosis, and, in some cases, severe delirium with autonomic instability (20).

Amphetamines

The use and abuse of methamphetamine (D-phenylisopropylmethylamine hydrochloride) (Fig. 12.2) and amphetamine (β-phenylisopropylamine) in the United States and other countries date back to the 1930s. From the 1960s through the 1980s, amphetamine derivatives ("designer amphetamines") developed a following. Illicit "chemists" had two goals in mind when modifying the structure of amphetamine: to avoid regulations and to induce effects such as hallucination. Some of their creations are well known (Table 12-2), for example, Ecstasy (MDMA), which has become especially popular as a "club drug"; others, such as para-methoxyamphetamine (PMA), have had waxing and waning popularity.

Because of the pleasure associated with their use, amphetamines are classified as "entactogens." Entactogens are generally believed to lack the major changes in perception and thought that are induced by hallucinogens, but they induce feelings of closeness, euphoria, and, for some, empathy with fellow partygoers (21). These effects are likely related to the drug's entactogen properties as well as its effects on seratonin, norepinephrine, and dopamine. Hallucinogenic properties of some amphetamine derivatives, methoxyamphetamines, have been described, including hallucinations and alterations in visual perception.

Props are associated with MDMA use in certain circles, for example, fluorescent light sticks and jewelry, mentholated ointments, and lollipops and infant pacifiers for mediation of the bruxism that can follow ingestion.

The most common route for ingestion of MDMA and related compounds is oral (through tablet, capsule, or drug-impregnated paper or sugar cube). It can also be taken intravenously, by nasal insufflation, and by smoking. Designer amphetamines in compressed pill format often have imprints such as cartoon characters or trademarks on one or both sides of the tablet. Websites such as www.dancesafe.org offer information about these imprints, but identification by this method is not definitive.

Detection Methods

Most hospital laboratories use the immunoassay technology to test for amphetamines. Some

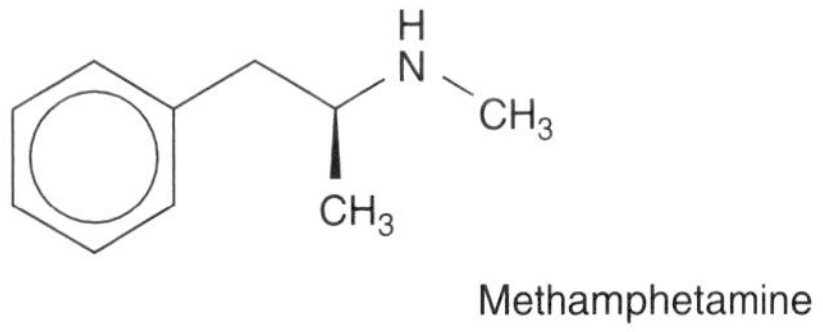

Methamphetamine

FIG. 12.2 Chemical structure of methamphetamine.

TABLE 12-2

STREET AND CHEMICAL NAMES FOR "DESIGNER" AMPHETAMINES

MDEA	*Street name:* Eve
	Chemical name: 3,4-Methylenedioxyethamphetamine
MDMA	*Street names:* Ecstasy, Adam, XTC, X, E, Lover's speed
	Chemical name: 3,4-Methylenedioxymethamphetamine
MDA	*Street name:* Love drug
	Chemical name: 3,4-Methylenedioxyamphetamine
DOB	*Street name:* Bromo-DMA
	Chemical name: 4-Bromo-2,5-dimethoxyamphetamine
2-CB	*Street names:* MFT, Venus, Bees, Nexus
	Chemical name: 4-Bromo-2,5-methoxyphenylethylamine
Methcathinone	*Street names:* Jeff, cat
DOM	*Street name:* STP (serenity, tranquility, peace)
	Chemical name: 4-Methyl-2,5-dimethoxyamphetamine
4-MTA	*Street name:* Flat liners
	Chemical name: 4-Methylthioamphetamine
PMA	*Street name:* 4-MA, death
	Chemical name: para-methoxyamphetamine
TMA-2	*Street name:* Zerox
	Chemical name: 2,4,5-Trimethoxyamphetamine

immunoassays do not react with all of the designer amphetamines and therefore give false-negative reports regarding the presence of amphetamine derivatives. Any amphetamine analysis must consider cross-reactions with products such as pseudoephedrine, ephedrine, phenylpropanolamine, and L-methamphetamine (22–24). EMIT has a monoclonal antibody component for amphetamine and methamphetamine and therefore can be selective for those compounds as well as 3,4-methylenedioxyamphetamine (MDA) and MDMA. The FPIA, radioimmunoassay (also used for blood and tissue analysis), CEDIA, and enzyme-linked immunosorbent assay might be limited by cross-reactivity to varying extents with MDA and MDMA. Since so many detection methods are available, and improvements to them are being made continuously, the clinician should confirm the sensitivity and specificity of the laboratory's analytic method before reaching a definitive conclusion about the results. Consultation with a forensic or clinical chemist should be considered. Case evaluation should include a review of the patient's legitimate medication use. For example, L-deprenyl (Selegiline), used to manage Parkinson's disease, is converted *in vivo* into L-methamphetamine and L-amphetamine but not into the D-enantiomers. This will present as a positive result on some amphetamine screens. The variety of amphetamines available makes the task of specific and rapid testing a challenge at best. The specific amphetamine can be typed definitively with GC/MS.

TLC is used in several commercially available systems, such as TOXI-LAB (Varian, Palo Alto, California). The accuracy of TLC in detecting amphetamine and methamphetamine is limited, however, because many of the sympathomimetic amines (pseudoephedrine, phentermine, ephedrine) have color characteristics similar to theirs. Techniques have been added to some TLC technologies to allow differentiation of selected amines.

Clinical Presentation

Methamphetamine Methamphetamine can be abused by multiple routes—intravenous, intramuscular, nasal, or inhalation. The medical consequences of intravenous, intramuscular, and transdermal (skin popping) injection are familiar to any clinician who treats intravenous drug abusers: local skin infections, abscess formation, endocarditis, and transmission of the viruses that cause hepatitis and the acquired immunodeficiency syndrome.

The clandestine manufacture of methamphetamine is a dangerous process, so if the user is also the producer, exposure to toxic chemicals should be considered as part of a patient's presentation to an emergency department. "Cooking" processes are posted on the Internet and are available from the "cooks" who will propagate recipes. Many start with a cold preparation containing ephedrine or pseudoephedrine. In an effort to control illicit manufacturing, some municipalities limit the amount of these preparations that can be purchased.

Other toxic chemicals involved in the production of methamphetamine include hydrochloric acid, red phosphorus, iodine, and alkalis (Table 12-3). Household members, especially children, can suffer consequences of the cooking process as result of inhalation of chemical fumes, chemical dermal burns, or thermal burns. A review of 507 admissions to a Kansas burn center during a 3-year period revealed that 34 patients were injured as a result of the use or manufacture of methamphetamine. Males predominated in the sample by a ratio of 10.3 to 1 (25). Laboratories have exploded (26). The manufacturing process can expose the user to contaminants in the chemicals used to derive the methamphetamine. Because lead acetate is used in some recipes, lead poisoning has been reported as a consequence of methamphetamine use (27,28). As in the cocaine trade, methamphetamine traffickers sometimes resort to body stuffing (swallowing the drug in an attempt to hamper a police officer's ability to connect it to the person) or body packing (transporting the drug by ingesting it or packing it in the rectum or vagina). These practices can have serious consequences if absorption occurs (29).

Concerns about the health consequences of methamphetamine abuse extend to local first responders. Most methamphetamine is produced locally rather than imported. In an evaluation of reports to the Hazardous Substances Emergency Events Surveillance System (26), 5 states reported 112 events associated with methamphetamine, in which 155 persons were injured. Half of those injured were firefighters, police officers, emergency medical services personnel, and hospital employees, and most of their injuries involved the respiratory system and the eyes. Hydrochloric acid and anhydrous ammonia were implicated in approximately one third of the cases (26).

Easily absorbed by multiple routes, methamphetamine has a long half-life and therefore potentially prolonged effects (>24 hours) (30–32). Clinical effects are a consequence of the ability of amphetamines to stimulate both central and peripheral adrenergic receptors. Consistent with this mechanism of action are hypertension, tachycardia, hyperthermia, agitation, euphoria, anorexia, psychosis, diaphoresis, mydriasis, tremor, and tachypnea. Other consequences include dysrhythmias, myocardial infarction, aortic dissection, vasospasm, seizures, and intracerebral hemorrhage. Prolonged agitation and/or hyperthermia can lead to metabolic acidosis and acute renal failure. Behaviors such as chronic repetitive task performance and bruxism are seen, as well as choreoathetoid movements (33,34). Necrotizing vasculitis with narrowing, beading of small to medium arteries, and necrotizing arteritis with multisystem organ involvement have been reported (35–38).

Acute treatment should address the symptoms of agitation, hyperthermia, and seizures and the consequences of end organ damage, aortic dissection, stroke, intracranial hemorrhage, or acute renal failure. External cooling and control of agitation with benzodiazepines are generally the first clinical considerations, followed by management of end organ effects. If hypertension does not respond to the control of agitation with benzodiazepines, some clinicians recommend the use of vasodilators such as nitroprusside or α-blockade drugs, for example, phentolamine. Amphetamine-induced psychosis has been shown to be responsive to dopamine antagonists such as haloperidol, but concerns about the effect of these agents on thermoregulation and seizure threshold lead some clinicians to start with benzodiazepines to control psychosis.

MDMA and Related Compounds The variety of modifications that have been made to the basic MDMA structure (Fig. 12.3) and all their subsequent derivations complicate the task of describing the clinical presentation of someone who has ingested these drugs. It is possible that those involved in the design of club drugs will continue to change the chemical structures, with untold clinical effects. Therefore, some generalities, based on what is known about MDMA, need to be applied in the attempts to describe the emergency department presentation of MDMA users and abusers.

TABLE 12-3

CHEMICALS OR PRODUCTS USED IN THE PRODUCTION OF METHAMPHETAMINE

Aluminum foil
Anhydrous ammonia
Coffee filters
Lithium batteries
Matchbook covers (for red phosphorus)
Road flares (for red phosphorus)
Pumice stones
Brake cleaner
Drain cleaner
Ephedra
Ethanol
Ether
Iodine
Methanol
Hydrogen chloride
Hydroiodic acid
Toluene
Vinegar
Starter fluid

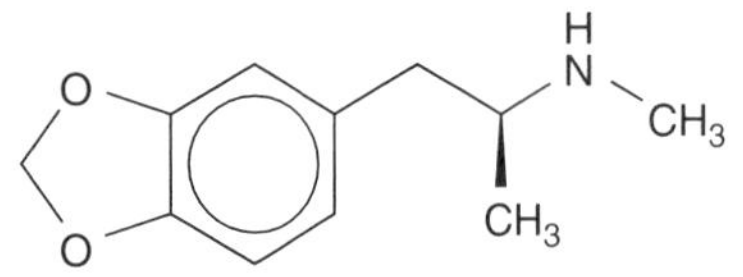

FIG. 12.3 Chemical structure of methylenedioxy-methamphetamine (MDMA, Ecstasy).

MDMA is typically sold as a tablet; related substances might be sold as a powder or on blotter paper. Adulteration with a variety of substances—caffeine, DXM, pseudoephedrine, or LSD (lysergic acid diethylamide)—has been reported (39,40). The buyer might believe that he or she is purchasing MDMA but end up with a related compound such as PMA or 2-CB.

Effects may appear as early as 30 minutes after ingestion and last for 8 hours (41). Feelings of distortion of time, anorexia, euphoria, insight, intimacy, and well-being are generally the user's goal (42). Trismus and bruxism, as can be induced by methamphetamine use, are undesired effects that lead some users to suck on lollipops or pacifiers (43). At low doses, MDMA has less of a stimulant effect than methamphetamine or dextroamphetamine, but this is countered by a more prominent serotonin release (44,45). The association between MDMA and serotonin release can lead to serotonin syndrome, the manifestations of which can include hyperthermia, autonomic dysfunction, hyperreflexia, clonus, mydriasis, rigidity, diaphoresis, agitation, pressured speech, delirium, and tremor (46). Along with supportive care, including temperature control, some role may exist for cyproheptadine in the management of serotonin syndrome (47).

Another consequence of the use of Ecstasy is liver injury. In a review of patients admitted to an intensive care unit in Spain, Ecstasy was considered the second most common cause of acute liver failure in patients under 20 years of age (48). Possible causes of liver dysfunction are an ischemic mechanism, hyperthermia, contaminants, or a destructive metabolite (49–52). A more specific mechanism might apply to individuals with low levels of debrisoquine 4-hydroxylase metabolic activity, potentially making them more vulnerable to toxicity (53).

MDMA is associated with a rise in antidiuretic hormone concentration, resulting in hyponatremia. Contributory factors include a hot dance club environment, intake of a large amount of water, and exertion (54–58). The long-term consequence of MDMA use is a growing question. A study of the effect of MDMA on human and animal brains suggests that the use of MDMA can lead to

5-hydroxytryptamine (5-HT) (serotonin) neurotoxicity (59). Other designer amphetamines might have different symptom expression. PMA, for example, is reported to have a more hallucinogenic effect and is associated with significant morbidity and mortality (60). Along with hallucinogenic effects, DOM (4-methyl-2,5-dimethoxyamphetamine) demonstrates more sympathetic stimulation.

Ketamine and Related Hallucinogens

Ketamine was developed during laboratory investigations for analogs of PCP, the reported advantages being lesser potency, shorter half-life, and (anecdotally) diminished emergence phenomena. Vetalar and Ketaset are the veterinary versions of ketamine. See Table 12-4 for the street and chemical names of ketamine and related compounds.

Because of ketamine's crystalline appearance, the drug can be mistaken for or passed off as methamphetamine or cocaine; ketamine is sometimes mixed with caffeine, MDMA, or ephedrine (61). In the Drug Abuse Warning Network databank of emergency department visits for reactions to multiple club drugs (http://dawninfo.samhsa.gov), ketamine is mentioned in 39% of cases. The liquid form of ketamine can be dried and then ingested orally, through nasal insufflation, or intravenously. This drug can be found on the Internet, packaged as capsule, powder, or tablet. It is abused in

TABLE 12-4
STREET AND CHEMICAL NAMES FOR KETAMINE AND RELATED COMPOUNDS

Ketamine	*Street names:* K, Special K, Cat Valiums, Vitamin K, kit-kat, super acid, jet
	Chemical name: 2-(2-chlorophenyl)-2-(methylamino)-cyclohexanone
	Trade names for pharmaceutical product: Ketalar, Vetalar, Ketajet
DMT	Dimitri
	Chemical name: N,N-dimethyltryptamine
5-MeoDMT	*Street name:* 5MEO
	Chemical name: 5-methoxy-dimethyltryptamine
5-MeO-AMT	*Street name:* Alpha-O
	Chemical name: 5-methoxy-α-methyltryptamine
5-Meo-DIPT	*Street name:* Foxy
	Chemical name: 5-methoxy-N,N-diisopropyltryptamine

conjunction with amphetamines, cocaine, and other club drugs (61) and is sometimes smoked as an additive to tobacco or marijuana. A review of 20 ketamine users in Scotland found that many experimented with a wide range of substances and tended to be young, well educated, and informed about the drug (62).

Ketamine's potential to induce changes in consciousness lends it to criminal intentions. Ketamine has been associated with drug-facilitated sexual assault, as have benzodiazepines, GHB, and the anticholinergic scopolamine (63). Ketamine's hallucinogenic properties are caused by its action on the N-methyl-D-aspartate (NMDA) receptor. In addition to dissociative effects, cognitive impairments are seen in ketamine users both immediately after use and 3 days later; delayed effects include schizotypal symptomatology (64).

Ketamine is readily available in the medical and veterinary communities. Because this drug is difficult to manufacture, most stores made available for abuse are really diverted medical and veterinary supplies. One attempt at diversion involved a phony recall letter to veterinary hospitals warning of a possible adverse effect from a lot of ketamine. The requested action was to forward the practitioner's name, office location, and batch numbers of the product; the presumed goal was diversion or robbery (65). Reports of abuse by medical personnel started to emerge soon after the drug's release (66). Dependence phenomena have been documented (67,68).

Detection Methods

Commercial immunoassays for ketamine are not readily available. Gas chromatography, flame-ionization detection, and mass selective detection are all considered possible detection methods for ketamine and its metabolites. Some laboratory authorities report cross-reactions between ketamine and PCP because of their structural similarity (Figs. 12.4 and 12.5) (69); others disagree (70). As for the other drugs discussed in this chapter, the emergency department physician's best action, given the changing technologies, is the confirmation of a test's strengths and limitations with its manufacturer (69,70). A liquid chromatography/mass spectrometry testing method can be utilized to detect ketamine, norketamine, and dehydronorketamine in urine (71). Many of these testing methods are time intensive. A simpler testing method using rapid electrospray ionization/mass spectroscopy for detection of ketamine in urine is now in development and appears to promise high sensitivity and specificity (72). Ketamine levels in blood can be measured by HPLC, although, again, this technology is not readily available for rapid clinical use (73).

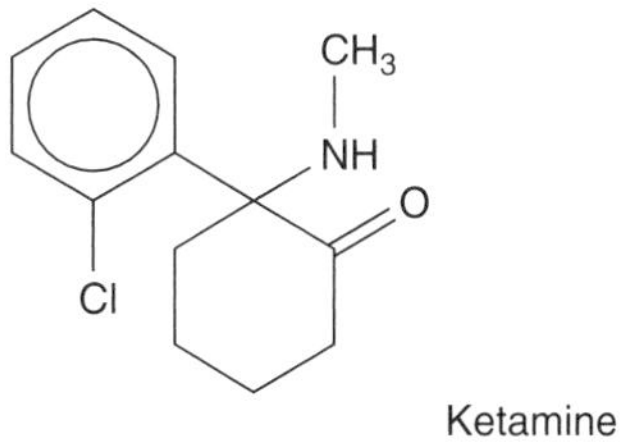

FIG. 12.4   Chemical structure of ketamine.

Clinical Presentation

Ketamine is used as a dissociative anesthetic. Its side effects are limitations for many clinicians, but they are, typically, attractions for the abuser: hallucinations, a dream-like state, the sensation of floating outside the body, "cosmic" experiences, body distortions, and loss of time comprehension (74, 75). Although most club drugs are used episodically, chronic ketamine use is well recognized in some settings, and tolerance to the drug is possible (74). Other reported effects in users include inability to speak, blurring of vision, and lack of coordination. Users might reduce the dose in response to these symptoms (76). Many effects of ketamine are believed to be similar to those of PCP, but ketamine is a much less potent agent. At its more extreme presentation, respiratory depression and coma have been seen. Motor effects include those associated with PCP as well as tremor, hyperactivity, myoclonic jerks, and catalepsy (77). Aspiration is considered a risk of ketamine-induced anesthesia, because of depression of laryngeal reflexes (78).

In a small series of ketamine abusers presenting to emergency departments, symptoms ranged from no complaint in half of the patients; others reported anxiety, palpitations, chest pain, confusion, vomiting, and memory loss. Tachycardia was the most common finding (detected in more than half of the series), followed by altered mental status, slurred speech, hallucinations, nystagmus, mydriasis, and hypertension (70). Another adverse effect reported by ketamine users is flashbacks.

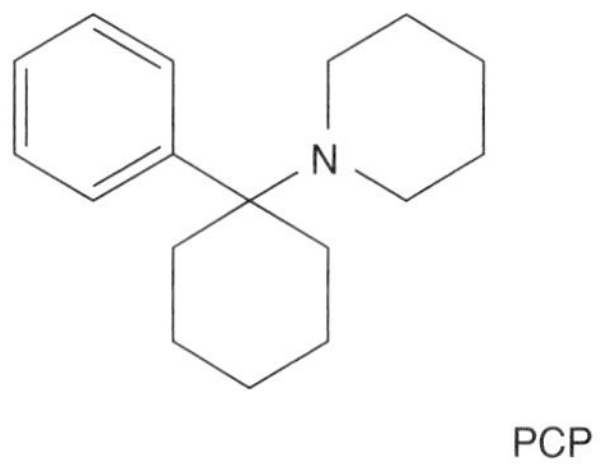

FIG. 12.5   Chemical structure of phencyclidine (PCP).

Dextromethorphan

DXM is a common ingredient of over-the-counter cold and cough medications, usually as the hydrobromide salt, and is therefore readily available in stores and on the Internet. It is abused by people seeking a PCP-like "high." The amount of DXM in cold/cough preparations varies: some products are primarily or only DXM and others combine DXM with acetaminophen, sympathomimetics, or antihistamines. CoricidinHBP (Schering-Plough Health Care Products, Inc., Memphis, Tennessee), an over-the-counter cough and cold medication, is available in several formulations with DXM. Its abuse has been reported with frequency in some communities (79,80). Ingestion of large doses of any DXM-containing product poses a great risk of a potentially toxic dose of the companion ingredient(s). Some abusers ingest up to 4 fluid ounces of cough syrup (81).

DXM is considered an opioid because of its propensity for opioid receptors. Its PCP-like effects on the NMDA receptor suggest a possible hallucinogenic effect and inhibition of the reuptake of serotonin. In high doses, it causes respiratory depression.

Metabolism might play a role in why some users become more symptomatic than others. In an evaluation of the ability to metabolize DXM, subjects classified as poor metabolizers (those deficient in the enzyme CYP 2D6) demonstrated greater psychomotor impairment, greater sedation, and dysphoria (82).

DXM is available as a powder, capsule, liquid, or tablet. The Internet is a frequent source of nonliquid forms of DXM. Most abuse occurs through the oral route. DXM could be more commonly abused than is recognized. In an evaluation of pills submitted to DanceSafe (www.dancesafe.org), DXM was second only to MDMA among most of the drugs most commonly identified in analysis (83). DXM has been known to cause false-positive results on PCP urine drug screens, but it is not believed to cross-react with the opiate immunoassay screens (84,85). In general, for the emergency department management of DXM effect/overdose, supportive care and the possible use of naloxone are appropriate (86).

Clinical Presentation

In high doses, DXM causes lethargy, excitability, tachycardia, ataxia, psychosis, nystagmus, diaphoresis, and hypertension. Reported psychological symptoms include increased perceptual awareness; altered time perception; tactile, visual, and auditory hallucinations; visual disturbances; and paranoia (87). Many of these effects probably stem from dextrorphan, the active metabolite of DXM, which is felt to bind to central nervous systems receptors (similar to the action of PCP) (88,89). Dextrorphan levels vary among individuals, depending on the host's metabolism, a possibility that might be related to vulnerability to addiction in general (88,89). Long-acting DXM preparations might prolong the release of dextrorphan, which would prolong the duration of symptoms (90). The effect of DXM on serotonin should raise concerns about serotonin syndrome (46).

As DXM is new to the drug abuse arena, routinely available laboratory testing platforms are not designed with DXM testing in mind. DXM has been reported as a false-positive result for PCP on urine screens (84). Consultation with a clinical chemist or other specialist should be considered if specific testing for DXM is required. Reported methods for detection include HPLC, liquid chromatography, and GC/MS (91–93).

SUMMARY

Drugs of abuse will continue to challenge the emergency physician. Some "newer" drugs of abuse are reviewed in this chapter, but novel compounds or changes in existing drugs will continue to task the emergency physician with identification of the patient's signs and symptoms. Advancing laboratory technology will be needed to keep pace with changing patterns of abuse. Specialists in toxicology and laboratory science can facilitate the identification of new drugs of abuse. By combining clinical presentation and, in some situations, confirmatory laboratory data, identification can be expected to improve.

REFERENCES

1. Fernando D. Fentanyl-laced heroin. *JAMA* 1991;265:2962.
2. *MMWR Morb Mortal Wkly Rep.* Scopolamine poisoning among heroin users—New York City, Newark, Philadelphia, and Baltimore, 1995 and 1996. *MMWR Morb Mortal Wkly Rep* 1996;45:457–460.
3. Langston JW, Ballard P, Tetrud JW, et al. Chronic parkinsonism in humans due to a product of meperidine-analog synthesis. *Science* 1983;219:979–980.
4. Osterhoudt KC, Henretig FM. Comatose teenager at a party: what a tangled 'Web' we weave. *Pediatr Case Rev* 2003;3:171–173.
5. Perry HE, Wright RO, Shannon MW, et al. Baclofen overdose: drug experimentation in a group of adolescents. *Pediatrics* 1998;101:1045–1048.
6. Crouch BI, Caravati EM, Booth J. Trends in child and teen nonprescription drug abuse reported to a regional poison control center. *Am J Health Syst Pharm* 2004;61:1252–1257.
7. Castelli M, Mocci I, Langlois X, et al. Quantitative autoradiographic distribution of gamma hydroxybutryic acid binding sites in human and monkey brain. *Brain Res Mol Brain Res* 2000;78:91–99.
8. Nelson T, Kaufman E, Klein J, et al. The extraneural distribution of gamma-hydroxybutyrate. *J Neurochem* 1981;37:1345–1348.
9. Elian AA. Determination of endogenous gamma-hydroxybutyric acid (GHB) levels in antemortem urine and blood. *Forensic Sci Int* 2002;128:120–122.

10. McCusker R, Paget-Wilks H, Chronister CW, et al. Analysis of gamma-hydroxybutyrate in urine by gas chromatography-mass spectrometry. *J Anal Toxicol* 1999;23:301–305.

11. Bortolotti F, DePauli G, Gottardo R, et al. Determination of gamma-hydroxybutyric acid in biological fluids by using capillary electrophoresis with indirect detection. *J Chromatogr B Analyt Technol Biomed Life Sci* 2004;800:239–244.

12. Meyers JE, Almirall JR. A study of the effectiveness of commercially available drink test coasters for the detection of the "date rape" drugs in beverages. *J Anal Toxicol* 2004;28:685–688.

13. Garrison G, Meuller P. Clinical features and outcomes after intentional gamma hydroxybutyrate (GHB) overdoses [abstract]. *J Toxicol Clin Toxicol* 1998;36:503–504.

14. Dyer JE. Gamma-hydroxybutyrate: a health food product producing coma and seizure-like activity. *Am J Emerg Med* 1991;9:321–324.

15. Chin RL, Sporer KA, Cullison B, et al. Clinical course of gamma-hydroxybutyrate overdose. *Ann Emerg Med* 1998;31:716–722.

16. Mason PE, Kerna WP II. Gamma hydroxybutyric acid (GHB) intoxication. *Acad Emerg Med* 2002;9:730–739.

17. Pretty IA, Hall RC. Self-extraction of teeth involving gamma-hydroxybutyric acid. *J Forensic Sci* 2004;49:1069–1072.

18. Sporer KA, Chin RLDyer JE. et al. Gamma-hydroxybutyrate serum levels and clinical syndrome after severe overdose. *Ann Emerg Med* 2003;42:3–8.

19. Couper FJ, Thatcher JE, Logan BK. Suspected GHB overdoses in the emergency department. *Ann Emerg Med* 2004;28:481–484.

20. Dyer JE, Roth B, Hyma BA. Gamma-hydroxybutyrate overdose. *Ann Emerg Med* 1991;9:321–324.

21. Kovar KA. Chemistry and pharmacology of hallucinogens, entactogens and stimulants. *Pharmacopsychiatry* 1998;31(Suppl. 2):69–72.

22. Cody JT, Schwarhoff R. Fluorescence polarization immunoassay of amphetamine, methamphetamine, and illicit amphetamine analogues. *J Anal Toxicol* 1993;17:23–33.

23. D'Nicuola J, Jones R, Levine B, et al. Evaluation of six commercial amphetamine and methamphetamine immunoassays for cross-reactivity to phenylpropanolamine and ephedrine in urine. *J Anal Toxicol* 1992;16:211–213.

24. Poklis A, Moore KA. Stereoselectivity of the TdxADx/FLx amphetamine/methamphetamine II immunoassay: response of urine specimens following nasal inhaler use. *Clin Toxicol* 1995;33:35–41.

25. Danks RR, Wibbenmeyer LA, Faucher LD, et al. Methamphetamine-associated burn injuries: a retrospective analysis. *J Burn Care Rehabil* 2004;25:425–429.

26. *MMWR*. Public health consequences among first responders to emergency events associated with illicit methamphetamine laboratories_selected states, 1996–1999. *MMWR* 2000;49:1021–1024.

27. Allcott JV, Barnhart RA, Mooney LA. Acute lead poisoning in two illicit users of methamphetamine. *JAMA* 1987;258:510–511.

28. Chandler DB, Norton RL, Kaufman J, et al. Lead poisoning associated with intravenous methamphetamine use—Oregon, 1988. *MMWR* 1989;38:830–831.

29. Kashani J, Ruba AM. Methamphetamine toxicity secondary to intravaginal body stuffing. *J Toxicol Clin Toxicol* 2004;42:987–989.

30. Cho AK. Ice: a new dosage form of an old drug. *Science* 1990;247:631–634.

31. Derlet RW, Heischober B. Methamphetamine: stimulant of the 1990's. *West J Med* 1990;8:105–108.

32. Derlet RW, Rice P, Horowitz BZ, et al. Amphetamine toxicity: experience with 127 cases. *J Emerg Med* 1989;7:157–161.

33. Klawans HL, Weiner WJ. The effects of d-amphetamine on choreiform movement disorders. *Neurology* 1974;6:312–318.

34. Rhee KJ, Albertson TE, Douglas JC. Choreathetoid disorder associated with amphetamine-like drugs. *Am J Emerg Med* 1988;6:131–133.

35. Boswick DG. Amphetamine-induced cerebral vasculitis. *Hum Pathol* 1981;12:1031–1033.

36. Citron BP, Halpern M, McCarron M, et al. Necrotizing angiitis associated with drug abuse. *N Engl J Med* 1970;283:1001–1003.

37. Davis GG, Swalwell CI. Acute aortic dissections and ruptured berry aneurysms associated with methamphetamine abuse. *J Forensic Sci* 1994;38:1481–1485.

38. Stoessl AJ, Young GB, Feasby TE. Intracerebral haemorrhage and angiographic beading following ingestion of catecholaminergics. *Stroke* 1985;16:734–736.

39. Graeme KA. New drugs of abuse. *Emerg Med Clin North Am* 2000;18:625–636.

40. Baggott M, Heifets B, Jones RT, et al. Chemical analysis of ecstasy pills. *JAMA* 2000;284:2190.

41. Schwartz RH, Miller NS. MDMA (ecstasy) and the rave: a review. *Pediatrics* 1997;100:705–708.

42. Morland J. Toxicity of drug abuse—amphetamine designer drugs (ecstasy): mental effects and consequences of single dose use. *Toxicol Lett* 2000;1123:147–152.

43. Smith KM, Larive LL, Romanelli F. Club drugs: methylenedioxymethamphetamine, flunitrazepam, ketamine hydrochloride, and gamma-hydroxybutyrate. *Am J Health Syst Pharm* 2002;59:1067–1076.

44. Callaway CW, Johnson MP, Gold LH, et al. Amphetamine derivatives induce locomotor hyperactivity by acting as indirect seratonin agonists. *Psychopharmacology* 1991;104:293–301.

45. De Souza EB, Battaglia G. Effects of MDMA and MDA on brain serotonin neurons: evidence from neurochemical and autoradiographic studies. *NIDA Res Monogr* 1989;94:196–222.

46. Boyer EW, Shannon M. The serotonin syndrome. *N Engl J Med* 2005;352:1112–1120.

47. Graudis A, Stearman A, Chan B. Treatment of the serotonin syndrome with cyproheptadine. *J Emerg Med* 1998;16:615–619.

48. Andreu V, Mas A, Bruguera M, et al. Ecstasy: a common cause of severe acute hepatotoxicity. *J Hepatol* 1998;29:394–397.

49. Sort P, Mas A, Salmeron O, et al. Recurrent liver involvement in heatstroke. *Liver* 1996;16:335–337.

50. Henry JA, Jefferys KJ, Dawlings S. Toxicity and death from 3,4-methylenedioxymethamphetamine ("ecstasy"). *Lancet* 1992;340:384–387.

51. Ellis AJ, Wendon JA, Williams R. Acute liver damage and ecstasy ingestion. *Gut* 1996;38:454–458.

52. Brown C, Osterloh J. Multiple severe complications from recreational ingestion of MDMA ("Ecstasy"). *JAMA* 1987;258:780–781.

53. Colado MI, Williams JL, Green AR. The hyperthermic and neurotoxic effects of 'Ecstasy' (MDMA) and 3,4 methylenedioxyamphetamine (MDA) in the Dark Agouti (DA) rat, a model of CYP2D6 poor metabolizer phenotype. *Br J Pharmacol* 1995;115:1281–1289.

54. Ajaelo I, Koenig K, Snoey E. Severe hyponatremia and inappropriate antidiuretic hormone secretion following ecstasy use. *Acad Emerg Med* 1998;5:839–840.

55. Holmes SB, Banerjee AK, Alexander WD. Hyponatremia and seizures after ecstasy use. *Postgrad Med J* 1999;75:32–33.

56. Henry JA, Fallon JK, Kicman AT, et al. Low-dose MDMA ("ecstasy") induces vasopressin secretion. *Lancet* 1998;325:1784.

57. Maxwell DL, Polkey MI, Henry JA. Hyponatremia and catatonic stupor after taking "ecstasy". *BMJ* 1992;307:1399.

58. Nuvials X, Masclan JR, Peracaula R, et al. Hyponatremic coma after ecstasy ingestion. *Intensive Care Med* 1997;23:480.

59. Ricaurte FA, McCann UD, Szabo Z, Toxicodynamics and long-term toxicity of the recreational drug, 3,4-methylenedioxymethamphetamine (MDMA, 'Ecstasy'). *Toxicol Lett* 2000;112–113:143–146.

60. Caldicott DG, Edwards NA, Kruys A, et al. Dancing with "death": p-methoxyamphetamine overdose and its acute management. *J Toxicol Clin Toxicol* 2003;41:143–154.

61. Ketamine Drug Facts. Available at http://www.ncadi. samhsa.gov/nongovpubs/ketamine. Accessed on April 1, 2005.

62. Dalgarno PJ, Shewan D. Illicit use of ketamine in Scotland. *J Psychoactive Drugs* 1996;28:191–199.

63. Negrusz A, Gaensslen RE. Analytical developments in toxicological investigation of drug-facilitated sexual assault. *Anal Bioanal Chem* 2003;376:1192–1197.

64. Curran HV, Morgan C. Cognitive, dissociative and psychotogenic effects of ketamine in recreational users on the night of drug use and 3 days later. *Addiction* 2000;95:575–590.

65. Office of Diversion, Press Release. Drug Enforcement Administration. Available at http://www.deadiversion.usdoj. gov/pubs/pressrel/vet_scam.htm. Accessed on August 31, 2005.

66. Ahmed SN, Petchkovsky L, et al. Abuse of ketamine. *Br J Psychiatry* 1980;137:303.

67. Arican FO, Okan T, Badak O, An unusual presentation from xylazine-ketamine. *Vet Hum Toxicol* 2004;46:324–325.

68. Moore NN, Bostwick JM. Ketamine dependence in anesthesia providers. *Psychosomatics* 1999;40:359–359.

69. Shannon MW. Recent ketamine administration can produce a urine toxic screen which is falsely positive for phencyclidine [letter]. *Pediatr Emerg Care* 1998;14:180.

70. Weiner AL, Vieira L, McKay CA, Ketamine abusers presenting to the emergency department: a case series. *J Emerg Med* 2000;18:447–451.

71. Moore KA, Skerov J, Levine B, Urine concentration of ketamine and norketamine following illegal consumption. *J Anal Toxicol* 2001;25:583–588.

72. Lua AC, Lin HR. A rapid and sensitive ESI-MS screen procedure for ketamine and norketamine in urine samples. *J Anal Toxicol* 2004;28:680–684.

73. Bolze S, Boulieu R. HPLC determination of ketamine, norketamine and dehydronorketamine in plasma with a high purity reverse phase sorbent. *Clin Chem* 1998;44:560–564.

74. Pal HR, Berry N, Kumar R, Ray R. Ketamine dependence. *Anaesth Intensive Care* 2002;30:382–384.

75. Jansen KL. Non-medical uses of ketamine. *BMJ* 1993;306:601–602.

76. Dillon P, Copeland J, Jansen K. Patterns of use and harms associated with non-medical ketamine use. *Drug Alcohol Depend* 2003;69:23–28.

77. McCarron M, Schulze BW, Thompson GA, et al. Acute phencyclidine intoxication: incidence of clinical findings in 1000 cases. *Ann Emerg Med* 1981;10:290–297.

78. Taylor PA, Towey RM. Depression of laryngeal reflexes during ketamine anaesthesia. *BMJ* 1971;ii:688–689.

79. Baker SD, Borys DJ. A possible trend suggesting increase abuse from Coricidin exposures reported to the Texas Poison Network: comparing 1998 to 1999. *Vet Hum Toxicol* 2002;44:169–171.

80. Simone KE, Bottie EM, Siegel ES, et al. Coricidin abuse in Ohio teens and young adults [abstract]. *J Toxicol Clin Toxicol* 2000;38:532–533.

81. Helfer J, Kim OM. Psychoactive abuse potential of Robitussin-DM. *Am J Psychiatry* 1990;147:672–673.

82. Zawertailo LA, Kaplan HLBusto UE, et al. Psychotropic effects of dextromethorphan are altered by the CYP2D6 polymorphism: a pilot study. *J Clin Psychopharmacol* 1998;18:332–337.

83. Baggott M, Heifets B, Jones RT, et al. Chemical analysis of ecstasy pills. *JAMA* 2000;284:2190.

84. Schier J, Diaz JE. Avoid unfavorable consequences: dextromethorphan can bring about a false positive phencyclidine urine drug screen. *Am J Emerg Med* 2000;18:376–383.

85. Storrow AB, Magoon MR, Norton J. The dextromethorphan defense: dextromethorphan and the opiate screen. *Acad Emerg Med* 1995;2:791–794.

86. Schneider SM, Michealson EA, Bouchek CD, et al. Dextromethorphan poisoning reversed by naloxone. *Am J Emerg Med* 1991;9:237–238.

87. Wolfe TR, Caravati EM. Massive dextromethorphan ingestion and abuse. *Am J Emerg Med* 1995;13:174–176.

88. Szelely JI, Sharpe LGJaffe JH, et al. Induction of phencyclidine-like behavior in rats by dextrorphan but not dextromethorphan. *Pharmacol Biochem Behav* 1991;40:381–386.

89. Tortella FC, Pellicano M, Bowery NG. Dextromethorphan and neuromodulation: old drug coughs up new activities. *Trends Pharmacol Sci* 1989;10:501–507.

90. Delvin KM, Hall AH, Smolinske SC, et al. Toxicity from long-acting dextromethorphan preparations [abstract]. *Vet Hum Toxicol* 1985;28:296.

91. Bendriss EK, Markoglou N, Wainer IW. High-performance liquid chromatography assay for simultaneous determination of dextromethorphan and its main metabolites in urine and in microsomal preparations. *J Chromatogr B Biomed Sci Appl* 2001;754:209–215.

92. Afshar M, Rouini MR, Amini M. Simple chromatography method for simultaneous determination of dextromethorphan and its main metabolites in human plasma with fluorimetric detection. *J Chromatogr Analyt Technol Biomed Life Sci* 2004;802:317–322.

93. Budai B, Iskandar H. Dextromethorphan can produce false positive phencyclidine testing with HPLC [letter]. *Am J Emerg Med* 2002;20:61–62.

SEROLOGY AND DNA EVIDENCE

13

ROSALIND BOWMAN ■
TERI J. LABBE ■
KIMBERLY A. MULLINGS ■

O nce a crime has been committed, law enforcement needs to determine what has happened (when, why, and how) and identify all parties involved. These questions can be answered by investigating closely, examining the crime scene, and analyzing the evidence recorded. Most, if not all, of these concerns can be resolved through a timely, methodical, and meticulous examination of the crime scene evidence.

Evidence, as defined by Encarta, is "the means by which disputed facts are proved to be true or untrue in any trial before a court of law." Physical evidence, as defined by Saferstein (1), is "any and all objects that can establish that a crime has been committed or can provide a link between a crime and its victim or a crime and its perpetrator." Testimonial evidence, obtained by skillfully interviewing witnesses to the crime and recording their eyewitness accounts, must be weighed for objectivity. It is of utmost importance that what could be physical evidence is recognized, documented, collected, and handled in the appropriate manner to ensure its integrity for forensic examination.

FORENSIC SEROLOGY

An investigation into a charge of sexual assault begins with examination of the primary crime scene, that is, the body of the victim. Specialized sexual assault evidence-collection kits are used by sexual assault forensic nurse examiners to provide the samples for forensic serologic analysis.

Forensic serology is the science that deals with the identification, isolation, and characterization of blood and bodily fluids from the victim, the suspect, and the environment of the crime scene for the purpose of comparison to known standards. These biologic substances, along with other trace evidence samples of hairs and fibers, may be transferred readily between the victim, the suspect, and the environment of the crime scene during the commission of the sexual assault. Sources of biologic evidence—blood, semen, saliva, urine, hair, teeth, bone, and tissue—give us deoxyribonucleic acid (DNA). Sources of trace evidence (e.g., fibers, hair, fur, paint, glass, gunshot residue, soil, explosives, and paper) must have known samples with which they can be compared.

Biologic evidence can be found in several common sites. Blood might be spattered about a scene in a pattern or found on a weapon, on clothing, or on other articles. Semen can be found in any body cavity (i.e., vagina, rectum, mouth, and colostomy opening), on clothes (particularly undergarments), on furniture, and on carpets and floors. Saliva can be found in bite marks, on cigarette butts, and on any part of the body that was licked or sucked. Other places to find saliva/DNA samples are envelopes, stamps, gum, sunglasses, phones, discarded food, and drinking containers. Epithelial cells on contact items such as gloves, caps, masks, lip balm, cosmetics, contact lens, earplugs, gags, cords, or shoelaces can also harbor DNA.

Serologic Testing

The forensic serologist evaluating the evidence from any crime scene has an advanced degree in the sciences and has completed on-the-job training programs, which are supplemented with continued education in specialized course work offered at the Federal Bureau of Investigation (FBI) and other government and private forensic laboratories.

The serologic examination of the sexual assault evidence-collection kit begins upon receipt of the kit. The examiner must ensure that the kit is submitted in compliance with laboratory protocols: evidence must be sealed properly and identified appropriately in regard to its attached laboratory request forms. If these conditions are met, the evidence chain of custody has been established. Acceptance of the kit for examination is documented by the signature of the examiner and the date on the evidence chain of custody form.

The kit is opened and its contents are inventoried. The individual envelopes containing samples to be tested are identified with information from the victim and are labeled as to the source: vaginal, oral, anal, and defined miscellaneous. A document that accompanies the kit indicates the results of the physical examination as well as the victim's testimonial evidence as told to the sexual assault nurse examiner.

Semen

The primary goal of the forensic serologic examination is to detect the presence of semen, as evidence of sexual activity, on the samples collected. The procedures used in this examination are predicated upon the biochemical interactions of the immune system: antigen to antibody and enzyme to substrate.

Semen is composed of seminal fluid and spermatozoa. Seminal fluid is a highly viscous fluid produced from the secretions of Cowper's gland, the prostate gland, and the seminal vesicles. It serves as both a carrier of the spermatozoa and a buffer of protection from the acidic environment of the vagina.

An alternate light source (e.g., an argon ion laser light or a mini crime scene scope, which uses filters for wavelengths of light in the range of 390–540 nanometers) is used by the serologist to locate suspected semen and saliva stains to be tested. Exposure to certain wavelengths of light excite flavins in the biologic stain, resulting in fluorescence against the substrate background.

Small sections of the samples are chemically tested for the presence of acid phosphatase, an enzyme found throughout the body, but most highly concentrated in secretions from the prostate gland. The results of this chemical testing are compared to a known semen standard. Samples that test positive for the presence of acid phosphatase are tested further by microscopic examination to visualize spermatozoa.

The average ejaculate contains 50 to 150 million sperm cells per mL, in addition to white blood cells and epithelial cells. Specialized staining allows the serologist to visualize the distinct regions of the spermatozoa: head or cell body, neck, midpiece, and tail section. Nucleated epithelial cells are also easily visualized against the other cellular background.

The serologist documents the detection of semen on the evidence samples that test positive for acid phosphatase as an indication of seminal fluid and that contain spermatozoa. Sections of these samples are retained for further characterization of the semen stain.

In some cases, the serologist is unable to visualize spermatozoa after detecting seminal fluid, especially if the victim bathed or douched before the medical examination. If the perpetrator's sperm is not found, he may have had a vasectomy or he may be a low sperm producer.

These samples are then tested for the presence of the prostate-specific antigen (P30), a large protein known to come from the prostate gland. The presence of semen is confirmed by the serologist in samples that test positive with commercial reagents containing anti-P30 antibodies through comparison with a known semen standard. Samples that test positive for the presence of both acid phosphatase and P30 are retained for further characterization through DNA analysis. Samples that do not test positive for either are not tested further. Additional testing for the presence of blood and saliva may be performed by the serologist on samples from the sexual assault evidence-collection kit.

Blood

Blood is a complex mixture of cells, enzymes, proteins, and other biochemical substances, which are used by the serologist for identification of an individual or animal. For conventional serologic and DNA analysis in sexual assault cases, a liquid whole blood sample is usually necessary. For forensic analysis, the collection of whole blood samples in an ethylene diaminetetracetate (EDTA) Vacutainer (lavender capped) is recommended. Whole blood samples must be refrigerated.

The use of bloodstain evidence provides an efficient means of collecting, transporting, and storing DNA blood samples. Most programs use cotton or filter paper cards of various thickness to collect bloodstain specimens from survivors. Unfortunately, as a result of deterioration of the specimen, conventional filter paper can produce inconsistent results after storage for as little as 6 months at ambient temperature (2).

A new option, the FTA-coated paper (Whatman plc, Middlesex, United Kingdom), was developed by Dr. Leigh Burgoyne and Dr. Peter Hallsworth at Flinders University of South Australia, in response to the need to transport specimens long distances (3). This paper is chemically impregnated to kill existing microorganisms in the blood sample collected and to trap DNA in a matrix, thereby stopping bacterial and environmental degradation of the specimen. It kills human blood-borne pathogens and prevents microbial decay of nonsterile blood and other biologic samples. It also inhibits nonmicrobial decay of DNA information, such as caused by oxidation, ultraviolet light, and an acidic environment. Ambient storage, even at high humidity, is possible for years without deterioration of the specimens.

A small section of a suspected bloodstained sample is subjected to a presumptive chemical test for the presence of blood. The results of the chemical testing are compared to a known blood standard. Evidence samples that test positive are further tested to confirm the presence of blood through microscopic visualization of heme-containing crystalline structures or with a commercial reagent kit containing human hemoglobin antibodies. Sections of these samples are retained for further characterization of the bloodstain. An antihuman hemoglobin reagent (antibodies to human serum produced by injection of human serum into an animal [rabbit or goat]) is used to demonstrate the presence of blood (hemoglobin) and the origin of the blood as human (4). Buccal cells have become the current option for collecting DNA standards from individuals for comparison with evidence. Buccal swabs provide the same genetic information as blood, while being less invasive when collected and less of a potential hazard to the people who handle the samples.

Saliva

Saliva is a mixture of water, mucus (cells, salts, glycoproteins), and the digestive enzyme salivary α-amylase. Small sections of suspected saliva stained samples are chemically tested for the presence of salivary α-amylase. The results of the chemical testing are compared to a known saliva standard. Specialized staining allows the serologist to visualize nucleated epithelial cells. Sections of these samples are retained for further characterization of the saliva stain.

Other Physical Evidence

Additional evidence samples for serologic examination may be recovered from the clothing of the victim and/or suspect or from the crime scene environment. The soil on a suspect's clothing and shoes may match the soil recovered or deposited at the crime scene. Fibrous items such as bedding, small rugs, and pillows can be used as sources of known fibers. Hair samples (head and pubic hair) are most often used for their intrinsic value in sexual assault cases because they possess identifiable characteristics regarding the origin from the body, racial group, and the manner in which the hair was removed. However, hair varies from one person to another within the same racial group. Hair may be recovered as individual shafts, portions of shafts, or as shafts with intact roots. Hair may be recovered from the scene of the incident; from objects at the scene; from clothing of the victim or suspect; or from a vehicle, weapon, or tool used in the crime. Hair found at a crime scene may corroborate the presence of the offender at the scene. In addition, the condition of the root may indicate whether hair was pulled out or naturally shed.

Documentation of Results

Upon completion of these examinations, the serologist uses an official laboratory report to document the results of all tests performed and which samples were consumed in analysis or retained for further characterization. The samples that test positive and are retained for further characterization through DNA analysis are packaged according to protocol. The contents of the sexual assault evidence-collection kit are returned to the kit, and the kit is properly resealed. The kit is released by the serologist into the custody of the evidence technician (with documentation on the evidence chain of custody form). The technician has the responsibility to transfer evidence to the evidence control section, where it remains in storage until presentation in court or until it is destroyed.

DNA ANALYSIS

In the past, further characterization of serologic samples positive for blood, seminal fluid, semen, and saliva consisted of ABO blood grouping and enzyme assays for erythrocyte acid phosphatase and/or phosphoglucomutase. These tests were time consuming and labor intensive and were of little value regarding the source of the evidence sample (is it from the victim or the suspect?). Scientific research has advanced analytic technology so that the DNA molecule can now be used as the standard for characterization of all biologic samples.

Forensic DNA testing was first demonstrated successfully through the use of "DNA fingerprinting," as developed by Alec Jeffreys in the sexual assault and murder case involving Colin Pitchfork. Jeffreys demonstrated that useful amounts of DNA could be recovered from old bloodstains and that forensic testing methods could be used for personal identification by comparing a known blood standard source to that of unknown evidence samples.

Restriction fragment length polymorphism (RFLP) DNA testing required high-molecular-weight and intact samples free from degradation. The usefulness of this procedure is limited because forensic samples tend to be at least somewhat degraded and yield only minute and fragmented segments of DNA. Short tandem repeat (STR) DNA testing was developed as a better alternative to address the requirements for characterization of samples typical of crime scene evidence.

Forensic STR DNA analysis utilizes nuclear DNA and compares genetic markers at 13 specific regions and a sex determinant. These 13 core locations provide a profile of genetic material left by the donor. The DNA profiles of the evidence samples are compared to the DNA profiles from the known victim and the known suspect. The results from STR DNA analysis are interpreted by an experienced DNA analyst as to inclusion, exclusion, or inconclusiveness. Evidence DNA profiles found to be inclusive are analyzed statistically as to the probability of frequency of occurrence.

Forensic STR DNA analysis involves the following steps:

- Isolation of nuclear DNA material from the substrate
- Purification of DNA from other cellular components
- Quantification of the extracted DNA
- Amplification of the extracted DNA through polymerase chain reaction (a multiplex DNA amplification utilizing commercial, fluorescently labeled DNA primers designed to identify and copy numerous polymorphic segments of template DNA in a single tube of cocktail mixture)
- Electrophoresis—separation of the fluorescently labeled DNA segments by the application of electrical current
- Data collection and electronic data recording
- Data interpretation

A report of the results of the analysis is submitted for technical and administrative review before release. Most laboratories allow 6 to 8 weeks to complete this process.

Mitochondrial DNA analysis is used in the examination of bones, teeth, and rootless hairs (that lack a follicular tag of nucleated cells) from degraded samples and samples from relatives of missing persons. Because mitochondrial DNA is inherited from the mother, it can be used to demonstrate a relation between a sample from an unknown person and a known standard of blood or buccal cells from the mother or a sibling. In contrast, nuclear DNA is inherited from both parents and is therefore used to demonstrate the uniqueness of an individual (5).

Forensic STR DNA analysis increased the number of DNA profiles available for comparison in forensic laboratories throughout North America. The Combined DNA Index System (CODIS) was developed by the FBI to assist law enforcement laboratories in comparing forensic evidence with DNA profiles nationwide. When used in conjunction with states that maintain databases of the DNA profiles of known convicted offenders, CODIS is a major investigative tool in the resolution of unsolved cases.

Similar to the forensic serologist, the DNA analyst has an advanced degree in the sciences and has completed on-the-job training programs supplemented with continued education in specialized course work offered at the FBI and other government and private forensic laboratories. In addition, the forensic community, in particular, the DNA Advisory Board, has established quality assurance standards for all forensic DNA testing laboratories that generate reports for the court and participate in CODIS. If a laboratory fails to remain in compliance with these quality assurance standards, it can be forced to stop DNA analysis and can be excluded from the CODIS program.

DNA analysis of sexual assault evidence samples begins upon receipt of the evidence as submitted by a serologist. The examiner must ensure that the submission complies with laboratory protocols: the evidence must be sealed properly and identified appropriately by the attached laboratory request forms. If these conditions are met, the evidence chain of custody has been maintained by the serologist. Acceptance of the submission for DNA analysis is documented by the signature of the analyst on the evidence chain of custody form.

The examiner opens the submission package and inventories its contents. The individual envelopes containing samples to be tested are identified with information from the victim and suspect and from the source of the evidence for comparison. Any specific concerns regarding the serologic analysis of the samples can be addressed by reading the associated serology case folder. A laboratory number specific to DNA analysis is assigned and the first in a series of laboratory forms that constitute the DNA case folder is completed. Maintenance of quality is mandatory and is documented throughout the DNA analysis. Most states have legislation requiring laboratories to reserve a portion of the evidence sample and the DNA isolated from it, when applicable, for independent examination at the request of the defendant.

A glossary of terms associated with DNA analyses and the reporting of their results is presented on the following pages.

GLOSSARY—DNA DEFINITIONS

A Designation of the purine base adenine; used in diagrams to represent a nucleotide containing adenine.

Adenine A purine base; one of the four nitrogen-containing molecules present in nucleic acids DNA and RNA; designated by the letter A.

Allele In classic genetics, one of the alternate forms of the gene at a particular locus. In DNA analysis, the term *allele* is commonly extended to DNA fragments of variable length and/or sequence that may have no known transcriptional product but are detected in a polymorphic system.

Allele Frequency The proportion of a particular allele among the chromosomes carried by individuals in a population.

AMP-FLP Amplified fragment length polymorphism.

Amplification Increasing the number of copies of a desired DNA sequence.

Amplification Blank A control consisting of amplification reagents without the addition of sample DNA; used to detect DNA contamination of the amplification reagents and materials.

Anneal The formation of double strands from two complementary single strands of DNA and/or RNA. In the second step of each polymerase chain reaction (PCR) cycle, primers bind or anneal to the 3′ ends of the target sequence.

Autoradiograph (Autoradiogram, Autorad) An image produced on a piece of film by radioactive or chemiluminescent material; a photographic recording of the positions on a film where radioactive decay of isotopes has occurred.

Autosome Any of the chromosomes other than the sex chromosomes X and Y.

Band/DNA Band The visual image representing a particular DNA fragment on an autoradiograph.

Band Shift The phenomenon in which DNA fragments in one lane of a gel migrate at a rate different from that of identical fragments in other lanes of the same gel.

Base Pair Two complementary nucleotides held together by hydrogen bonds; base pairing occurs between adenine (A) and thymine (T) and between guanine (G) and cytosine (C).

C Designation of the pyrimidine base cytosine; used in diagrams to represent a nucleotide containing cytosine.

Chromosome The structure by which hereditary information is physically transmitted from one generation to the next; the organelle that carries the genes.

Controls Tests performed in parallel with experimental samples and designed to demonstrate that a procedure worked correctly.

Cytosine A pyrimidine base; one of the four nitrogen-containing molecules in the nucleic acids DNA and RNA; designated by the letter C.

Degradation The breaking down of DNA by chemical or physical means.

Denaturation The conversion of helical, double strands of DNA to single strands by heat or chemical reagents. Denaturation by heat is the first step of each PCR cycle.

Deoxyribonucleic Acid (DNA) The genetic material of organisms, usually double-stranded, composed of two complementary chains of nucleotides in the form of a double helix; a class of nucleic acids characterized by the presence of the sugar deoxyribose and the four bases adenine, cytosine, guanine, and thymine.

Diallelic Referring to DNA variation showing only two forms with a frequency of more than 1%.

Differential Extraction A stepwise extraction procedure designed to separate intact sperm heads from lysed sperm and other cell types. The separation generally results in an enrichment of sperm DNA in one cell fraction relative to the other cell fraction. The fractions can be analyzed individually.

DNA Contamination The unintentional introduction of exogenous DNA into a DNA sample or PCR reaction prior to amplification.

Enzyme A protein that is capable of speeding up a specific chemical reaction but that itself is not changed or consumed in the process; a biologic catalyst.

Ethidium Bromide An organic molecule that binds to DNA, fluoresces under ultraviolet light, and is used to identify DNA.

Extension The covalent linkage of deoxyribonucleoside triphosphates in a template-directed manner by DNA polymerase. Linkage is in a 5′ to 3′ direction starting from the 3′ end of bound primers. PCR primers are extended one nucleotide at a time by a DNA polymerase during each PCR cycle.

G Designation of the purine base guanine; used in diagrams to represent a nucleotide containing guanine.

Gametic (Phase) Equilibrium The state at loci on different chromosomes when the allele at one locus in the gamete varies independently of that at the other loci; in gametic (phase) disequilibrium, a specific allele at one locus is associated with an allele at another locus on a different chromosome with a frequency greater than expected by chance.

Gel Semisolid matrix (usually agarose or acrylamide) used in electrophoresis to separate molecules.

Gene Frequency The relative occurrence of a particular allele in a population.

Genetic Drift Random fluctuation in allele frequencies.

Genome The genetic constituent of an organism, contained in the chromosome; the total genetic makeup of an organism.

Guanine A purine base; one of the four nitrogen-containing molecules present in the nucleic acids DNA and RNA; designated by the letter G.

Human Leukocyte Antigen (HLA) Protein–sugar structures on the surface of most cells, except blood cells, that differ among individuals and are important for acceptance or rejection of tissue grafts or organ transplants; the locus of one particular class, HLA DQ, is used for forensic analysis with PCR.

Hybridization The process of complementary base pairing between two single strands of DNA and/or RNA.

Kilobase (KB) Unit of 1,000 base pairs of DNA or 1,000 bases of RNA.

Locus, Loci The site on a chromosome where a gene or a defined sequence is located.

Marker A gene with a known location on a chromosome and a clear-cut phenotype that is used as a point of reference in the mapping of other loci.

Membrane The matrix (usually nylon) to which DNA is transferred during the Southern blotting procedure.

Molecular Weight Size Marker A DNA fragment of known size, from which the size of an unknown DNA sample can be determined.

Multilocus Probe A DNA probe that detects genetic variation at multiple sites in the genome; an autoradiogram of a multilocus probe yields a complex, stripe-like pattern of 30 or more bands per individual.

Nucleotide A unit of nucleic acid composed of phosphate, a five-carbon sugar (ribose or deoxyribose), and a purine or pyrimidine base.

PCR Cycle The PCR cycle consists of three steps: (i) denaturation of the template, (ii) annealing of primers to complementary sequences at an empirically determined temperature, and (iii) extension of the bound primers by a DNA polymerase.

Polymerase Chain Reaction (PCR) An enzymatic process by which a specific region of DNA is replicated during repetitive cycles.

Polymorphism The occurrence, in a population, of more than one allele or genetic marker at the same locus, with the least frequent allele or marker occurring more frequently than can be accounted for by mutation.

Primers Small oligonucleotides complementary to the 3′ ends of the target sequence. A pair of primers specifies the boundaries of the region being amplified during the PCR.

Probe A fragment or sequence of DNA that hybridizes to a complementary sequence of nucleotides in another single-strand nucleic acid (target).

Purine The larger of two kinds of bases found in DNA and RNA; a nitrogenous base with a double-ring structure, such as adenine or guanine (compare pyrimidine).

Pyrimidine The smaller of two kinds of bases found in DNA and RNA; a nitrogenous base with a single-ring structure, such as cytosine, thymine, or uracil.

Quality Assurance Those planned or systematic actions necessary to provide adequate confidence that a product or service will satisfy the given requirements for quality.

Quality Audit A systematic and independent examination and evaluation to determine whether quality activities and results comply with planned arrangements and whether these arrangements are implemented effectively and are suitable to achieve objectives.

Quality Control The day-to-day operational techniques and the activities used to fulfill requirements of quality.

Quality Plan A document setting out the specific quality practices, resources, and activities relevant to a particular product, process, service, contract, or project.

Reagent Blank Control All reagents used in the test process minus any sample; used to detect DNA contamination of the analytic reagents and materials.

Recombinant DNA Fragments of DNA from two species, such as a bacterium and a mammal, spliced into a single molecule.

Restriction Enzyme A bacterial enzyme that recognizes a specific palindromic sequence of nucleotides in double-stranded DNA and cleaves both strands; also called restriction endonuclease.

Restriction Fragment Length Polymorphism (RFLP) The variation occurring in the length of DNA fragments generated by a specific restriction enzyme; a technique that uses single-locus or multilocus probes to detect variation in a DNA sequence according to differences in the length of fragments created by cutting DNA with a restriction enzyme.

Ribonucleic Acid (RNA) A class of nucleic acids characterized by the presence of the sugar ribose and the pyrimidine uracil, as opposed to the thymine of DNA.

Serology The discipline concerned with the immunologic study of body fluids.

Serum The liquid that separates from blood after coagulation.

Single-Locus Probe A DNA probe that detects genetic variation at only one site in the genome;

an autoradiogram that uses one single-locus probe; usually displays one band in homozygotes and two bands in heterozygotes.

Somatic Cells The differentiated cells that make up the body tissues of multicellular plants and animals.

Southern Blot The process by which DNA is separated by electrophoresis, transferred from the gel to an immobile support (e.g., nitrocellulose or nylon), and bonded onto the support in single-strand form for hybridization.

Stringency The conditions of hybridization that increase the specificity of binding between two single-strand portions of nucleic acids, usually the probe and the immobilized fragment. Increasing the temperature or decreasing the ionic strength results in increased stringency.

Substrate Control Unstained material adjacent to or representative of the area on which the biologic material is deposited.

T Designation of the purine base thymine; used in diagrams to represent a nucleotide containing thymine.

Tandem Repeats Multiple copies of an identical DNA sequence arranged in direct succession in a particular region of a chromosome. See Variable Number of Tandem Repeats.

Thymine A pyrimidine base; one of the four nitrogen-containing molecules present in DNA; designated by the letter T.

Uracil A pyrimidine base in RNA.

Variable Number of Tandem Repeats Copies of a DNA sequence arranged in succession in a chromosome.

SOURCES FOR GLOSSARY

Dean RL, Long T. DNA typing: RFLP vs PCR or (What are all these initials for?). *A DNA primer for prosecutors*: Maryland State's Attorneys Association, June 21, 1998.

National Research Council. Committee on DNA technology and forensic science. *DNA technology and forensic science*: Washington, DC: National Research Council, 1992.

REFERENCES

1. Saferstein R. *Forensic science handbook*. Englewood Cliffs, NJ: Prentice-Hall, 1982.
2. Burgoyne L. *Technical information: long-term storage of DNA using the FTA gene guard system*. Bedford Park, Australia: Flinders University of South Australia, 1989.
3. Williamson P, Seim S, Wiessner L, et al. *Automation of in situ DNA sample preparation for PCR using the FTA DNA collection system and Rosys laboratory workstation*: American Biotech Laboratories, December 1995.
4. Hochmeister MN, Budowle B, Sparkes R. et al. Validation studies of an immunochromatographic 1-step test for the forensic identification of human blood. *J Forensic Sci* 1999;44(3):597–602.
5. Isenberg AR, Moore JM. Mitochondrial DNA analysis at the FBI laboratory. *Forensic science communications*, Vol. 1, No. 2. Washington, DC: DNA Analysis Unit II, FBI, July 1999.

SUGGESTED READINGS

Budowle B, Smith J, Moretti T, et al. *DNA typing protocols: molecular biology and forensic analysis*. Natick, MA: BioTechniques Books, Eaton Publishing, 2000.

Butler JM. *Forensic DNA typing: biology, technology, and genetics of STR markers*, 2nd ed. San Diego, CA: Academic Press, 2005.

DNA forensics. Oak Ridge, TN: U.S. Department of Energy Office of Science, Genome Management Information System, 2004. Available at www.ornl.gov/sci/techresources/Human_Genome/elsi/forensics.shtml. Accessed on October 24, 2005.

FBI laboratory: DNA analysis units I and II. Washington, DC: Federal Bureau of Investigation, Available at www.fbi.gov/hq/lab/org/dnau.htm. Accessed on October 24, 2005.

Federal Bureau of Investigation *FBI laboratory serology unit protocol manual*. Washington, DC: U.S. Government Printing Office, 1989.

Fisher BAJ. *Techniques of crime scene investigation*, 7th ed. Boca Raton, FL: CRC Press, 2003.

Gaensslen RE. *Sourcebook in forensic serology, immunology and biochemistry*. Washington, DC: U.S. Government Printing Office, 1983.

Olesen K. *pDRAW32: DNA analysis software (freeware)*. AcaClone software. Available at www.acaclone.com. Accessed on October 24, 2005.

Rudin N, Inman K. *An introduction to forensic DNA analysis*, 2nd ed. Boca Raton, FL: CRC Press, 2001.

14

■ DONALD E. STEINHICE

When a sexual assault case is reported, it is almost always first reported to the police or another law-enforcement agency. Although law enforcement may be the first notified, the investigation of sexual assault requires teamwork involving the sexual assault forensic examiner (SAFE), the crime laboratory, prosecutors, and other agencies.

In most cases of sexual assault, a uniformed police officer is the first person in the criminal justice process encountered by the victim. The first officer to respond to a call involving rape has a great responsibility, as few crimes rely so heavily on physical evidence as rape. The officer's first responsibility is to the victim and her condition. The officer should be mindful of the trauma, both physical and emotional, that the victim has incurred. In crimes of rape/sexual assault, most victims are females.

MEDICAL NEEDS OF THE VICTIM

The first police officer arriving at the location of a reported sexual assault must ascertain the victim's condition. If the victim is injured, the priority is to have her taken immediately to the nearest hospital. This need may create a dilemma if the nearest hospital does not have the capabilities to perform the detailed sexual assault/rape examinations that are needed to support the criminal aspects of the case. However, the primary concern must be the well-being of the victim, even if some evidence may be lost in the process of treating her. Under no circumstances should officers or investigators overlook the victim's treatment needs. If the victim is transported to a hospital in an ambulance, the officer should accompany her to the medical facility. This may become important months later if a criminal case goes to trial, because the defense attorney could use a chain-of-custody argument. The officer should attempt to ascertain if the victim has washed or changed clothing in the time since the assault occurred. If the assault involved licking, kissing, or biting, the forensic examiner must be informed of those acts. The examiner will then be able to perform the proper examination in an attempt to make the proper recoveries.

If the victim is a child, the officer must ensure that a parent or guardian is present at the treatment facility. No person who may be a suspect should be near or have contact with the child while the examination is being performed. Because of the inability of most young victims to testify, the role of the SAFE becomes especially important. Physical evidence and medical findings are essential to subsequent testimony. The responding officer should notify the investigating officer as soon as possible so that he/she can respond to the victim.

After assessing the medical needs of the victim, with the appropriate action taken, the officer's next area of concern should be the suspect. The officer should obtain as much information as possible from the victim, as quickly as possible, and should relay it to other law-enforcement personnel, who can begin looking for the suspect or for a vehicle if one was taken from the victim. However, the primary officer/investigator should not conduct a detailed interview of the victim. The detailed interview should be conducted the following day or several days after the incident. The passage of time allows the victim to calm down and think about the incident in greater detail than was possible shortly after it occurred. The reactions of rape victims vary: the emotional and psychological reactions are as different as the victims. When the physical examination is completed, the officer should ask the victim to write down what she remembers as it comes to mind, in preparation for the forthcoming interview.

Many sexually assaulted victims know or are acquainted with the suspect (1–3). In these cases, the officer/investigator has more time to gather and disseminate a description of the suspect than when an unknown suspect is being sought.

LOCATING AND PRESERVING THE CRIME SCENE

The responding officer must ascertain from the victim where the assault took place. The victim may be found or met at a site other than where the crime occurred. In many cases, information obtained from the victim greatly assists in locating and processing the crime scene. Once the site is identified, the primary officer must ensure that the crime scene is preserved. Unlike eyewitness evidence, physical evidence located in a crime scene can never be intrinsically wrong. The evidence located and properly collected at a crime scene can make the difference between a guilty or not-guilty verdict.

In a rape or other sexual assault investigation, the victim's body may hold evidence of the crime. Evidence must be collected from the victim with the same care, caution, and proper methodology as used at the scene. Medical personnel must be accurate in recovering physical evidence from the victim and in marking and documenting the containers, envelopes, and other packaging used to collect and protect the evidence. When the police officer or investigator receives the evidence from the medical personnel, he or she must ensure that all evidence is marked correctly and initialed by the person who collected the items. Rape evidence kits are now used in most emergency departments where sexual assault victims are examined.

During the forensic examination, if the victim is wearing the same clothing as at the time of the assault, it will be taken and submitted for analysis. Officers should arrange for replacement clothing, if possible, through family or a friend of the victim. If the assault took place in the victim's home, the crime scene should not be disturbed to gather replacement clothing.

The officer should be trained in interviewing to elicit sensitive information from the victim, as in situations in which anal, oral, or other assaults occurred. The officer must give this information to the SAFE, so that any possible evidence may be recovered. The officer may try to ascertain whether the victim is experienced enough to know if penetration or ejaculation occurred. If possible, the officer should ask the victim when the last consensual sexual activity occurred and with whom.

The crime scene must be protected and preserved so that the evidence is not lost, moved, altered, contaminated, or destroyed. The officer responsible for protecting the scene must make certain that only persons necessary for the investigation enter the scene. A command post should be established away from the scene. The scene should have one point of entry and one exit. A crime scene log must be maintained, listing the names and assignments of those who enter the scene.

Officers must have a working knowledge of processing a crime scene: from the initial photographing or videotaping by the mobile crime lab technician, to sketching of the scene, to collection of all items known to be or thought to be evidence.

If the crime occurred at night, the scene should be processed and then reexamined in daylight hours as soon as possible. Alternate light sources should be used at the scene, such as ultraviolet lights and lasers for possible deoxyribonucleic acid (DNA) samples and other evidence. If the crime scene is enclosed in a building, the points of entry and escape should be processed.

In some cases, the victim may feel that she has been the victim of a drug-facilitated sexual assault. If this type of assault is suspected, the officer should attempt to determine when it occurred and when the victim last voided her bladder. Urine provides evidence of the presence of drugs; therefore, if voiding becomes necessary, any clean empty container may be used to collect a specimen. The officer should record the date, time, and location of the collection. The officer should have the crime lab photograph and collect all possible evidence of the administration of a drug to the victim, for example, glasses (with and without residue), crystalline material, pills, vomit, excrement, cigarette butts, or napkins. If the victim states that she urinated while under the effects of the drug, efforts should be made to recover items that her urine contacted, for example, clothing, bedding, a car seat, or the ground, in an effort to identify the drug used.

If the victim and the suspect met on the Internet, the officer/investigator should contact a computer forensic investigator for assistance. The victim's computer should be secured until the computer forensic investigator has concluded his/her investigation for a possible connection to the suspect.

If the suspect is located, a search warrant should be obtained for any computers he has used. Those computers should be secured until the computer forensic investigator has concluded the investigation and collected any information about attempts to contact the victim's friends or chat room associates.

REPORTING

Field Notes

The primary officer, and other officers on the scene, must maintain legible, accurate field notes. These notes should answer the six basic questions that must be answered in every type of case:

- WHO (victim, suspect, witnesses)
- WHAT (nature of crime)
- WHERE (location of the scene)
- WHEN (date, time; occurred, reported)
- HOW (way in which the crime was committed)
- WHY (reasons for the offense)

Within each of these primary questions are numerous related questions. The officer should attempt to answer as many of these as possible in the field notes. These notes are the primary information source for the officer's detailed offense report of the incident. They are very important at all stages of the investigation and the prosecution of the suspect. The following pertinent information should be documented:

- The date and time of the call
- How the call was received
- Time of arrival
- Met by whom?
- Was the victim alone?
- What was the physical appearance and mental condition of the victim?
- Was there obvious injury?
- Did the assault happen at the location of the call? If not, where and how did the victim get to the location of the call?
- Was a vehicle used or taken?

Officers and investigators should use one notebook for each sexual assault case and keep that notebook with the case folder. This avoids information of other cases being mixed in with this investigation.

Formal Reports

Officers must prepare detailed, thorough, accurate reports documenting the offense that was committed. These reports become the basis for everything that happens in the case, from the initial reporting through the investigation. Incomplete or incorrect reports can be the reason for a suspect not being identified or for the case being lost in court. The reporting officer must never rush through the reporting aspects of duty. As a general rule, short sentences and short paragraphs make the report much easier to understand and less likely to be misinterpreted by the reader. Officers should also keep in mind, particularly in rape/sexual assault cases, that the fewer formal medical terms they use, the better. Doctors and nurses will use the medical terminology in their reports. The reporting officer should state the doctor's determination, such as "the victim had injuries to her vaginal and rectal area, indicative of rape." The formal medical report will give all other necessary details.

Additional Reports

The primary officer or the investigating detective is responsible for coordinating and collecting reports from the other units involved in the case, that is, from the mobile crime lab, the trace analysis lab, the DNA analysis, and the hospital. All documents should be collected and placed in the case folder, which is used as the primary repository for the incident. The case folder should also contain printed copies of any photographs taken in the case.

In some jurisdictions, copies of all laboratory reports, photographs, drawings, and sketches are sent directly to the prosecutor or state attorney's office at the same time they are sent to the case investigator. It is the responsibility of the investigator to make certain that all parties have the same documents.

INVESTIGATION

Most detectives and investigators have been police officers for several years and therefore have developed the necessary level of experience and ability to conduct detailed investigations. Essential qualities of an investigator are listed below:

- The investigator must be patient: good investigations often take time to develop and bring to a successful outcome.
- A good investigator must be thorough: in many investigations, even the smallest detail can make the difference as to whether the case is solved or remains open.
- Some would argue that luck plays a large part in the success of a detective or investigator. At times there is an element of luck, but more often cases are solved by inductive reasoning and the open-minded approach an investigator brings to the case.

- Detectives and investigators must be confident and well disciplined.
- They must refrain from being opinionated. Tunnel vision can end an investigation before it starts.

A rape/sexual assault investigator must be compassionate, understanding, and sensitive. The investigator must elicit as much detail as possible about the incident without causing additional emotional distress for the victim. From the preliminary stages through the trial of the defendant, the detective/investigator must build and maintain a solid professional relationship with the victim that is, above all, reassuring. The victim must be reassured that she is important, respected, and supported by the investigator and the entire criminal justice process.

The rape/sexual assault investigation begins with the first officer on the scene and continues until the suspect(s) is apprehended and tried. The detective/investigator assigned to the case will initially make certain the crime scene is processed correctly by the mobile crime lab personnel. If it is learned that items such as cell phones, ATM cards, or a vehicle was taken in the offense, the investigator must notify the proper technical services so that the items may be traced and their use recorded.

In most agencies, the detective/investigator meets the victim at the hospital where the rape examination is being done. This is the time when the victim's trauma and emotions are still very intense. The initial interview should be made after the detective/investigator has received the basic information from the first officer(s) on the scene. As previously mentioned, the detective/investigator should not conduct a lengthy and detailed interview at this time. If the investigator is a man, he may wish to have a female investigator present to help the victim feel more at ease; however, this should be the victim's decision. The investigator must not interfere with or interrupt the medical examination. In fact, it may be better for the investigator to wait and get preliminary medical findings from the hospital staff before interviewing the victim. This is not to be confused with the previously mentioned suggestion that the primary officer obtain basic information from the victim about the incident and the suspect.

As is the case with all types of criminal investigations, the detective must look at all the evidence. This includes the victim's statements, any witness information, suspect statements, and the physical evidence that is known in the case. The totality of these data with proper interpretation by the case investigator will lead to a successful conclusion.

DEOXYRIBONUCLEIC ACID/COMBINED DNA INDEX SYSTEM (DNA/CODIS)

Evidence recovered by the SAFE may reveal a DNA profile. This profile and the related evidentiary item must be kept in a secure/stable location that ensures the integrity of the evidence. This evidence and profile information may be kept for years, until a profile is obtained from a person whose DNA matches the evidence recovered.

The SAFE knows that the chain of custody is paramount in all cases. When defense attorneys cannot challenge the evidence, they will try to attack how the evidence was obtained and stored. They will also challenge the chain of custody, how the evidence was stored, and whether it was properly marked and recorded. In the crime scene triangle, we must attempt to connect the victim, the crime scene, and the suspect (Fig. 14.1). In all crimes, the theory of transfer is utilized. It is thought that the suspect(s) brings something to the scene and takes something from the scene, even if it is only a footprint or dust.

Notes taken and reports prepared by the SAFE are very important. At the conclusion of the examination of a sexual assault victim, all the recovered clothing and rape kit evidence are recorded, marked, and signed by the SAFE and then given to the police. The police then submit the evidence to the evidence custodial agency used by their department. This is the start of the chain of custody of the items. If any of those items reveals evidence of DNA after the laboratory has examined them, it is noted that the SAFE has essentially recorded history. The DNA will show that two items or people made contact in the past. Every time evidence is moved or examined, it must be signed for, with the date and time recorded.

Forensic biology that brought us DNA analysis has greatly assisted law enforcement in the search for the truth. Prior to DNA analysis, specimens were typed only by RH blood type groups and ABO groupings. The recent use of DNA in investigations has identified suspects in many older unsolved cases and has excluded persons who were accused. The fact that evidence such as this is so very important mandates that reports, notes, and chain of custody always be complete. Because of this

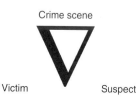

FIG. 14.1   The crime scene triangle.

technology, many agencies have instituted cold-case investigations in an effort to solve cases and give victims some closure.

The Federal Bureau of Investigation (FBI) Laboratory's Combined DNA Index System (CODIS) blends forensic science and computer technology into an effective tool for solving violent crimes. CODIS enables federal, state, and local crime labs to exchange and compare DNA profiles electronically, by linking crimes to each other and to convicted offenders using forensic and offender indexes.

CODIS generates investigative leads when biologic evidence is recovered from a crime scene. The forensic index contains DNA profiles from crime scene evidence. The offender index contains DNA profiles of individuals convicted of sex offenses and other violent crimes. Many states are expanding legislation to include other felonies in which a suspect is required to give a DNA specimen. Matches made among profiles in the forensic index can link crime scenes together, possibly identifying serial offenders. On the basis of a match, police in multiple jurisdictions can coordinate their investigations and share the leads they developed independently. Matches made between the forensic and offender indexes provide investigators with the identity of the perpetrator(s). After CODIS identifies a potential match, qualified DNA analysts in the laboratories contact each other to validate or refute it.

THE SUSPECT

The perpetrators of crimes of violence, including rape/sexual assault, are discussed in Chapter 1. In this chapter, we limit our discussion to what the detective/investigator should and must do from the investigational perspective.

If a suspect is arrested almost immediately after the crime has been committed, the investigator must make certain that all clothing the suspect is wearing is seized and submitted as evidence. Certainly, all preservation-of-evidence procedures must be followed, and the items must be submitted to the laboratory for examination. As a general rule, it is not necessary to obtain a court order or a search-and-seizure warrant to collect the suspect's clothing when an immediate arrest has been made, but departmental rules and regulations must be followed to avoid problems when the case goes to trial.

The suspect must be advised of his constitutional (Miranda) rights before any interrogation is conducted. The exception held valid by the courts is that if the suspect voluntarily talks about the case, without having been asked by the police, the remarks are admissible in trial. To be on the safe side of the law, it is usually wise to advise the suspect of his rights and to have him read, understand, initial,

and sign an explanation-of-rights form, documenting that he waived his rights, before beginning any formal interrogation. An interview of an individual who is not yet a suspect does not require that Miranda rights be given.

When interrogating a suspect, the investigators should have already established a firm working knowledge of the crime scene and the condition of the victim. Open-ended questions should be asked, and the suspect should be allowed to answer without interruption. Even when the detective/investigator knows the suspect is being less than honest, it is more productive to let him tell "his story" and then use that information later in the interrogation. All statements made by the suspect must be documented, because they can be crucial evidence for use during the trial.

The interrogation should be conducted in an area that is private, quiet, and free from interruption. The room should be empty except for a table and chairs. If an audiotape or a videotape of the interrogation is being made, the suspect must state on the tape that he is aware of the taping and has been advised of his constitutional rights, which he has waived.

Some agencies require that two investigators conduct the suspect interrogation. It is recommended that one investigator ask the questions while the other takes notes of what the suspect says, highlighting any inconsistencies that can be used later in the interrogation. If the suspect writes his statement or confession, it should be expressed in his own words. It is unlikely that a suspect would actually state, "When I arrived at the scene, my intent was to sexually assault the victim." The suspect should not be coached. Even the perception that the suspect was led in his statement can have a devastating negative result in court.

During the interrogation of the suspect, everything the detectives/investigators do should be documented. If the suspect is taken to the bathroom, given food or a drink, or allowed to stand and walk around the room, it must be documented. In addition, if the suspect is photographed or if a laboratory test such as buccal swab test is conducted, the times when it began and when it was completed must be documented. All of this information must be kept in the case folder.

Upon completion of the interrogation, the suspect should be photographed before being transported to the detention facility to show his condition and appearance at the time of the interview. If the suspect is to be immediately charged with the crime, all charging documents should be prepared and the suspect then transported to the detention facility. When the suspect is sent to the detention facility, an institution photograph of him should be taken and placed in the case folder.

INVESTIGATIVE INTERVIEW WITH THE VICTIM

The investigative interview with the victim should be conducted as soon after the examination and initial report as possible, but at a time when the victim is ready for this discussion. The interview should be held in a place that is private and comfortable. While the interview is being conducted, there should be no interruptions. The primary investigator and one other investigator should be present. If the victim indicates that she would like a female investigator, then it should be arranged if possible. The primary interviewer should compassionately, skillfully, and professionally attempt to obtain information about the incident. The second investigator should take detailed notes.

The victim should be told that the purpose of the interview is to gather information that will assist in the investigation. Once the interview is started, the investigator should not interrupt the victim while she is answering, but let her finish and then follow-up with appropriate questions. If the victim made notes of what she remembered since the initial report and forensic examination, she should be allowed to state what she remembers. Many times this is where new information is learned. If the victim would like to have a person with whom she is comfortable close by, outside the room, that should be arranged, but the interview is for the victim. All other people with information about the assault should have a separate interview. The notes should indicate if the victim is given something to drink or eat or if she goes to the bathroom. Once all the information is obtained and exchanged, the investigator should thank the victim and any support persons for their time and assistance. The lines of communication should remain open throughout the entire legal process.

If any bruises or injuries have become more visible since the initial assault, new photographs of the injuries should be taken before or at the conclusion of the interview, not during the interview.

THE PROSECUTION

Case preparation for trial is a critical part of the investigation. It is the time when the detective/investigator reviews all the facts of the case with the prosecuting attorney. The pretrial process varies from jurisdiction to jurisdiction. Essentially, it is the time the case moves to the next tier of the criminal justice process. Everything that was done in the case will be reviewed. From the report of the first officer on the scene of the assault to the last report that has been written, the prosecuting attorney must see everything.

This is usually when the victim and the prosecutor meet for the first time. Because of the unique nature of sexual crimes, many jurisdictions have a specific unit in the prosecutor's office that handles these cases. Generally, this group of attorneys has been selected not only for their legal ability but also for their ability to make the victim comfortable during the trial.

It is extremely important that the primary detective/investigator work with the prosecutor at this stage of the case. Months may have passed since the incident occurred. The victim might show signs of emotional trauma induced by the assault. When the prosecutor and the victim meet, they will exchange information. The prosecutor will try to calm the victim, if necessary, and prepare her for the legal process. Information provided by the victim will be helpful to the prosecutor in placing the proper charges against the suspect. The meetings are actually an exchange of information, as the prosecutor explains the legal process to the victim and attempts to answer any questions the victim may ask. If the victim knows the suspect, she should be made aware that the defense will raise the issue of consent. Means of communication are set up between the prosecutor, the investigating officer, and the victim for use throughout the investigation. More than one meeting may be necessary, so open lines of communication are important from the beginning of the process in preparation for the impending trial.

The prosecutor and the SAFE should have a pretrial conference for each case. When the SAFE testifies about her examination of the victim, she will most likely state what kind of medical equipment was used. A photograph of the equipment and lamps used during the examination will make her explanation easier to understand. If the prosecutor has not contacted the forensic nurse examiner by the time she receives a summons, it is recommended that she contact the prosecutor to set up an interview.

Not all sexual assault cases go to trial. During the investigative process, many things may be revealed that may lead to a criminal case, which cannot be tried (e.g., additional evidence that may not lead to the suspect or certain things that may rely on the truthfulness of a witness and/or victim). The legal process is a search for the truth in the matter on trial.

When the case goes to trial, it is as if the state is on trial, because the state must prove beyond a reasonable doubt that the suspect is guilty of the charges. The defendant is always innocent until proved guilty.

SUMMARY

The police are the first representatives of the criminal justice system to interact with the victim of rape/sexual assault. The victim's initial encounter with the first officer and investigator will have a lasting effect. Professional law-enforcement personnel have a duty to do everything possible to help the victim. From obtaining immediate medical attention through the prosecutorial process, officers must make certain they are compassionate and sensitive to the victim. The officers' attitude must help the victim understand that they are concerned but that they also have a mandate to gather information and facts, which may at times make her more uncomfortable. The victim has to know that the officers' ultimate goal is to search for the truth and, if possible, secure the arrest and conviction of the person(s) responsible for the crime. For the police to do less would only make the rape/sexual assault victim feel further victimized.

REFERENCES

1. Bachman R, Coker AL. Police involvement in domestic violence: the interactive effects of victim injury, offender's history of violence, and race. *Violence Vict* 1995;10(2): 91–106.
2. Tjaden P, Thoennes N. *Prevalence, incidence, and consequences of violence against women: findings from the National Violence Against Women Survey.* U.S. Department of Justice, National Institute of Justice, November 1998. Available at http://ncjrs.org/pdffiles/172837.pdf. Accessed on July 20, 2005.
3. Stermac LE, Du Mont JA, Kalemba V. Comparison of sexual assaults by strangers and known assailants in an urban population of women. *CMAJ* 1995;153(8):1089–1094.

SUGGESTED READINGS

The FBI's Combined DNA Index System Program. Available at www.fbi.gov/hq/lab/codis/brochure.pdf. Accessed on July 20, 2005.

Fisher BAJ. *Techniques of crime scene investigation*, 6th ed. Boca Raton, FL: CRC Press, 2000.

Geberth VJ. *Practical homicide investigation*, 3rd ed. Boca Raton, FL: CRC Press, 1996.

Ogle RR Jr. *Crime scene investigation and physical evidence manual*, 2nd ed. Vallejo, CA: Robert R. Ogle, Jr., 1998.

Spitz WU, Fisher RS. *Medicolegal investigation of death*, 2nd ed. Springfield, IL: Charles C. Thomas Publishers, 1992.

SEXUAL ASSAULT AND THE CRIMINAL JUSTICE SYSTEM

15

SHARON A. H. MAY ■

"Innocent until proven guilty," the cornerstone concept of the American criminal justice system, embodies constitutional principles designed to achieve a delicate balance between the maintenance of certain societal interests and the protection of individual civil rights. The government has the responsibility of seeing to the people's general welfare, which encompasses their health and safety. At the same time, the government must safeguard the individual's liberties, particularly when that individual is accused of a crime.

The Bill of Rights, comprising the first ten amendments to the US Constitution, provides substantive and procedural due process for the individual charged with a crime. Substantive due process requires that the law be fair, equitable, and unambiguous. Procedural due process guarantees appear in the Fourth through the Eighth Amendments. The Fourth Amendment prevents the government from searching and seizing unreasonably. The Fifth Amendment ensures that a person cannot be forced to incriminate or bear witness against himself. That same amendment protects an individual from being tried (being put in jeopardy) twice for the same crime. From the Sixth Amendment comes a citizen's right to know the charges against him, the right to be represented by counsel, and the right to have a speedy and public trial by an impartial jury.

SEX OFFENSES

The American legal system evolved from the English system of justice. Common-law crimes came from a series of specified offenses deemed to be crimes against the king. Rape and sodomy were in that series. Over time, however, American legislatures realized that a number of other sexual crimes were not covered by the common-law definitions of and punishments for rape and sodomy. Currently, the phrase "sex crime" typically embodies a broad spectrum of sexually related or sexually motivated crimes.

Some state laws divide sexual assaults by degrees and impose greater punishment when specific aggravating circumstances are involved, such as using a weapon; inflicting strangulation, suffocation, or serious bodily harm; or being aided or abetted by other perpetrators. State laws have broadened to make criminal the touching or penetration of a victim's various body parts by foreign objects or by a perpetrator's various body parts. There are statutes that address sexual child abuse by household members, strangers, and those with temporary care or custody. Other laws involve the sexual exploitation of children, which covers sexual gratification of the perpetrator without a requirement that the child be physically touched or harmed. Sex crimes also include incest, obscenity, public nudity, and child pornography.

The law is constantly changing to expand and clarify definitions of criminal acts, alter requirements of proof, and increase punishment. Most often, such changes result from actual cases or incidents, which, because of an unforeseen hole in an existing law, cannot be prosecuted. In recent years, lawmakers have been challenged by changes in technology that strain typical criminal definitions and alter one's view of personal privacy. One example is in the area of child pornography. Because of legal requirements for identifying a specific victim, child pornographers can thwart investigation and may escape prosecution by creating photographs of nude children from body parts of several (even adult) individuals rather than taking a picture of a single identifiable child victim.

OVERVIEW OF THE CRIMINAL JUSTICE SYSTEM

While basic constitutionally constructed and protected procedures within the criminal justice system remain constant from state to state, each state has established specific differences. Therefore, this discussion of the criminal justice system is undertaken with the understanding that the particulars of the criminal process and procedure depend on the geographic location of the crime.

The prosecution and punishment of a sexual assailant or predator require the effective interplay of multiple components of the criminal justice system. Law enforcement, the judicial branch of government, and the corrections system each play a significant role in identifying, prosecuting, and processing criminals effectively and fairly. The first component of the criminal justice system, law enforcement, serves as the charging and investigative arm of the criminal system. Police officers, investigators, or law enforcement agents interview victims, witnesses, and suspects; pursue leads to identify the alleged perpetrator(s) of a crime; and make arrests. Crime lab technicians collect, analyze, and preserve tangible evidence and generate a report of their findings. Prosecutors review the evidence gathered by police and various experts, evaluate the sufficiency of the case against an accused, and consider whether to proceed to trial. Assuming that the decision is to go forward, the prosecutor prepares and presents the evidence to the trier of fact. Police and prosecutors exercise significant discretion in performing their duties, ideally guided by constitutional, statutory, and departmental requirements.

The courts represent the judicial branch and have the authority to hear facts and evaluate evidence within an accusatorial and adversarial legal model. In this model, the state must prove beyond reasonable doubt that the defendant committed the crime. Criminal proceedings are presided over by a judge, who must ensure that the substantive and procedural rules are upheld by the prosecution and defense.

During a jury trial, the judge decides what facts can be presented to the jury, maintains order, and instructs the jury as to the law. Depending upon the jurisdiction, the judge or the jury determines the sentence.

A not-guilty verdict means that a defendant must be released from the charges for which he was tried. A defendant convicted after a trial has the automatic right to an appeal. However, a defendant who pleads guilty may appeal on very limited grounds.

ILLUSTRATION OF THE CRIMINAL JUSTICE PROCESS

As informative as the abstract may be, it is helpful to put the theory into a practical application. Consider the following scenario and commentary. A jogger is raped and beaten while running in the park. A man walking his dog happens upon the injured jogger, who blurts out what just occurred. The man calls for help. Uniformed police arrive on the scene and glean just enough information to determine the nature of the attack and to initiate standard investigative procedures, including broadcasting a description of the perpetrator and how he left the area. An ambulance transports the victim to the nearest hospital staffed by a forensic nurse examiner team. At the scene, police officers cordon off the scene to prevent the contamination or destruction of valuable evidence. Mobile crime lab technicians scour the crime scene, searching for physical evidence that might show that a crime occurred and who committed that crime. Physical evidence includes fingerprints, hair, clothing fibers, body fluids, and any items that may contain trace evidence linking the assailant to the crime. Police officers canvass the area and interview potential witnesses.

At the hospital, the victim's medical history is documented. In addition, the forensic nurse examiner gathers information about what happened in order to treat the victim appropriately and to know what type of samples to collect. After the medical evaluation and treatment, detectives from the sex crimes unit interview the victim and obtain a more detailed description of the events. The victim spells out what transpired before, during, and after the assault. What the assailant did before might provide clues about whether the victim was randomly selected or targeted. Specific acts committed during and after the attack may link the perpetrator to other similar crimes. The police learn the exact nature of the sexual assault to decide what charges to bring if an arrest is made. The victim is asked whether force, threats, or weapons were used during the attack. Small bits of information blossom into significant clues about the perpetrator's identity.

INVESTIGATION

Crucial to any investigation of a sexual assault is the cooperation of the victim. As evidenced in the above scenario, important details known only to the victim can lead directly to the assailant. Building a strong case brings that assailant into court. Why then do some victims withdraw from the criminal investigation? Telling total strangers repeatedly about what happened and using graphic terms is embarrassing and extremely uncomfortable. A victim may become reluctant after realizing that participation in the criminal process is not necessarily limited to testimony at trial. The victim may be asked to present evidence to a grand jury and testify at a preliminary hearing or a pretrial motion. The major court appearance will require the victim to face the accused and point him out to the trier of fact. The prospect of the whole process can be overwhelming.

Some victims analyze and reanalyze whether they caused or contributed to the assault. They fear being judged and not being believed. Some victims of sexual assault perceive insensitivity from the criminal justice system and law enforcement personnel. Efforts have been made to make the process more accommodating to the victim to encourage prosecution. For example, rape shield laws have been enacted to exclude mention of a rape victim's sexual history, unless the previous sexual activity involved the defendant or could explain the victim's injuries or pregnancy. Police departments around the country have created speciality units staffed with professionals who have a special interest and expertise in investigating sex crimes. Prosecutors refer sexual assault victims to support programs. Nevertheless, victims are not convinced, and perhaps rightly so, that old attitudes have disappeared. At a training class on sexual assault, one small-town police officer remarked, "If a woman goes to a place where her mother or husband said not to go and something happens to her, it isn't rape."

Occasionally, victims alleging sexual assault are asked to take a polygraph test. In some situations, such a request may be appropriate. Lie detector devices can be effective investigative tools, particularly when the evidence does not add up and the case has stalled. However, such devices should never be used as blackmail. A victim should not be instructed to submit to a lie detector device as a prerequisite for the investigation to continue.

The police will expand their investigation to include possible witnesses, especially the first person to have contact with the victim after the assault. The victim's sudden, unsolicited statement to the dog walker in the scenario is a powerful piece of evidence. In some jurisdictions, the first report of a sexual assault (i.e., the statement of the victim to a third party) is admissible at trial. A statement made by an out-of-court declarant offered in court to prove the truth of the matter asserted is hearsay. Ordinarily, hearsay is not admissible, but there are exceptions. An excited utterance, such as one made by the newly injured sexual assault victim, to the first passerby or a police officer may be admissible in court. This excited utterance is deemed trustworthy because the statement is likely made under stressful circumstances, when the speaker has not had time to fabricate the remark.

At various stages of the investigation, the detectives reevaluate their case. Eyewitness accounts of the crime, witness descriptions of suspicious people in the area, the victim's own account, forensic evidence from the crime scene, and medical evidence from the sexual assault get reviewed. All of this information is used to identify an accused person and to develop the prosecution's case.

ARREST

In the assault scenario, several days pass after the attack on the jogger. Police on routine patrol near another small city park hear a woman scream. A citizen runs up and reports noticing a suspicious man, oddly dressed considering the season. The citizen saw the man hastily emerge from among the trees and toss an object into the bushes. Acting on this information, the officers search the bushes and recover a knife. The broadcast on the police radio band brings other officers to the area, and a search for the man begins. Within minutes, a man matching the description given by the citizen is stopped a few blocks from the park. The police ask the man for identification and want to know why he is in the area. He says he does not have any identification and claims to live near the park.

In the meantime, other officers locate the intended female victim. Her description of the assailant sounds very much like the description from the broadcast. The intended victim is taken to where the police are interviewing the oddly dressed man. She shouts, "That's him! He attacked me with a knife!" The man is arrested.

The law supports the actions of the police in this scenario. They have reason to believe a violent crime is occurring or is about to occur. The observations of the citizen coupled with the police officers' independent observations are reason enough to stop the man and ask him basic questions about who he is and why he is there. The US Supreme Court case of *Terry v. Ohio*, 392 US 1 (1968), and its progeny give police the authority to stop a citizen in the manner set forth in the scenario. In addition, when the police have a reasonable belief based on specific and articulable facts, the officers may conduct a limited search of outer clothing to discover a weapon. The courts examine the totality of the circumstances and then weigh the individual's Fourth Amendment protection from unreasonable searches and seizures against an officer's safety.

The identification made by the intended victim established probable cause for the arrest. Furthermore, it is likely that a pretrial challenge to the one-on-one identification would not be successful. Such "show up" identifications are not deemed to be impermissibly suggestive.

Typically, police read a suspect his Miranda rights immediately, although the rights are not required until a custodial interrogation takes place. Blurts made by a suspect who has not been asked a question and has not been advised of his/her rights may still be ruled admissible. Responses to questions asked before the advice of rights or after a request for legal counsel are likely to be excluded at trial. If a suspect's statement is obtained illegally, other incriminating information or tangible evidence that was unearthed on the basis of that statement cannot be presented at trial. Such evidence is considered "fruit of the poisonous tree" and must be excluded. (See *Wong Sun v. United States*, 371 US 471 [1963].)

The scenario arrest is warrantless because the suspect was apprehended at the scene of the crime on the basis of evidence or observation that supports a determination of probable cause. Since a felony was allegedly committed, the police were not required to request a warrant from a judge. Had the crime been a misdemeanor, the police could arrest without a warrant only if the crime had been committed in their presence. When the police do not witness the commission of the misdemeanor, the victim must go before a judicial officer, file charges, and take an oath that the allegations are true.

When a suspect is not apprehended contemporaneously with the crime, the victim or witnesses may be asked to view a photo array or attend a lineup. In either of these identification procedures, the police and prosecutors must ensure that the "filler" individuals share very similar physical characteristics and clothing with the suspect. To do otherwise makes the procedure impermissibly suggestive and taints the identification, making it inadmissible at trial. When identification is to be made using a photo array, the police must follow strict departmental procedures, including using either all-color or all-black-and-white photographs. During a physical lineup, the participants may be asked by the police to repeat certain statements allegedly made during the commission of the crime. This allows the victim to hear the voice of the alleged perpetrator and may be the sole basis for identification when the victim or witness did not get a good look at the assailant.

The lineup is conducted in a manner and place that prevents the suspect from seeing the witness.

BOOKING

After being arrested by the police, the suspect is transported to the police station or a central pretrial holding facility for booking. Booking is a police administrative process, which essentially records specific information about the suspect and the nature of the crimes committed. When booked, the suspect is fingerprinted and photographed. In jurisdictions using modern technology, the suspect places each finger on a glass, where his prints are read and recorded by the computer. His photograph is taken in color by a digital camera. Police check a national database for outstanding warrants on the defendant. Those warrants can act as detainers, a mechanism for holding a suspect even if the charges that gave rise to the present arrest are dropped. Typically, a suspect is permitted to make one phone call following the booking process.

In serious crimes against persons, such as sexual assault, a suspect may also be photographed to document his overall appearance and particular physical characteristics. The photo memorializes his clothing, which may fit the description of what was worn during the crime. The suspect's clothing may be confiscated and carefully packaged so that valuable trace evidence is preserved. Blood droplets, fibers, and natural products may link the suspect to the victim and/or the crime scene. In addition, police will take close-up shots of any injuries, which may be consistent with the victim's account of the crime.

After booking the suspect, police may get a court order to collect certain evidence from the suspect's body. For example, in a sexual assault, a forensic nurse examiner may extract head and pubic hairs and bodily fluids. Police are required to obtain a search and seizure warrant to get such samples from a suspect.

COMPLAINT

The police officer or detective files a complaint, the initial charging instrument. The complaint contains a statement of the facts, demonstrating the existence of probable cause and forming the basis of the offense charged. When a warrant is requested, the complaint is presented to a judge in support of the warrant. In a warrantless arrest, the complaint serves as the charging document at the initial appearance or preliminary hearing.

PROSECUTOR

The prosecuting attorney, whose proper title may be district attorney, state's attorney, attorney general, or

United States' attorney, represents the government in all criminal cases within his or her jurisdiction. While the prosecutor confers with police to review and assess the adequacy of evidence, the decision whether to proceed with the case rests with the prosecutor. The prosecutor evaluates the weight and admissibility of the evidence, the credibility of the witnesses, and the overall impression the victim will make on the trier of fact. Further, the prosecutor must be convinced that the case against the defendant can be proved beyond reasonable doubt. At any time before the case concludes, the prosecutor may withdraw or reduce charges. In some situations, the prosecutor and the defense may negotiate a plea.

The prosecutor may find it necessary to delay bringing the case into court and order the suspect's release for the moment. Statutes of limitations, which set a specific time frame during which a charge can be brought, vary from state to state and crime to crime. Sexual offenses may have no statute of limitations or may have a set period for charging, depending on the jurisdiction.

The strength of a criminal case may deteriorate at any given moment. Prosecutors are able to combat some problems by utilizing evidence rules or state laws. For example, witnesses change their stories or refuse to cooperate. State evidence rules may allow the prosecutor to admit a witness' taped statement as substantive evidence after the witness has recanted on the stand.

In an assault and attempted murder case tried in the State of Washington, the prosecutor introduced into evidence a taped statement of the defendant's wife. The statement was made during interrogation by the police and was presented to show that the stabbing was not done in self-defense. The wife decided to invoke her marital privilege and so refused to repeat her statements at trial. The husband was convicted and he appealed on the ground that his Sixth Amendment right to confront his accusers had been violated. The US Supreme Court ultimately decided the case. In *Crawford v. Washington*, 541 US 36 (2004), the justices agreed with the defendant and ruled that statements that are testimonial in nature are admissible only when the declarant is unavailable and the defendant has had an opportunity to cross-examine the witness.

The holding in *Crawford* is having a significant impact on the prosecution of criminal cases. To facilitate trying sexual and physical child abuse cases, several states passed "tender years" of child hearsay statutes, which allowed a young child's account of abuse to come into evidence through a doctor, nurse, school principal, teacher, or social worker. The child hearsay statutes provided that, although the child was available, the prosecutor could avoid traumatizing the child by bringing out the victim's

account through these other witnesses. This practice is no longer possible in light of the *Crawford* ruling.

In some cases, the prosecutor may decide not to prosecute. That decision may be based on the weight of evidence presently available, the emotional condition of the victim, the lasting negative effects of a trial on the victim, and other factors. The key points that a prosecutor must keep in mind are that the state will get only one shot at the defendant and that the state must be able to prove the defendant guilty beyond reasonable doubt.

Today's prosecutors have found it necessary to add a new tactic to their presentation of evidence to the trier of fact. They have to make certain the jurors are not evaluating the state's case using the television version of criminal investigation. Television medical examiners and lab technicians have Einstein intellects, solve crimes using fake science, investigate the crime, build the case, and interrogate the suspect in a half-lit room without advising him of his Miranda rights or having a lawyer present. Jurors watch this on television four to five times a week and come to believe through sheer repetition that what they are seeing is true. In contrast, real medical examiners perform the autopsy and prepare a protocol, which never states that the deceased died between 1:00 and 1:30 a.m. because there is no reliable scientific way to determine time of death. A real lab technician can enlarge a photograph of the possible murder weapon. However, he cannot and will not pour plaster of Paris in the murder victim's stab wound to determine the type of weapon used, because that cannot be done. In the real world, the roles of each component in the system are clearly defined. Real law enforcement personnel mesh the case facts with findings from the medical examiner and the lab technicians and build the case. The police arrest the suspect and advise him of his rights. Wise prosecutors make certain that throughout the trial they dispel the myths and defuse the impact of television.

INITIAL APPEARANCE

Within a reasonable time after the arrest, the accused must be taken before a judicial officer. At this proceeding, the judicial officer verifies the identity of the accused, informs him of the charges, and explains his right to counsel and to a preliminary hearing. If the defendant's charge is a felony, a preliminary hearing date is set. States vary on the time frame for that hearing, which could occur within 10 to 30 days of arrest.

The judicial officer then determines the defendant's eligibility for pretrial release on the basis of such factors as the defendant's criminal record, the seriousness of the crime, the threat to public safety, the defendant's ties with the community, and his record of appearing for trial previously. The pretrial status of the accused is also affected by whether the judicial officer finds probable cause. If the judicial officer is a judge, the defendant may be ordered to do certain things, including reporting to pretrial release staff regularly or not having contact with the victim prior to trial. Bail can be revoked if this order is violated or if the defendant commits certain crimes while awaiting trial.

PRELIMINARY HEARING

After the initial hearing before a judicial officer, in more than half the states, a felony defendant is afforded another hearing. The preliminary hearing is a determination by an independent magistrate as to whether there is probable cause to allow the state to charge a felony defendant. Probable cause examines the likelihood that a crime was committed and that the defendant is the perpetrator of that crime.

At the preliminary hearing, the state presents witnesses whose testimony provides the probable cause for the arrest of the defendant. Hearsay is permitted. This means that a police officer may testify as to what the victim and other witnesses said, the crime lab's conclusions, and the doctor's report. The defendant or his attorney may ask questions of the state's witnesses. However, because the hearing is not a determination of guilt or innocence, the defense does not call witnesses to refute the charges. If the preliminary hearing judge determines that sufficient evidence exists to hold the accused or if the accused waives his right to the preliminary hearing, the state files a criminal information. This is simply another type of charging document.

The prosecutor makes the decision whether to use a preliminary hearing or a grand jury for the probable cause determination. The state does not have to present every piece of evidence that will be used at trial; it must demonstrate only that there is sufficient probable cause. When the probable cause mechanism is a preliminary hearing, the defense gets to hear a sampling from the state's case.

Some jurisdictions, such as California, tend to use the preliminary hearing more frequently than the grand jury. Amazingly, California voters passed a referendum on the length of preliminary hearings. The vote came after the year-long preliminary hearing in the famous McMartin Day Care Center child abuse case. Apparently, the voters felt that the process was too costly, particularly because no charges were ever brought against the owners or staff of the day-care center.

GRAND JURY

In the alternative, the state may opt to present evidence of probable cause before a grand jury, which is a panel of citizens meeting in closed and secret probable cause proceedings. The prosecutor calls witnesses and presents evidence in support of probable cause. Hearsay is permitted. A defendant is not entitled to be present but may choose to testify. If he does so, it is without the presence of his attorney. The attorney may be consulted as necessary by the defendant but cannot be inside with the grand jury. It is very unusual for a defendant to testify before the grand jury, because defense attorneys are keenly aware of the inherent dangers of doing so. For example, Captain Jeffrey MacDonald, whose conviction for the 1970 murder of his wife and children was the subject of the book *Fatal Vision*, opted to testify before the grand jury. Later he was never able to overcome some serious contradictions between that testimony and his testimony at the trial.

The grand jury is empowered with broad investigative powers, including the power to compel witnesses to appear, to have witnesses testify under oath, and to compel witnesses to produce records and documents. Once the prosecutor has finished presenting evidence, the grand jury deliberates in secret and decides by a majority vote whether to indict. When an indictment is handed down, the grand jury issues an arrest warrant if the accused has not already been apprehended.

Some authorities contend that a grand jury will "indict yesterday's newspaper" if the prosecutor says so. However, not all grand juries merely rubber stamp the prosecutor's will. Grand jurors have been known to "no bill" cases involving citizens such as business owners who tired of being victimized, took the law into their own hands, and killed intruders intent on stealing. Grand jurors have declined to indict men charged with having sexual relations with underage females whose general behavior and sexual conduct far exceeded their years. Given that the grand jurors' discussions and votes are held behind a closed and locked door, the precise reasons for such "no bills" remain unknown.

ARRAIGNMENT

At a proceeding called an arraignment, an accused person is presented to a judge to hear a reading of the formal criminal information or grand jury indictment. The defendant is informed of his right to an attorney if one has not already been obtained. The court appoints a counsel if the accused is unable to afford legal representation. There is no constitutional right to a separate arraignment proceeding. A defendant can be arraigned on the same day as his scheduled trial. Some jurisdictions arraign the accused separately to ensure the defendant will have a counsel on the appointed trial date, thereby avoiding delays. Arraignment can also be used to make the filing of pertinent motions a part of the court record.

At the arraignment, the defendant may enter one of five pleas: not guilty, guilty, *Alford, nolo contendere* (no contest), or not criminally responsible plea. The first two types of pleas are self-explanatory and commonly understood. The third stems from a Supreme Court case, *North Carolina v. Alford*, 400 US 25, 91 Sup Ct 160 (1970), which held that a defendant may acknowledge the sufficiency of the government's case to convict without admitting guilt. Instead, the defendant only wishes to take advantage of the plea bargain. Although the defendant maintains his innocence, the court treats the *Alford* plea as if it were a guilty plea. So long as the state provides a statement of facts that satisfies all the elements of the crime, the court will find the defendant guilty.

A *nolo contendere* plea is not an admission of criminal conduct. The court has the discretion to allow or disallow the use of this plea. Once accepted, the court treats this plea in the same manner as a guilty plea and can sentence accordingly. As is true with a straight guilty plea, a defendant gives up the right to complain about procedural defects in his case. One other unique feature of a *nolo contendere* plea is that it cannot be used against a defendant in a subsequent civil proceeding. The most famous *nolo contendere* plea in Maryland history was that of US Vice President Spiro T. Agnew, who was accused of crimes committed while he was the governor of Maryland. Eventually, Agnew was forced to resign as Vice President.

Another variety of guilty plea is "not criminally responsible." Use of this plea is an admission by the defendant that he has committed the crime, but he contends that because of a mental illness or defect he was unable to understand the criminality of his conduct and was unable to confine his behavior to the requirements of law. Unless the government agrees with the assessment that the defendant was not criminally responsible, the case proceeds to trial.

When a defendant enters a guilty, *Alford*, or *nolo contendere* plea, the judge must make certain that the accused is entering that plea freely, voluntarily, knowingly, and without coercion. The defendant must respond to a series of specific questions to demonstrate that he understands the rights he is waiving and the effect of the plea. Once the record is made and the court is satisfied the plea is entered voluntarily and knowingly, the state recites a statement of facts indicating the evidence that would have been presented against the defendant at a trial. If the facts are sufficient and support the charges, the court will find the defendant guilty.

The judge may reject the plea if he concludes that the defendant does not understand what he is doing,

has been unduly influenced, or has been subjected to duress. A not-guilty plea is then entered and the case proceeds to trial.

DISCOVERY

The attorneys on both sides learn more about the case through a process called *discovery*. Criminal discovery permits the exchange of information between the prosecution and the defense. The defense learns the nature of the evidence the government has collected. Sometimes before but often after arrest, the suspect has been required to undergo a variety of examinations, including blood and saliva, deoxyribonucleic acid (DNA), and hair sample analysis. Results of those tests, the existence of physical evidence, hospital records, conclusions of experts, and any evidence tending to show the innocence or lessen the culpability of the defendant are turned over to the defense. The defendant informs the government of any alibi witnesses who will be called. In some states, such as California, discovery must be completely open, meaning that both sides must disclose everything that may be presented at trial. In other states, however, discovery may be so restricted as to permit surprises at trial.

In some jurisdictions, defendants charged with crimes in which bodily fluids may have been exchanged can be ordered by the court, upon the victim's written request, to undergo human immunodeficiency virus (HIV) testing before trial or after conviction. Health department officials counsel the victim and defendant regarding repeated testing and the interpretation of the results. The test results are not disclosed to the counsel or the court and cannot be used at trial or sentencing. Consequently, there is no discovery issue related to HIV test results.

PRETRIAL MOTIONS

Between the arraignment and the trial, the prosecuting attorney and the defense attorney make several court appearances and argue various motions. Such motions include challenges to the validity or sufficiency of the charging document, requests for discovery, and motions to suppress evidence allegedly obtained illegally by the police.

Pretrial rulings can end a criminal case. For instance, if the court grants a defense motion to suppress the use of seized drugs in a drug possession case, the prosecution has no choice but to dismiss the charge. Possession, the key element of the charge, cannot be shown because the seizure and subsequent analysis of the drugs cannot be mentioned to the trier of fact.

PLEA NEGOTIATIONS

Plea negotiations may occur at any stage prior to the entry of a verdict, even while the jury is deliberating. In less complex cases, the negotiations may occur at arraignment. The defendant is likely offered the best deal he will ever get at that stage. On occasion, adverse pretrial rulings for one of the parties crystallize the strengths and weaknesses of a case. Miraculously, discussions about a possible guilty plea take place.

Usually both sides compromise during plea negotiations. The defendant agrees to plead guilty if the government will reduce the charges, call lesser counts, recommend a lesser sentence, or agree not to proceed with other yet uncharged cases. The prosecutor should discuss the plea with the victim but does not have to abide by his or her wishes. The court must approve the plea agreement. Individual judges differ on whether it is appropriate for them to get involved in plea negotiations.

Generally speaking, the public tends to be less than enthralled with plea-bargaining. Citizens decry "giving away the courthouse" and releasing the criminals back into the city streets. However, those who work within the system in large urban areas recognize good reasons to work out cases short of trial. It is physically impossible to take every case to trial. Impaneling juries is difficult. In the past, notices for jury service were sent to registered voters; however, because of dwindling voter registration, cities now also draw from the list of licensed drivers. Even so, jurors find all sorts of reasons to get out of jury service. Others simply do not show up for court. At the other end of the process is the problem of insufficient prison space for those who are sentenced to jail time. Plea-bargaining becomes the solution to these problems.

DEFENDANT AND DEFENSE COUNSEL

The Sixth Amendment right to counsel took on new meaning in the US Supreme Court case of *Gideon v. Wainwright*, 372 US 335 (1963). Gideon had allegedly broken into a poolroom with the intent to commit a misdemeanor, that is, a minor crime. He asked the trial court to appoint an attorney for him. The judge refused, citing Florida law that provided counsel only to indigent defendants charged with capital crimes. Gideon represented himself, was convicted, and was sentenced to 5 years. His case made its way to the US Supreme Court, which held that indigent defendants forced to represent themselves were being denied a fundamental right guaranteed to them through the Fourteenth Amendment. Following the *Gideon*

ruling, many states, although not all, funded public defender offices to meet the needs of those who could not afford a single attorney, let alone a "dream team."

A criminal defendant must be present at all critical stages of the criminal process. He is entitled to have his attorney present as well. Critical stages include lineups, preliminary hearings, pretrial motions, and the trial. The role of the defense counsel is to provide effective representation of the defendant and to ensure that the government acts within the law and presents a fair case to the trier of fact.

At trial, the burden of proof is always on the state to prove an accused guilty beyond reasonable doubt. Consequently, a defendant does not have to present a defense. He is not required to refute the state's evidence nor must he testify during the trial. If the defendant opts to remain silent, the defense counsel may ask the court to instruct the jury that the defendant's silence does not imply guilt.

An accused can raise defenses and attack the state's case in a variety of ways. He can simply deny the charges, point the finger at another possible perpetrator, or present an alibi. A defendant can also chip away at the state's case by challenging the credibility of lay witnesses and the opinions of experts. This can be done through cross-examination and the presentation of the defense's own lay and expert witnesses.

Prior to trial, the defendant may ask to take a polygraph test to demonstrate his innocence. The results of that test may influence the prosecutor's willingness to proceed against the defendant. In most jurisdictions, however, the results of a polygraph test as well as a defendant's willingness or refusal to take one is inadmissible in a criminal court because courts generally are not convinced of the reliability of truth-verification devices. The courts look to see whether a particular device or technology has gained acceptance in the scientific community. Although a few jurisdictions permit introduction of polygraph evidence, truth-verification devices are still not widely accepted in the scientific community.

TRIAL

The Sixth Amendment guarantees a defendant the right to a trial by an impartial jury. Individual states codify which crimes or, more accurately, which sentences trigger a defendant's right to a jury trial. When imprisonment for more than 6 months may result, this requirement has been interpreted as an absolute right in some jurisdictions.

The defendant elects whether to be tried by a court or by a jury. If he chooses a jury trial, the defense and the prosecutor select individual jurors through a process called *voir dire*, a French term meaning *to bring forth the truth*. The court and the attorneys question jurors about their prior knowledge of the case, their familiarity with the defendant or witnesses, pretrial publicity, personal incidents or prejudices, and anything else that may cause them not to be fair and impartial. The court must be satisfied that the jurors will fairly and impartially evaluate the evidence. First, jurors are "struck for cause" by the court on the basis of verbalized reasons given by counsel for both sides. One reason might be a juror's admitted inability to be fair and impartial because his religion prohibits him from sitting in judgment of others. Next, the attorneys exercise what are called peremptory challenges. The attorneys may remove the jurors without stating a reason on the record. Each side gets a set number of peremptory challenges, with the defense usually getting more challenges than the state. There is no requirement that each side exercise all of its peremptory challenges.

After the jury is selected, the jurors take an oath to well and truly try the defendant. With that oath, jeopardy attaches in a jury trial. In a court trial, jeopardy attaches when the first witness is sworn. The attachment of jeopardy signifies the state's one opportunity to try the defendant on the particular charge under the specific facts of the case. For example, if the defendant is acquitted of raping Jane Doe on May 11, 2005, the state cannot try him again on that same charge. To do so would violate the defendant's constitutional right against double jeopardy.

During opening statements, the attorneys outline their theories of the case and establish what the evidence will show. Defense counsel has the option of speaking directly after the prosecutor or can reserve remarks until the start of the defense's case. Some states, such as Connecticut, do not permit opening statements.

The state presents its case-in-chief first because the state has the burden of proof. Typically, although not always, the victim is the first witness and is followed by others who have information to present to the trier of fact. Defense counsel may cross-examine a state's witness as to basis of knowledge, credibility, bias, and other relevant issues. Cross-examination can be painstakingly thorough to highlight weaknesses in the witness's testimony.

At the conclusion of the state's case, the defense moves for a judgment of acquittal on the basis of the insufficiency of the evidence presented by the state. If the motion is granted on all counts, the trial ends and the case is dismissed. If the motion is denied, the case proceeds. The defense may then present a case if it chooses. The defense may offer evidence to challenge the prosecution's case and generate reasonable doubt. A defendant's right to remain silent includes his right not to be called by the state, not to testify in the defense portion of

the case, and not to present any evidence. Knowing the burden of proof is on the state to prove the defendant's guilt, the defense counsel may decide not to present a defense if the prosecution's case is glaringly weak.

The most common defense in sexual assault cases is consent. Defendants have been known to deny culpability and even any connection to the victim during the early stages of the case. However, when DNA results prove that the defendant had sexual contact with the victim, suddenly the defense becomes consent.

At the conclusion of the defense's case, the prosecution may present rebuttal evidence, but only if the defense presents a case. The rules of evidence require that rebuttal must refute evidence developed during the defense portion of the trial. During rebuttal, the state may not present newly discovered or previously omitted evidence that is not a direct response to evidence presented by the defense.

When all the evidence has been presented, the defense renews its motion for judgment of acquittal in the hope of gaining a dismissal of some or all charges. Next, either the court will instruct the jury or the counsel will deliver their final arguments. Procedural rules differ among the states as to the order of closing arguments. Jury instructions may or may not precede closing arguments. Also, in some states, the state argues first and last, whereas other jurisdictions allow only one argument per side.

Jury deliberations by the entire panel, excluding alternates, are held in private. Generally, the verdict must be unanimous as to guilt or innocence. Procedural rules may allow a less than unanimous verdict so long as both sides agree to that. If the jury is unable to return a verdict, the court will declare a hung jury. That panel is dismissed and the state has the option of trying the case for as many times as it takes to reach a unanimous verdict.

If the jury finds the defendant not guilty, the decision is final and the verdict may not be appealed. The not-guilty verdict does not necessarily indicate that the defendant was innocent. It signifies that the state did not prove its case beyond reasonable doubt. (The not-guilty verdict could also indicate the jury's desire to nullify the law that applied in the defendant's case.) After the acquittal, the defendant is released. He may not be retried on the same charge because of the protection against double jeopardy.

Regardless of the verdict in the state case, the defendant may be tried anew in federal court if the same acts break a federal law. This dual jurisdiction is not deemed a violation of the double jeopardy provision. For example, state and federal courts have concurrent jurisdiction in bank robbery cases. The state court may try a defendant on robbery under state law. Because banks fall under federal protection, the same defendant can face federal robbery charges as well. As a practical matter, however, this is not done often. In concurrent jurisdiction situations, federal and state authorities will confer as to which jurisdiction will prosecute. One factor that might be considered is which jurisdiction has stiffer penalties. Another factor might be that one jurisdiction classifies a particular act as criminal while the other jurisdiction does not. Occasionally, federal authorities will initiate charges because a federal jury composed of citizens from throughout the state is more likely to convict on certain crimes than a local jury panel.

If the verdict is guilty, the defense usually submits a motion for new trial, alleging that some procedural error occurred, that the verdict was against the weight of evidence, or that the defendant did not receive a fair trial. Such motions are often not successful. The motion is frequently set on the same day as sentencing. If the motion is denied, the judge proceeds to sentencing. When a new trial motion is granted, the state must decide whether to try the defendant again.

SENTENCING

Judges possess the ultimate authority for imposing sentences. In the case of felonies, the judge orders a presentence report. The report summarizes the criminal's personal and social background, criminal history, adjustment to probation and institutionalization, employment, health, and mental stability. Often included in the report is a victim impact statement. The purpose of the presentence report is to assist the judge in pronouncing an appropriate sentence by presenting aggravating and mitigating circumstances while incorporating the public policy goals of retribution and rehabilitation. The judge has some restrictions imposed by the criminal code, such as minimum and maximum sentences. Nevertheless, the court retains a significant degree of flexibility in considering sentences. Generally the judge may impose a suspended sentence, a fine, probation only, a split sentence combining jail and probation, or straight incarceration. In death penalty cases, the defendant chooses whether he wants the judge or the jury to decide if the sentence should be death or life.

POSTCONVICTION PROCEDURES

A defendant can exercise several rights following conviction, all of which have strict filing deadlines. After being sentenced, a defendant typically petitions the sentencing judge to modify the sentence. Presumably, the court made a very reasoned decision as to sentencing in the first place. Consequently, there would have to be a significant basis for reducing

or modifying the sentence. It seems unlikely that an incarcerated defendant could present adequate justification to support a modification.

The court can build the possibility of modification into the original sentence. For instance, a youthful offender or a defendant with no prior adult record may be encouraged to complete very specific tasks or fulfill certain conditions by a particular date. Once those have been completed, the court converts the disposition into probation before judgment (PBJ). The court strikes the guilty finding in favor of the PBJ. The advantage of a PBJ is that the defendant has no conviction of record. Having a clean record helps one's prospects of attaining higher education, financial aid, and employment.

Some jurisdictions permit a defendant to have his sentence reviewed by a panel of judges, not including the original sentencing judge. This fresh set of eyes may take a different position as to disposition. Maryland rules allow defendants sentenced to 2 or more years to petition for a three-judge panel review within 30 days of the sentencing. That panel, which can consult the original sentencing judge, has the authority to lower the sentence, keep it the same, or even raise it. Once filed, the petition cannot be withdrawn. Needless to say, defense attorneys vigorously discourage such petitions.

The primary mechanism of postconviction relief is appeal. Defendants have an automatic right to appeal their convictions after a full trial. Appropriate issues for appellate review include the admissibility of evidence, the instructions given to the jury, prosecutorial misconduct, and other procedural rulings. Defendants who plead guilty may appeal or ask for permission to appeal on very limited grounds. The judge and counsel make a careful, thorough record of the guilty plea proceedings to ensure that a defendant knows all the rights he is waiving. By entering the guilty plea, the defendant gives up his right to object to most errors and to raise defenses.

Some states have a statutory process called *postconviction relief* for defendants who qualify to utilize the statute. Postconviction relief is a collateral attack on the verdict and provides relief on limited grounds, such as incompetence of trial and appellate counsel. Should postconviction relief be granted, the defendant may receive permission to file a belated appeal, a belated reconsideration of sentence, or even a new trial.

Once a defendant convicted in state court exhausts all possible state appeals and remedies, he can apply for federal *habeas corpus* ("you have the body") relief. The state postconviction process must be completed within 5 years of sentencing. The petition for federal *habeas corpus* relief must be based on constitutional issues.

INCARCERATION

Newly sentenced defendants go through a classification process. Correctional authorities decide whether a prisoner should be housed in a minimum, medium, or maximum-security facility. Also, placement may vary depending on what special programs a prisoner might need such as drug treatment, psychiatric services, medical treatment, sex offender counseling, or basic educational programs.

Incarceration, not surprisingly, does not automatically end a prisoner's criminal behavior. Crimes that occur within the prison walls may be handled through internal administrative proceedings or referred to state or local prosecutors. Prisoners convicted of escape or crimes against correctional officers and other inmates are often given sentences consecutive to whatever time was already being served.

PAROLE

Depending on the state's sentencing system, prisoners are given either a mandatory release after serving their time or a discretionary release on the basis of the decision of the parole board. In most states, the parolee is required to remain under supervision until his sentence would have expired. States vary in their laws concerning when a prisoner is eligible for parole and the crimes to which parole may apply. State law may provide that prisoners receive a set number of days off their sentence each month for good behavior. A prisoner's release date is calculated immediately upon his arrival at the prison. The warden makes it clear that the prisoner may lose good time as punishment for infractions. Penal authorities argue that good time is a necessary and valuable carrot to encourage positive behavior by prisoners.

State laws further set forth when or whether a prisoner can be paroled. Someone sentenced to life in a prison in Virginia, for example, will spend his or her remaining days on earth behind bars. By contrast, a Maryland prisoner under a life sentence becomes eligible for parole after serving 15 years minus 5 good-time days off per month. If the Parole Board recommends that a prisoner serving life should be released, the governor's signature is required to make that happen. Only when the prosecution serves notice of an intention to seek life without parole can a Maryland judge impose that sentence.

DEATH PENALTY

Furman v. Georgia, 408 US 238 (1972), is a *per curiam* (unanimous) US Supreme Court decision ruling that the death penalty could not be applied "sparsely, selectively, and spottily." Furman, Jackson, and Branch, the three defendants who were the subject of the case, were all African Americans. Furman, who was tried in Georgia, had psychiatric issues and had, at one point, been deemed incompetent to stand trial for murder. Jackson, also convicted in Georgia, got the death penalty for murdering a white woman. Jackson was of average intelligence and had no mental health problems. He had previously been convicted of auto theft. While on escape from a work gang, Jackson was charged with burglary, auto theft, and battery. Branch was convicted of rape in Texas. He was of borderline intelligence and had received the equivalent of $5\frac{1}{2}$ years of grade school education. The Supreme Court held that the death penalty in these three cases amounted to cruel and unusual punishment, in violation of the Eighth and Fourteenth Amendments, in that the decision to execute was not made fairly. The Court charged state legislatures to pass laws that are "evenhanded, nonselective, and nonarbitrary."

State lawmakers responded by rewriting the death penalty statutes. One consequence of *Furman* was that defendants convicted of rape could no longer be executed.

SUGGESTED READINGS

Allison JA, Wrightsman LS. *Rape: the misunderstood crime.* Thousand Oaks, CA: Sage Publications, 1993.

Bailey FL, Rothblatt HB. *Investigation and preparation of criminal cases.* Rochester, New York: The Lawyers Co-operative Publishing Company, 1970.

Cole GF. *The American system of criminal justice*, 7th ed. Pacific Grove, CA: Brooks/Cole Publishing Company, 1995.

Hall R. *Rape in America: a reference handbook.* Santa Barbara, CA: Clio, 1995.

Hall DE. *Criminal law and procedure*, 4th ed. Albany, New York: Delmar Publishers, 2003.

Hohenhaus S. Patterned injury and court testimony in a sexual assault. *J Emerg Nurs* 1998;24: 614.

Hohenhaus S. SANE legislation and lessons learned: sexual assault nurse examiner. *J Emerg Nurs* 1998;24: 463–464.

Hrones S, Czar C. *Criminal practice handbook*, 2nd ed. New York: Mathew Bender, 1999.

Lowey AH, LaFrance AB. *Criminal procedure arrest and investigation.* Cincinnati, OH: Anderson Publishing, 1996.

McGregor MJ, Le G, Marion SA, et al. Examination for sexual assault: is the documentation of physician injury associated with the laying of charges? A retrospective cohort study. *Can Med Assoc J* 1999;160 (11) : 1565–1569.

Maryland Community Crime Prevention Institute. Available at www.dpscs.state.md.us/aboutdpscs/pct/ccpi. Accessed on May 4, 2005.

Paquin GW. Legal aspects of acquaintance rape. In: Wiene VR, Richards AL, eds. *Intimate betrayal. Understanding and responding to the trauma of acquaintance rape.* Thousand Oaks, CA: Sage Publications, 1995: 88–107.

Pentilla A, Karhumen PJ. Medicolegal findings among rape victims. *Med Law* 1990;9: 725–737.

Reed M. The judicial system and laws. *Sexual assault forensic examiner training manual.* University of Maryland, Department of Surgery, Division of Emergency Medicine, 1998; Sec. 7: 1–59.

Selkin J. *The child sexual abuse case in the courtroom*, 2nd ed. Denver, CO: James Selkin, 1991.

Soules MR, Stewart SK, Brown KM, et al. The spectrum of alleged rape. *J Reprod Med* 1978;20 (1) : 33–39.

Stuckey GB, Roberson CR, Wallace H. *Procedures in the justice system*, 7th ed. Upper Saddle River, NJ: Prentice-Hall, 2003.

Temkin J, ed. *Rape and the criminal justice system*. Brookfield, WI: Dartmouth Publishing Company, 1995.

United States Constitution *West Virginia sexual assault legal guide*. Available at www.lectlaw.com/files/sex11.htm. Accessed on May 4, 2005.

16

TESTIFYING

SHARON A. H. MAY ■

ROLE OF THE SEXUAL ASSAULT HEALTH CARE EXAMINER

The sexual assault health care examiner, be it a physician, nurse, physician's assistant, or forensic nurse examiner (FNE), is frequently the first health care practitioner to have contact with the sexual assault victim in the aftermath of the attack. In addition to attending to the emotional needs of someone who is understandably distressed and distraught over a vicious, dehumanizing, and demoralizing event, the health care practitioner is responsible for assessing the extent of injury and providing the necessary treatment and support for the acute injuries and anticipated health hazards. Although the first priority is directed at identifying physical and psychological injury and rendering medically indicated therapy, the practitioner's responsibilities necessarily extend to the collection of evidence and the accurate recording of the victim's history, physical findings, and the results of laboratory and radiographic studies. The ability to prosecute the assailant may hinge on the accuracy and precision of assembling the historical data, physical findings, and crucial forensic evidence. Deficient or defective intervention by the practitioner at the preliminary stage of this investigative process can lead to the inability to charge an alleged attacker criminally or the failure to convict a defendant. Similarly, the effective collection of pertinent forensic evidence can potentially exculpate an innocent suspect.

Consequently, the indispensable role of the practitioner after a sexual assault encompasses two distinct duties: (i) the irrevocable legal duty to render reasonable medical care and (ii) a professional duty to gather evidence that will help authorities determine whether a crime has been committed and establish the identity of the perpetrator. Ultimately, the practitioner must be prepared to report the sexual assault examination findings in a professional and unbiased manner to an official fact-finding tribunal. Understanding that the practitioner bears an enormous responsibility to the victim and to the society at large, the practitioner must be intensely vigilant and attentive to detail in handling sexual assault cases to ensure that competent and reliable decisions can be achieved regarding the criminal disposition of cases.

Effective involvement of the health care practitioner in sexual assault cases requires a fundamental understanding of the process and procedure of criminal prosecution. When an individual has allegedly committed a criminal act or is under suspicion for committing a criminal act, the police and prosecutors investigate and possibly bring charges against the suspect. If there is sufficient probable cause to arrest and if there is a viable case, the prosecutor will charge. (In general, prosecutors have the discretion as to whether any charges should be filed against a suspect.) Critical to placing charges is a full understanding of the facts. The police and prosecutors must interview the witnesses and especially the victim to determine exactly what happened. The facts will determine what charges can be lodged. For example, if the perpetrator used a weapon as opposed to threatening the victim verbally, use or possession of a deadly weapon would be an appropriate charge. In a sexual assault case, use of a deadly weapon qualifies the suspect for being charged with an aggravated sexual assault such as rape in the first degree. A typical penal code states that a person is guilty of rape in the first degree if the person engages in vaginal intercourse with the victim by force or threat of force, without the consent of the victim, and employs a deadly or dangerous weapon, inflicts suffocation or strangulation, or is aided and abetted by others or if the person commits the act during the course of a burglary. To convict the defendant, the prosecution must prove each and every element of any crime on which a defendant is tried. Failure to prove any individual element can result in a defendant being convicted of a lesser included crime or being acquitted altogether. For instance, if the State does not present evidence that a weapon was actually used, the defendant may be convicted only of rape in the second degree. The State's burden is to prove the accused guilty beyond reasonable doubt.

The gravamen of most sexual assault charges is proving that the victim did not consent. In the absence of clear evidence of physical force, the victim's physical helplessness, or the victim's mental defect to show lack of consent, the prosecution's task becomes much more challenging. Without such probative evidence, the prosecution must rely on the testimony and credibility of the victim, the attendant circumstances of the crime, and the perception of the defendant's lack of credibility to build a case. In many cases, the forensic evidence collected, observed, and interpreted by qualified health care practitioners is pivotal to the prosecution of a sexual assault case.

The defense attorney attempts to counter or neutralize the prosecution's case by attacking weaknesses. This is accomplished through cross-examination of the state's witnesses or by offering contradictory evidence during the defense portion of the trial. One of the defense's objectives is to demonstrate that the prosecution has failed to present evidence of each element of the crime. The defense attorney may argue that his or her client could not have committed the crime because of an alibi that places the defendant at another location at the time the crime was perpetrated. Alternatively, the defendant may assert that the victim consented.

THE FORENSIC NURSE EXAMINER AS EXPERT WITNESS

The evidence presented at the trial may be complex, technical, and beyond the comprehension of the average juror. Therefore, professionals who possess the requisite level of expertise and good communication skills are indispensable in the legal process. The presence of the expert witness helps the jury understand and connect the evidence to make a measured inference that the defendant committed the crime. An expert witness, in contrast to a lay witness, is permitted to express an opinion on relevant issues pertaining to the facts and falling within his or her professional expertise. The expert must be able to render the opinion to a "reasonable degree of medical certainty."

The lay witness, on the other hand, may testify only to what he or she saw, heard, felt, or smelled. The lay witness must have direct knowledge of the event rather than secondary knowledge. The lay witness is not qualified to express an opinion or speculate about the meaning of certain testimony. However, the lay witness can testify to ordinary observations, such as the statement "the car was going fast." The expert witness is needed to say how fast the car was going or whether the speed was reasonable and prudent for that particular location.

The sexual assault examiner or health care practitioner is routinely called to testify as to the medical findings. Many jurisdictions have certified FNEs as experts for judicial purposes. In one nationally publicized sexual assault investigation in New York City, evidence was submitted to the grand jury to determine whether the accused perpetrators would be indicted for the crime. The evidence included the testimony of the doctors who examined the victim, the testimony of Federal Bureau of Investigation (FBI) experts who analyzed the forensic evidence gathered from the rape kit, and other physical evidence gathered during the investigation. The grand jury received testimony from two forensic pathologists who had reviewed the FBI reports and the medical reports concerning the victim's condition. Forensic psychiatrists formulated opinions and testified to the likelihood that a sexual assault was committed, on the basis of a review of the medical records. Using the evidence supplied during that proceeding, the grand jury declined to indict the alleged attackers.

To determine how to treat the patient, the examining health care practitioner asks the victim questions about the attack. The examining practitioner's testimony as to what the victim related during the examination is technically hearsay, which is generally inadmissible. However, the examiner may be permitted to testify concerning historical information under an exception to the hearsay rule. A treating practitioner may testify as to what the victim/patient said, so long as it is relevant to the treatment of the medical or psychological condition. If the victim told the physician or nurse that she was bitten several times on her back and that her arm was twisted, the physician or nurse may testify to this statement. Generally, the physician is not permitted to testify to statements of identity or culpability. If the victim stated, "John, my friend's brother, forced me to the ground and assaulted me," the portion of the statement that identifies the assailant could possibly be inadmissible. As a practical matter, identification can be elicited through the victim's direct testimony at trial.

The examining practitioner may testify as to the mental state of the victim upon arrival at the health care facility. The victim's demeanor may be important in categorizing the response as consistent or not consistent with a traumatic event. Obviously, this assessment is prone to subjectivity and therefore may not be a reliable determinant. The trier of fact must decide what weight to give any observations regarding the mental state of the victim.

The testimony of the practitioner about the examination and laboratory results and the victim's statements concerning physical force or injury may prompt the jury to decide that the sexual encounter was not consensual. Clearly, any complaints of pain and any corroborative evidence of injury, such as abrasion, bruises, bite marks, lacerations, bleeding, sprains, strains, broken bones, closed head injuries, penetrating trauma, or injury to the genitalia, perineum, or rectum, bolster the probability that the act was not consensual.

In the absence of persuasive physical evidence, the practitioner's impression of the victim's demeanor, state of mind, affect, or emotional status during the examination may or may not help the trier of fact to decide whether there was a sexual assault. A tearful, excited, angry, withdrawn, anxious, or distraught patient could have experienced some traumatic event other than a sexual assault. On the other hand, a patient displaying just the opposite demeanor could have been sexually assaulted. Therefore, an attempt to categorize or label a particular response as consistent or inconsistent with a sexual assault is fraught with danger. The sexual assault examiner should be familiar with the spectrum of recognized posttraumatic responses accompanying a sexual assault and should be able to articulate those varied responses in front of the trier of fact.

CONSTRUCTING THE MEDICAL REPORT

The medical record should contain a variety of information. A sexual assault victim may be transported to the emergency department or some other health care facility by ambulance or in the automobile of a friend, family member, or stranger; the victim may have walked to the nearest facility. The method of transport should be documented in the medical record. After a preliminary trauma assessment, a comprehensive history is obtained. This history should include the following information:

- A description of the incident
- Location where the assault took place
- Identity of the assailant, if known
- Home and workplace of the assailant, if known
- Method by which the assailant left the scene
- Whether a weapon was used to coerce the victim
- Whether drugs or alcohol were used before or during the attack
- Whether the patient had changed clothes, showered, voided, or douched since the incident
- Complaints of pain or injury
- Date of the victim's last consensual intercourse
- Date of the victim's last menstrual period
- Any birth control measures used

Physical examination includes a survey of the entire body for evidence of physical injury. Gynecologic and genital examinations of a female are mandatory unless the victim refuses. An anal examination must be included to document the presence or absence of penetration injuries. The increasing use of a colposcope with a camera attachment to assist in gathering forensic evidence is having enormous implications in providing relevant evidence in a prosecution. A Wood's lamp may be used to identify semen stains on the victim. A swab of the external genitalia, the cervix, and the anal canal may reveal motile sperm.

A clinician or FNE will be asked to report in painstaking detail any findings that corroborate or dispute that the sexual assault took place. In this role, the examiner is providing firsthand impressions as an expert witness. The examiner records the victim's complaints and photographs physical findings. The victim's history, physical examination, studies, and lab results are introduced through oral testimony and medical records.

Recognizing the intensity with which the medical report will be scrutinized, the examiner must address the evaluation and management of a sexual assault victim with an unrelenting compulsion. A complete examination and management are indicated. Meticulous medical record documentation constitutes the foundation of the medical evidence presented at trial. All records and materials are transmitted to the prosecuting attorneys and turned over to the defense. Medical records, including those created by other physicians in addition to those performing the initial rape examination, may be introduced into evidence. Any notes written by the examining physician will be included as part of the medical record. Therefore, the medical record must be neat, understandable, accurate, and consistent. The record will be used to refresh the practitioner's memory and will be combed extensively by the defense to uncover shortcomings in the evaluation.

CHAIN OF CUSTODY

The forensic evidence collected by the examiner may provide the most powerful evidence in identifying the suspect or perpetrator of the crime. Each item must be meticulously collected and maintained. Samples, which can deteriorate, need to be preserved properly. Handling of the evidence must be documented accurately to establish and safeguard the integrity and competence of the evidence. The examiner must demonstrate that evidence was gathered, preserved, sealed, and stored in such a manner as to prevent tampering. Documentation should include the name of the law enforcement official who received the rape kit and any other collected evidence, along with the date and time of that receipt.

SUBPOENA

A subpoena strikes fear in the hearts and minds of men, women, and physicians who recognize that as a result of this written instrument they have temporarily lost free will. For those unfamiliar with the power of a subpoena, it is no more threatening than a traffic citation. A frequent response to the subpoena is to ignore it. Both approaches should be erased from a witness's mind.

A subpoena is a written legal document issued by a court at the request of a party to a civil or criminal legal proceeding. The subpoena directs a named witness to appear at a designated place for a designated reason. A subpoena is issued under court authority and directs the witness to obey and respond to the order. If the witness fails to comply with the subpoena, he or she may be arrested. Furthermore, subpoenaed witnesses who have moved out of state are not relieved of their responsibility to appear. Every state has procedural mechanisms that allow the court where the witness resides to demand that the witness show cause why he or she should not appear in the requesting state. A properly executed and properly served subpoena cannot be ignored.

A subpoena issued by a court of competent jurisdiction must be served upon the person named or to an agent authorized by appointment or by law to receive service for the named person. The subpoena may be served by a sheriff or by a person who is not a party and who is at least 18 years old. Some states may have specific rules that allow service by mail.

The top of the subpoena identifies the case. A criminal case is captioned as State v. John Doe. A civil case is captioned Smith v. Brown. The names may mean very little to the named witness. In most cases, FNE personnel will have had contact with only the victim, whose name is not on the subpoena in a criminal case. The subpoena will give the date and time on which the witness is commanded to appear. The place, including a room number, should be printed on the subpoena. In addition, the document should indicate whether the state, plaintiff, or defense is calling the witness to testify. The expert witness should contact that party to verify specifically which case is going to trial and what is expected.

A subpoena for records requires the production of certain documents, such as medical records. The person to whom this type of subpoena is directed may not necessarily be required to appear, but may only need to produce the documents on a designated date at a particular place. A *subpoena duces tecum* requires the summoned witness to appear on the given date and bring certain specified documents or objects. Again, any witness who receives a subpoena of any variety should contact the summoning party for further information and instruction.

ORIENTATION OF THE COURTROOM

One bit of information that the subpoenaed witness can get by contacting the summoning party is an orientation of the courtroom. Courtroom designs vary, but a prototypic form tends to prevail. The judge's bench is situated in front of the courtroom and elevated, giving the judge a view of the entire space. The witness box is generally to the left or right of the judge's bench, but it may be on a lower level. There are tables for the prosecution and defense. The jury box is located perpendicular to the judge's bench. The party with the burden of proof sits at the table nearest the jury box. In a criminal case, the prosecution sits closest to the jury. In a civil case, the plaintiff sits closest. Generally, on the other side of the bar is spectator seating (criminal defendants are entitled to a public trial).

Additional courtroom personnel sit in front of the judge's bench. The courtroom docket clerk notes procedural steps on the court file and keeps track of tangible evidence. The stenographer often sits close to the witness box to record the testimony verbatim. A sheriff or other law enforcement official typically sits between the judge and the attorney's tables, poised to dissuade outbursts from the displeased or rambunctious and to take custody of prisoners.

In front of the witness box, there is sometimes a podium, which the attorneys may be required to use when examining witnesses and addressing the jury. When the attorneys are confined to the podium, they usually have their trial notes before them as a guide.

The courtroom atmosphere is typically stern and sterile. An expectation exists that all the participants comply with courtroom decorum and demonstrate the utmost respect for the process. A health care practitioner serving as expert witness, although respected for her expertise, receives no preferential treatment in the process of seeking the truth. The judge, prosecution, or defense may vigorously challenge the expert.

QUALIFYING AS AN EXPERT

The advent of the FNE as a specialist has advanced the capacity to collect and preserve evidence to assist with the prosecution of assailants and, in some instances, the exoneration of the falsely accused or the erroneously implicated. While facilitating the psychological, physical, and medical needs of the victim, the FNE has been trained to collect forensic evidence according to correct chain of custody procedure. The quality of evidence collection is tremendously high because the FNE is focused and performs sexual assault examinations regularly. Because of the skill and expertise of the nurse, FNEs have been qualified as expert witnesses in most of the jurisdictions in which they serve.

Through the process called *voir dire* ("speak the truth"), the attorneys ask a series of questions to demonstrate and test a witness's expertise. If the witness is being called by the state, the prosecutor will ask the witness about employment, duties, education, training, professional experience, and the number of works published. In addition, the FNE will be asked how many sexual assault examinations she has done either independently or with the aid of another practitioner. Finally, the prosecutor will elicit whether the witness has ever qualified as an expert in sexual assault forensic examination previously, and if yes, how many times and in which courts.

Defense counsel may, if he or she so chooses, *voir dire* the witness. Very specific questions about sexual assault, studies in the field, definitions of terms, and the use of certain techniques or medications may be asked in the hope that the witness will get stumped on something. Once the questioning by both sides is concluded, the prosecutor then offers the witness as an expert in the field of sexual assault forensic examination. Opposing counsel may object. Depending on the answers given by the witness, the court may or may not declare that the witness is an expert.

The decision to request qualification should not be made when the witness is on the stand. A denial of the state's motion to qualify may undermine the case and will most certainly diminish the witness and the prosecution in the eyes of the jury. Well before the trial date, the witness and the party calling that witness need to discuss whether the witness will actually be treated as an expert, that is, be allowed to render a scientific or medical opinion. At the outset, the attorney should be given a copy of the witness's resume. This alerts the attorney to the appropriate areas that ought to be covered during *voir dire*. The attorney should be made aware of how many times the witness has in fact qualified as an expert and where. If the pending case represents the first time, the attorney will assess whether it is even appropriate to attempt qualification. The decision to offer a witness as an expert is based on the education, training, years of experience in the discipline, amount of experience, and knowledge of the discipline.

TESTIFYING ON DIRECT EXAMINATION

Testifying can be a terrifying experience. Obviously, with time, practice, and experience, the encounter becomes less intimidating. Like any other experience in which the individual has to perform before an audience, preparation is the best antidote for anxiety surrounding an anticipated courtroom appearance.

Because the stakes are high, the practitioner should expect to undergo an interrogation about the medical findings by both the prosecution and defense. Both will want to meet with the clinician before trial to review the evidence and the testimony. This is an important exercise for the witness and the attorney. The practitioner should take the initiative by contacting the attorney who issued the summons (usually the prosecutor). The practitioner, especially one with limited or no experience as a witness, never wants to appear in court unprepared.

For the witness to achieve success, first and foremost, he or she must have a command of the facts. The examiner should have a thorough knowledge of the circumstances of the assault; the history, including physical complaints; and the physical findings, particularly from the genitalia examination. Laboratory results and radiographic studies should be memorized. The expert witness must be thoroughly familiar with her testimony, which means significant time has to be spent before the trial reviewing the medical record and anticipating questions. The expert should study and prepare for the presentation as if preparing for an examination or a formal lecture. The expert witness will greatly impress the jury with a smooth presentation. The witness should sound as though the label "expert" is accurate.

Once mastery has been achieved regarding the facts of the case, the witness must be able to communicate the salient information to the jury in a credible and unbiased manner. The expert witness is reminded that her role is not to take sides but to convey her findings to the jury objectively and allow the jury to make a decision on the basis of the credibility of the evidence delivered. The expert witness may be asked whether the evidence suggests that a physical assault took place. The witness should answer this question within the limits of his or her medical judgment.

It is critically important that the witness tell the truth and not feel obligated to help one side or the other. This means that social biases and prejudgments must be divorced from the oral testimony. The oral communications should reflect a clinical approach devoid of emotion or embellishment. Direct questions should be answered systematically and methodically. The expert must speak loudly and clearly so that all the jurors can hear without straining. The expert should explain answers in simple, easy-to-understand language. The sexual assault practitioner should avoid using slang or profanity. A trial is not the time to entertain the jury with a few well-placed jokes or punch lines. The witness should use a natural voice with an even and smooth delivery and not attempt to dramatize or reach a theatrical, Perry Mason–like climax. It is important to make eye contact with the examining attorney and the judge, as appropriate. The expert witness should appear confident, competent, professional, and courteous to all counsel. The witness must not argue or pontificate with the attorneys.

The expert witness will be asked a series of questions, which will develop a pattern of facts that the prosecution is asserting. The witness must listen to the questions intently and answer as concisely and precisely as possible. The witness should remember his or her answers because on cross-examination, those answers will be revisited and likely challenged. A frequent ploy is for the defense attorney to misstate an answer in an effort to confuse the witness and the jury. Consequently, the witness should listen closely to the question. It may be necessary to reassert a prior response in a self-assured yet nonbelligerent manner. A witness who has misspoken should not be afraid to say so and should correct the error.

The witness's courtroom decorum is equally important because the jury may judge the credibility of the witness by simple observations such as dress, mannerisms, voice quality, and delivery. As a consequence, the witness must engage in conduct that will enhance credibility rather than diminish it. Attire for a courtroom appearance should respect the formality and seriousness of the event.

The following pointers may be helpful. The witness should sit upright and face the person asking the questions. Because the testimony is recorded, the witness should avoid covering his or her mouth. All answers must be verbal. Nods cannot be recorded by a stenographer and may not be discernible on a video. In addition, the witness should not eat or chew gum while on the stand. Nervousness is natural, but the witness should make every effort to appear calm. A few deep breaths should help limit a halting speech pattern. Usually, as the testimony progresses, the witness will begin to relax. The witness needs to control his or her temper no matter how irritating the counsel becomes.

Occasionally, the counsel may ask the expert witness to leave the witness box and either approach the jury or move closer to the audiovisual equipment. The witness might do this when demonstrating how something occurred or while using an item to explain a particular point. For instance, the witness may use an enlarged diagram of the female genitalia to show exactly where the victim's injuries were located. Such demonstrations must be planned in advance by the expert in consultation with the attorney who calls the expert.

CROSS-EXAMINATION

Cross-examination frequently is the true measure of a lawyer's trial skills. After one side has presented a witness to recite evidence to bolster its case, the opposing counsel is given an opportunity to clarify or dismantle the testimony. The goal of the defense in a criminal case is to plant doubt in the minds of the jury concerning the witness, the testimony, or the other evidence presented. The defense counsel wants to damage the expert witness's credibility. Even when the defense counsel readily agrees to the witness's qualification as an expert, counsel may still ask questions designed to attack the witness. In fact, the defense's strategy may be to diminish the witness's efficacy by demonstrating the expert's lack of knowledge. Defense counsel may attack the way the examination was performed or the way the evidence was collected. The defense attorney may also challenge the conclusions drawn from the evidence by eliciting admissions that contradict the principal conclusions made by the expert. The defense tries to discredit the expert or lead the expert to provide an opinion helpful to the defendant.

On cross-examination, the witness must be particularly attentive to the questions asked. The attorney may be pleasant, courteous, nonthreatening, and conciliatory at the outset to lull the witness into a false sense of security. The next series of questions will go to the heart of the matter. Unlike direct examination, cross-examination consists almost exclusively of leading questions, which characteristically contain the answer within the question and can usually be answered with a simple "yes" or "no." For example, "Isn't it true that the injuries sustained by the victim could have been caused by vigorous intercourse?" The intent of such a question is to provide a plausible explanation other than force for the victim's injuries.

To reduce the likelihood of falling prey to tricky questions, the witness must listen very carefully to each component of a question. If an individual part of the question is incongruous or inaccurate, the witness should point that out immediately. This forces the attorney to revise or retract the question. Furthermore, the witness should take care to answer only what is asked. Waxing eloquent with long, scholarly explanations provides the opposition with fodder to dismantle the expert's findings and opinions. Opposing counsel may attempt to short-circuit answers that go beyond "yes" or "no." The court may admonish the cross-examiner to allow the witness to complete the answer. If not, the longer explanation may be elicited by the State on redirect.

Hypothetical questions present various combinations of facts and circumstances similar to or distinctive from the facts of the pending case. The expert is asked to draw a conclusion. "Suppose a woman has been using drugs and drinking alcohol before the incident. Isn't it possible that she would not recall accurately and precisely everything that happened?" Before answering, the witness must make certain that the hypothetical question is factually consistent and contains enough facts for a reasonable conclusion to be drawn.

The witness should take as much time as necessary before answering and have the question repeated if necessary. A thoughtful answer requires some measuring and deliberation. A response given too quickly may be erroneous or unclear. At the same time, a protracted pause before an answer is given raises suspicion in a juror's mind that the expert lacks knowledge or that the answer is fabricated. A witness must always answer questions truthfully. It is appropriate for the witness to admit that he or she does not know the answer, cannot recall a particular fact, needs to have the question repeated, does not understand what is being asked, or needs to consult the records. However, overuse of any answer can irritate the jury and diminish the witness's credibility. The witness, unless an objection is sustained, must answer every question.

Finally, boilerplate jury instructions include the advice from the court that the jury may use a witness's manner of testifying to evaluate his or her credibility. This means that the manner of speaking, words used, demeanor, presence or lack of ease, and even facial expressions of the witness are appropriate factors to determine whether an expert is credible. Another jury instruction advises the jurors to view the expert's testimony as they would the testimony of any other witness. The jurors may believe all, some, or none of the expert's testimony. The expert witness should keep these instructions in mind while testifying.

ACKNOWLEDGMENT

The author acknowledges the contributions of DePriest W. Whye, Jr., MD, JD, to the chapter published in the first edition.

SUGGESTED READINGS

Allison JA, Wrightsman LS. *Rape. The misunderstood crime.* Thousand Oaks, CA: Sage Publications, 1993.

Bailey FL, Rothblatt HB. *Investigation and preparation of criminal cases.* Rochester, New York: The Lawyers Co-operative Publishing Company, 1970.

Ceci SJ, Hembrooke H, eds. *Expert witness in child abuse cases.* Washington, DC: American Psychological Association, 1998.

Ernoehazy W, Murphy-Lavoie H. *Sexual assault.* www.eMedicine .com, November 7, 2005. Available at http://www.emedicine .com/emerg/topic527.htm. Accessed on November 22, 2005.

Hall R. *Rape in America. A reference handbook.* Santa Barbara, CA: ABC CLIO, 1995.

Hohenhaus S. Patterned injury and court testimony in a sexual assault. *J Emerg Nurs* 1998;24:614.

Hohenhaus S. SANE legislation and lessons learned. *J Emerg Nurs* 1998;24:463–464.

Hrones S, Czar C. *Criminal practice handbook,* 2nd ed. New York: Mathew Bender, 1999.

McGregor MJ, Le G, Marion SA, et al. Examination for sexual assault: is the documentation of physician injury associated with the laying of charges? A retrospective cohort study. *Can Med Assoc J* 1999;160:1565–1569.

Paquin GW. Legal aspects of acquaintance rape. In: Wiene VR, Richards AL, eds. *Intimate Betrayal. An understanding and responding to the trauma of acquaintance rape.* Thousand Oaks, CA: Sage Publications, 1995:88–107.

Pentilla A, Karhumen PJ. Medicolegal findings among rape victims. *Med Law* 1990;9:725–737.

Poynter D. *The expert witness handbook. Tips and techniques for the litigation consultant.* Santa Barbara, CA: Para Publishing, 1997.

Reddington FP, Kreisel BW, eds. *Sexual assault: the victims, the perpetrators, and the criminal justice system.* Durham, NC; Carolina Academic Press, 2004.

Reed M. The judicial system and laws. In: Jackson C, ed. *Sexual assault forensic examiner training manual,* Sec. 7, Baltimore, MD: University of Maryland, Department of Surgery, Division of Emergency Medicine, 1998;1–59.

Report of the Grand Jury Concerning the Tawana Brawley Investigation. Court Online Legal Documents. Available at http://www.courttv.com/archive/legaldocs/newsmakers/ tawana/part1.html. Accessed on November 22, 2005.

Selkin J. *The child sexual abuse case in the courtroom,* 2nd ed. Denver, CO: James Selkin, 1991.

Taslitz AE. *Rape and the culture of the courtroom.* New York: New York University Press, 1999.

Temkin J, ed. *Rape and the criminal justice system.* Brookfield, WI: Dartmouth Publishing Company, 1995.

Warner CG, ed. *Rape and sexual assault: management and intervention.* Germantown, MD: Aspen Publishers, 1980.

West Virginia sexual assault legal guide. 'Lectric Law Library. Available at http://www.lectlaw.com/files/sex11.htm. Accessed on November 22, 2005.

17

■ WILLIAM S. SMOCK
■ PATRICK E. BESANT-MATTHEWS

A good photograph . . . is one which conveys to the observer something which he has not seen, known, or thought of before.

—*Andreas Feininger, photojournalist, 1906–1999*

To the list of individuals who take pictures—professionals who do so for a living and amateurs who do so for fun—must be added occupational, semiprofessional, and functional photographers.

Emergency physicians and nurses fall into this last category. The health professional in an emergency department (ED) may use photography as often as once a week or daily but may have never had the benefit or luxury of any formal photographic instruction. The purpose of this chapter is to inform and educate the emergency physician and nurse on the principles and practices of forensic photography in the ED.

WHY USE PHOTOGRAPHY IN THE EMERGENCY DEPARTMENT?

We use photography in the ED because a well-composed picture is worth *at least* a thousand words. In the ED, photography is generally used for one of two reasons: forensic or educational. The term *forensic photography* implies that the photograph, when properly obtained, may be used in legal proceedings (1). Traditionally, the use of forensic medical photography has been limited to crime scene locations and autopsy suites.

Now, and with ever-greater frequency, forensic medical photography is finding its way into EDs in the United States. Cameras, both digital and film, are being used to document wounds on individuals who survive their injuries. This change is being brought about primarily by the development of new fields of expertise, such as sexual assault nurse examiner (SANE) programs, child abuse and domestic violence units, and clinical forensic medicine programs, and as part of residency and nurse training.

The reasons for employing a camera to aid in addressing the forensic needs of living patients in the ED are numerous and include the following:

1. To record and document injuries and evidence that cannot be preserved indefinitely or left untouched, given the treatment that is medically indicated.
2. To act as a future reference or aid to memory.
3. To document lesser features and details of a situation that would not otherwise be practical or important for the purpose of medical treatment.
4. To permit the court and jurors to see things as they were and, in effect, check the testimony being presented to see if it makes sense in context.
5. To document injuries or conditions, and to record what they looked like before and after medical treatment.
6. To demonstrate malice or criminal intent.
7. To show the condition of evidence or injuries at the time of discovery or examination.
8. To demonstrate the absence of injury or alleged findings.

9. To illustrate and supplement the written medical record.
10. To teach nurses, medical students, and residents.

From the standpoint of photography's educational merits, the rationale is self-evident. The ability of the emergency physician or nurse to photographically document a patient's injury, wound, lesion, or rash or to obtain a radiograph will ensure that the patient's information can be shared with other health care professionals for educational purposes.

CONSENT FOR FORENSIC PHOTOGRAPHY

After death, the patient capitulates the right of refusal and the investigating agency makes decisions and follows an accepted course of practice; however, living persons and patients must give consent for photography, unless they are unconscious, under arrest, and/or there is a court order for pictures to be taken, or unless they are photographed from a public place, such as a street or sidewalk. The physician or nurse is obligated by law to obtain consent, either implied or informed, from the living patient before photographs are taken for educational or forensic purposes. Informed consent involves explaining to the patient the purpose of taking the forensic or educational photograph. An awake and alert patient may refuse to be photographed, just as a patient may refuse to undergo a medical procedure or test. The health care provider must explain the reason for the photograph and the associated risks and benefits, if any. When approached in a respectful and polite manner, most patients permit the photographic documentation of their injuries or wounds, especially when it can be of benefit to their criminal case. Likewise, most patients agree to have their lesions, injuries, or rashes photographed for educational purposes when it is explained that future students will benefit from their generosity. The consent form (Fig. 17.1) must become part of the patient's permanent medical record.

Implied consent is a legal construct used to secure consent from an individual who is unconscious or so seriously injured as to be incapable of comprehending the consent request or responding to it. Consent in this context is construed as a course of action that a reasonably prudent person would adopt. A reasonably prudent person would allow the photographic documentation of injuries when the photographs will aid in the subsequent evaluation and treatment.

The photographic documentation of injuries may be vital to the conviction of those individuals who perpetrated a crime or inflicted a wound. Conversely, such documentation may help ensure that suspects are not wrongfully charged (2). For example, when an unconscious victim of an assault presents with a soot-covered gunshot wound (Fig. 17.2), the physician may obtain photographs on the basis of the assumption that a reasonably prudent person would permit photographic documentation of injuries or evidence that would be destroyed or altered in the course of medical treatment (Fig. 17.3). When implied consent has been used, the physician must obtain consent from either the patient or the next of kin at some later time.

Hospitals may include consent-for-photography language on operative consent or admission forms (Fig. 17.4), such as, "I consent to photographing of the operation/procedure, including portions of the body for medical, scientific, or educational purposes, provided my identity will not be revealed by the pictures or the descriptive text accompanying them" (3). If photography language is not included in the routine surgical consent form, then a separate form with wording similar to the above is required. Wording may vary slightly from state to state (such as in Louisiana, where slightly different laws exist because of the French influence many years ago). The text of the consent form must be reviewed and approved by hospital administration.

The following is an example of a draft for a separate consent to medical photography form:

In connection with the medical services that (name of patient, child, or ward) is to receive at (name of hospital), I hereby consent that photographs, videotapes, motion pictures, or illustrations may be made of him/her by members of the staff or other personnel working with or for the hospital, or any hospital staff member, for the following uses and subject to the following conditions: (a) photographs, or excerpts therefrom, may form part of the medical record or be used for illustrative purposes in lectures and medical publications, being shown, published, and republished in any manner that the hospital and medical staff shall deem proper; (b) best efforts will be made to prevent or limit personal identification and recognition. I expect no compensation or other remuneration. This consent as to any use of the said photographs, videotapes, motion pictures, or illustrations shall act to expressly release from liability the photographer, videographer, or illustrator, the attending physicians, the hospital and affiliated corporations, the authors, editors, and publishers, if any, and their officers and members.

The form should include the name of the physician or nurse and be signed and dated by the patient. If the patient is unable to sign, an authorized representative of the patient or the next of kin should sign the consent form.

University of Louisville Hospital

Medical Record No.

Name

PHOTOGRAPH/INTERVIEW CONSENT

Unit/Bed

Date	Unit	Name of Patient

I, _____ ; authorize the party named

below to photograph, video tape and/or interview _____

while a patient at University of Louisville Hospital. I release University of Louisville Hospital from any and all liability

which may arise from the use of these photographs, tapes or interviews. I waive all rights I may have for any claims

for payment in connection with any exhibition, televising or publication of said photographs.

X	TYPE OF CONSENT	YES	NO
	1. Interview		
	2. Photograph		
	3. Video Taping		

Please indicate location where photographs/tapes will be stored (cannot be stored in Medical Records)

X	PURPOSE OF CONSENT	YES	NO
	1. Public Relations Purposes (newspapers, radio, television)		
	2. Legal Purposes		
	3. Educational Purposes		
	4. Personal Reasons		

Name of Person Conducting Photo/Taping/Interview Session	Title of Person		
Name of Organization Being Represented			
Address of Organization	City	State	Zip Code	Telephone No. ( )
Signature of Patient/Legal Guardian	Date	Relationship to Patient	
Witness	Title		Date

ULH/600-113(10/96)

FIG. 17.1 Sample consent-for-photography form from the University of Louisville Hospital. The consent form becomes a permanent part of the patient's medical record. The photographer should also maintain a copy for his/her records.

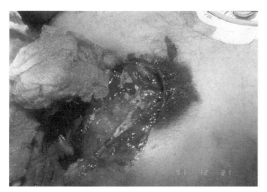

FIG. 17.2 The soot on this close-range shotgun wound is short-lived. It will be removed when the wound is scrubbed in preparation for debridement and closure (see color plate).

ADMISSIBILITY AND SUBSTANTIVE EVIDENCE

To be accepted as evidence in a court of law, a photograph, either digital or on film, must be an accurate and objective depiction of its subject (4–9). The photographer and the photograph must be able to withstand legal challenges as to authenticity, integrity, and credibility, or the judge has an obligation to disregard it as demonstrable evidence (4–9).

A photograph is usually not substantive evidence. This means that a photograph cannot be submitted in court as evidence and stand alone without an

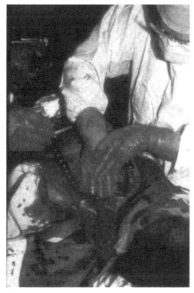

FIG. 17.3 Opening the chest wall alters a wound's size and characteristics. If possible, wounds and fragile evidence should be documented before surgical intervention.

advocate for it. Someone is going to have to verify it and attest to it and say that they either took it or saw it taken. The court will expect to hear from the advocate presenting the photograph that it is indeed a fair and accurate representation of the situation at the time it was taken.

A photograph will probably be admitted as evidence by a judge if:

1. It shows the original appearance or findings and "fairly and accurately depicts" what the health professional saw.
2. It assists in the identification or characterization of the wound or injuries.
3. It is not unduly gruesome or inflammatory.
4. It is of sufficient value to warrant its inclusion.
5. It will aid the court or jury in obtaining an intelligent or dispassionate evaluation or conclusion.
6. It is well composed, and most of the picture area is filled with the wound or injury in question.
7. The feature or wound is clearly visible.
8. It is nicely exposed and about the right color.
9. It is in focus.
10. It has a small ruler in the plane of the wound, to show the wound size (in inches and/or centimeters) (Fig. 17.5).
11. The image corresponds closely to the verbal description given by the emergency physician or nurse.
12. It does not contain extraneous matter such as surgical instruments or bloody dressings (Fig. 17.6).

The nurse or physician must also be ready for legal challenges regarding the admissibility of the photographs. The questions and challenges may include the following:

1. Exactly where and when the photograph was taken.
2. Exactly what the photo depicted (use lay terms for the benefit of the court, attorneys, and jurors).
3. The exact anatomic location (supplement with lay terms).
4. The type of camera and film used.
5. If filters were used on the lens.
6. Whether the photograph was obtained by informed or implied consent.
7. Where the film was developed and if it represented the hospital's standard protocol.

The use of digital cameras in the ED for forensic purposes has been accepted by US courts (7). Digital images present another set of potential special challenges for their admission into evidence and will be discussed in detail in the section on digital photography in this chapter.

Consent:

The above has been explained to me by Dr. _____. I have had a chance to ask questions and I have the information I need to make a decision about this procedure. I consent to this procedure. I agree to let the hospital use or dispose of tissue removed from me. I consent to photographing of the operation/ procedure including portions of the body for medical, scientific, or educational purposes provided that my identity will not be revealed by the pictures or descriptive text accompanying them. **I have answered the doctor's questions about my health truthfully.**

I would like a copy of this consent form.   ☐ YES   ☐ NO

_____   _____   _____
        Patient's Signature   Date   Time

Witness and/or Interpreter:

_____   _____   _____ _____
    Witness to Patient's Signature   Interpreter   Date   Time

0919001 (11/99)   (OVER)

FIG. 17.4 Operative consent form, which includes language about intraoperative photography for educational purposes.

A photograph with potentially inflammatory content will be challenged. If a photograph is so gruesome and "inflammatory" (4) that it may cause "undue prejudice" (5) toward the accused on the part of the jury, the judge may exclude it from evidence.

Suppose that an elderly woman seen in the ED suffered a severe vaginal laceration from a sexual assault and the accused assailant is on trial. The emergency physician who examined the patient is testifying about the victim's injuries. The physician describes lacerations (a blunt force, torn, crushing injury) of the vaginal wall, consistent with forced vaginal penetration. The district attorney or commonwealth attorney, who called the treating physician as a witness, produces a photograph (Fig. 17.7) and asks, "Doctor, do you recognize this photograph?" The physician replies, "Yes, it was taken in the ED. The photograph depicts the victim's vaginal laceration." After asking several more questions of a legal nature, the lawyer shows the photograph to the defense attorney, offers the photograph in evidence, and hands it to the judge. The defense attorney rises and says that he objects to the

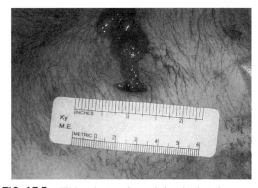

FIG. 17.5 This photo of an abdominal stab wound from a single-edged blade is nicely composed, with the ruler parallel to the wound. The scale is in the plane of the wound and accurately depicts the size of the wound.

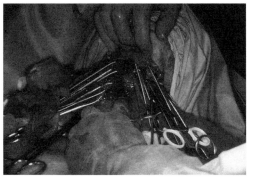

FIG. 17.6 The presence of extraneous surgical instruments and bloody dressings detracts from the significance of this photograph.

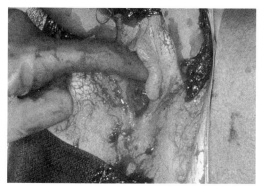

FIG. 17.7 A large vaginal laceration resulting from sexual assault. The presence of blood and the graphic nature of the injury resulted in the judge ruling the photograph inflammatory and not admissible (see color plate).

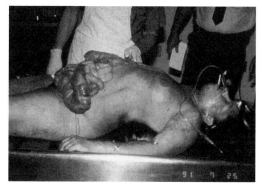

FIG. 17.8 Photographs taken from a distance are important for an overview or general shot but may not be admissible in court on the grounds that they are not specific, detract from the significance of the injury, or include unnecessary information.

introduction of the photograph. His principle concern is that its introduction will be prejudicial to his client. The judge, whose role it is to see that the trial is conducted according to the accepted rules of law, proceeds to examine the photograph and its suitability for use as evidence. The judge sustains the objection and the photo is not admitted on the grounds that the severity of the laceration and the presence of blood would be inflammatory and prejudicial.

In general, a judge probably will *not* admit a photograph if any of the following conditions apply:

1. The composition is absurd because the photograph was taken at such a distance from the wound that the wound occupies only a fraction of the image. The remainder of the image area is taken up with parts of the resuscitation or autopsy table, on which are a number of potentially offensive and objectionable items, such as bloody sponges, dressings, pools of partly dried blood, scissors, or clumps of hair (Fig. 17.8).
2. The wound is out of focus and hard to see.
3. The picture is overexposed and "washed out." There is a reflection of the on-camera flash in the middle of the wound. The color is not right. There is a distracting greenish reflection of the overhead fluorescent lights in the metal surface of the resuscitation table.
4. Poor "scale" technique is used:
   a. Only a section of a plastic ruler is used, cut so that numbers begin at 2 on the inch side and 5 on the centimeter side.
   b. An equipment maker's name is seen on the scale.
   c. The scale is covering part of the wound.
   d. The scale is not in the plane of the wound but at an angle to it, meaning that because part of the wound is nearer the camera than the scale,

any measurement derived from it will be in error by several percentage points.
5. The physician has just described the wound as being vertical, and clearly it was vertical with respect to the standard anatomic position, but the wound appears horizontal in the photograph.
6. The photograph was not taken at 90 degrees to the wound, causing perspective distortion (Fig. 17.9).

A recent Kentucky ruling determined that "there was no reason to exclude photographic evidence by claiming the photographs were unduly gruesome when the crime itself was brutal and gruesome. The Commonwealth cannot be prevented from proving the commission of a crime that is by its nature heinous and repulsive. Gruesomeness of the photographs alone cannot be the basis for the exclusion of such evidence" (4).

BASIC FORENSIC PHOTOGRAPHY

The physical care of the patient is always paramount. As important as they are, photographic documentation and evidence collection are secondary concerns. In practice, it is possible to perform forensic photographic evidence collection without compromising patient care (2).

Emergency physicians and nurses who intend to take forensic photographs should have some basic working knowledge of photographic theory. Even if providers are utilizing a "point-and-shoot" camera, they need some background information to understand what goes into making an acceptable forensic photograph. For the purposes of discussion, the author assumes that the reader will be using a 35-mm single-lens reflex (SLR) camera with film or an SLR digital camera. The *35-mm* camera is so named because the film it uses is 35 mm wide.

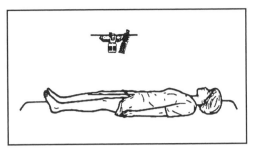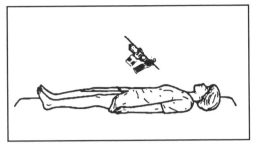

FIG. 17.9   The emergency department photographer should maintain the lens at 90 degrees to the subject. Angles less than 90 degrees introduce perspective distortion, which renders the scale inaccurate. (Reprinted from Smock WS. Forensic photography. In: Stack L, Storrow A, Patton D, eds. *Physician's handbook of clinical photography.* Philadelphia, PA: Hanley & Belfus, 2000, with permission.)

Lens Characteristics

The lens is a clear window of glass, or high-tech plastic, made and positioned so as to gather and focus light onto the light-sensitive film or an electronic sensor inside the camera when the shutter is opened. The lens controls the magnification of the object photographed and other characteristics (sharpness, contrast, color, etc.) of the image. In conjunction with the shutter, it also controls the amount of light that reaches the film or light–sensitive device.

The focal length of a lens is the distance from a point called the optical center to the point behind the lens at which rays of light from a distant subject are brought to a focus. If a lens brings rays of light from a distant object to a focus in a distance of 50 mm (just under 2 in.), then this is the focal length of the lens. In effect, it is the magnifying power of the lens.

If one takes the 50-mm lens off the camera and replaces it with another that has a focal length of 100 mm (just under 4 in.), then the subject will appear twice as large in the viewfinder and on the film. It is as though we put a telescope on the camera and made everything look nearer. We see less of the subject in the viewfinder but what we do see appears twice the size. Ignoring various technicalities of optics, people frequently refer to such a lens as a telephoto.

Now suppose we replace the 50-mm lens with another that has a focal length of 24 mm (just under 1 in.) and look through the viewfinder again. We will see a much wider field, with more things in the field of view, but each object appears about half the size. We are now using what is called a wide-angle lens.

So you can either stand at a distance of 4 ft and photograph the whole upper part of a patient on a stretcher with your 50-mm lens, or you can put on your 105-mm lens and, from the same working distance, concentrate on the head of an injured person, which is now about twice as big in the viewfinder as it was before.

The value of a "longer" lens (longer or greater focal length) is that it gives you more distance to work with. In surgery or in the ED, a 200-mm lens (instead of a regular 50-mm) will enable you to:

1. Stand four times as far away from the patient and get the same size image,
2. Stand at the same distance but get an image four times larger, or
3. Stand twice as far away and get twice as large an image, simultaneously.

In general, there is a direct relation between focal length and working distance. If you double the focal length, the camera-to-subject distance doubles for the same image size. If your work entails extensive close-up photography, you should buy a lens that is specially designed for that purpose. These "macro lenses" are designed to give:

1. Excellent sharpness in the close-up range, including sharpness from edge to edge of the image, not only at the center.
2. Flat undistorted fields, meaning no curved lines when copying graph paper, diagrams, and printed matter.
3. Excellent contrast.
4. The ability to focus down to half life size, or even life size, without any additional attachments.

In fact, the best macro lenses are so good that they will resolve more detail than those that many ordinary films can record (Fig. 17.10). They are also very good for general subject matter. As you might expect, they tend to be more expensive because they are sold in smaller numbers, but for EDs where a significant amount of close-up work will be done, they are well worth the cost.

Macro lenses are available in three focal length ranges:

1. 50 to 60 mm, excellent for copying flat materials.
2. 100 to 105 mm, a very popular range (there are a few at 90 mm) with twice the working distance.

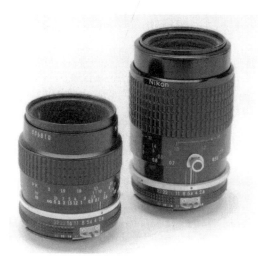

FIG. 17.10 Micro-Nikkor 55-mm, f/2.8, and Micro-Nikkor 105-mm lenses permit the emergency department photographer to take close-up photographs with good depth of field.

These are great for general patient, injury, and autopsy photography. If in doubt, this is the type you should buy first, unless a very large part of your work involves copying flat objects or similar tasks.
3. 180 to 200 mm. These lenses are a bit more specialized. They are understandably popular with nature and wildlife photographers who want to leave subjects, such as insects, undisturbed or need to keep their distance from dangerous animals. They are also excellent for operating room photography and for patient photography (e.g., when one does not want to get too close to a nervous child or to a recent victim of sexual assault).

In general, a macro lens with a longer focal length—say 100 mm—will enable you to obtain the same image from twice as far away as a 50-mm lens or twice the image size from the same distance. In biomedical and forensic work, their increased working distance is invaluable under the following circumstances:

1. In the operating room over the surgeon's shoulder.
2. During the sexual assault examination for close-up documentation of vaginal or rectal injuries.
3. In the ED when an incoherent patient in restraints is trying to hit you.
4. At a crime scene, enabling you to "reach" the hair and blood on the windshield of the vehicle while resting your arms on the back of the front seat.
5. In an outdoor setting, facilitating the recording of evidence on the ground with a minimum of kneeling and bending over.

A zoom lens offers continuously variable magnification (focal length). Zoom lenses have a collar or ring that can be turned, or slid lengthways, thereby moving the lens elements to give the image the magnification you desire.

Aperture

Now that the meaning of focal length is understood, lens aperture becomes quite easy because the f/- numbers are derived from the effective aperture and the focal length of a lens. In theory, if a lens has an opening of 2 in. and it brings parallel rays to a focus at a distance of 4 in., then its aperture is $\frac{2}{4}$ or, as photographers say, f/2. Likewise, if a lens has a 1-in. opening and brings light to a focus at a distance of 4 in., it has an aperture of $\frac{1}{4}$ or f/4. This is the reason the size of the hole admitting light and the amount of light that gets through a given lens go down as the f/- number goes up, and vice versa.

What the ED photographer should know is simply that every time you move from one full f/- number to another, the amount of light entering the camera is halved or doubled, depending on the direction you are going.

Shutter Speeds

The fact that lens apertures move in steps of two is equally important because when you look at your camera you will see that the shutter speeds also go up and down in steps of two. Examine your shutter speed control. It reads something like 2, 4, 8, 15, 30, 60, 125, and so on, which is an abbreviation for $\frac{1}{2}$, $\frac{1}{4}$, $\frac{1}{8}$, $\frac{1}{15}$, $\frac{1}{30}$, $\frac{1}{60}$, $\frac{1}{125}$, and so on, of a second.

Exposure

Now we are in a position to control the amount of light reaching the film or the electronic sensor of a digital camera, by adjusting either the size of the aperture or the time the shutter is open. In particular, we have the option of trading lens aperture against shutter speed. For instance, if we double the amount of light coming through the lens and cut the shutter time in half, we will end up with the same amount of light reaching the film.

This is one of the most basic and useful concepts in photography. Suppose there is enough light to get a proper exposure with a shutter speed of $\frac{1}{125}$ second and a lens opening of f/8. By simply doubling the aperture (f/8 to f/16) and halving the shutter speed ($\frac{1}{125}$ to $\frac{1}{60}$), we can still obtain the correct exposure.

For all practical purposes, any of the above combinations will admit the same amount of light, so we can now choose whatever pair we desire. This gives us flexibility and control.

If we wish to "catch" or "stop" a moving object such as a high jumper, it would be desirable to use a short shutter opening of $\frac{1}{1,000}$ second or less with a big lens opening, whereas if we wanted to create a blurred, artistic image of water coming over a waterfall, we might choose $\frac{1}{2}$ second or longer with a small lens opening.

Now you see why understanding that lens aperture and the shutter speeds progress in steps of two is so valuable. Simply stated, we use whatever combination of aperture and shutter time we need to obtain the photograph we want.

Shutter Priority

Shutter priority means that you select the shutter speed for the job at hand, and the camera will calculate the right lens aperture at the moment you make the exposure.

■ Use this mode when you have to control action, for instance, to freeze moving cars on a freeway with a short shutter time or to blur the water of a waterfall by the use of a longer opening.
■ Be alert to the possibility that if the shutter is open for only a short period and the lens opens, the depth of field may be too shallow.

Aperture Priority

Aperture priority means that you select the lens opening to give you the depth of field you require, and the camera will determine the proper shutter time when you make the exposure.

■ Use this when it is important to use a small aperture for greater depth of field or a large aperture to throw a background out of focus, and thereby emphasize a nearer subject.
■ Be alert to the possibility that a long shutter opening may blur anything that moves during the exposure.

Program

Some cameras allow the user to select a "program" setting. This means that the camera has been pre-programmed by the manufacturer to choose between shutter speeds and apertures, depending on the distance of the subject and the amount of light available when the camera is used. For instance, the manufacturer is likely to have programmed the camera to avoid very long shutter openings, during which the hands of the user might shake and thereby smear the image. All will be well with the "program" setting if, and only if, the subjects being photographed match the built-in instructions reasonably well.

Depth of Field

Depth of field is determined by the size of the aperture set on the lens (the f/- number). The depth of field indicates the nearest and farthest distances between which things will appear acceptably sharp or in focus.

If the close-up lens is wide open at f/4.0 and you focus on a subject 5 ft away, the lens will yield a sharp focus from approximately 4 ft, 11 in. to 5 ft, 1 in. If you change the aperture to f/22 and again focus on a subject at 5 ft, the lens will yield a sharp image from approximately 5 ft, $7\frac{1}{2}$ in. to 5 ft, 5 in. That is to say, as the aperture becomes smaller, the lens provides a greater depth of sharpness, called *depth of field*, in front of and behind the point at which the lens is theoretically in perfect focus. This has great practical value. We can use a wide aperture to capture an image separate from its surroundings or a small aperture to get the surroundings sharp on the near and far side of the focal image.

Although it may seem at first glance that we should always keep the lens closed down to get the greatest depth, this is not necessarily true. At small apertures, there may be loss of sharpness due to a physical effect called *diffraction*. Also, at small apertures, one has to compensate for lack of light with a faster (more sensitive) film or longer exposures (risking the blur caused by camera motion). At very wide apertures, optical shortcomings (lens aberrations) may reduce sharpness.

In summary, the following should be remembered regarding lenses:

1. The focal length of a lens is in essence its magnifying power. The smaller/shorter the focal length, the wider the angle the lens will "see." Conversely, the larger/longer the focal length, the nearer and bigger objects will appear.
2. Moving from one full f/- stop to another will double or halve the amount of light that reaches the film, depending on the direction you are going in.
3. As the f/- number increases, the amount of light that can reach the film decreases and vice versa.
4. Smaller apertures (larger f/- numbers) yield greater depths of acceptable sharpness than larger apertures (smaller f/- numbers).

Lighting

Lighting is the key to photography. Anyone can take a reasonable photograph if the lighting is good, but not when it is bad. You must devote some thought to light and to how it behaves. A general principle is to mimic or add to existing light or to create your own lighting according to your preference and the kind of subject.

Photographic lighting is the practical and artistic application of scientific principles:

■ There must be enough light to expose the film or the charge-coupled device (CCD)/complementary metal-oxide semiconductor (CMOS).
■ The color of the light should be right for the film or American Standards Association (ASA) rating (see in the subsequent text) selected for the CCD/CMOS.
■ Contrast (range of brightness between the darkest shadows and the brightest highlights) should be within the capability of the film.

Roughly speaking, the brightness range that can be handled is approximately 1,000:1 for the eye, approximately 100:1 for the film, approximately 30:1 for new video systems, and approximately 20:1 for old video systems. Translated, this means that the film can, at best, handle a brightness range of approximately $6\frac{1}{2}$ f-stops. Normally a ratio of 3:1, 4:1, or 5:1 is the best.

In the ED and in a forensic setting, we too must be concerned about lighting. Flash is convenient, but we must control it, get the exposure right, eliminate unwanted shadows, and draw attention to the subject.

When living persons are your subject matter and the flash is too close to the lens, you may see the phenomenon called *red eye*. Simply stated, light travels into the eye of a person, picks up the color of blood at the retina, and is reflected back to the camera lens. It is prevented by making the pupil of the eye close down and/or moving the light source away from the line along which the lens of the camera sees. Many of the newer cameras have a red-eye reduction mode. This provides up to 15 flashing bursts to reduce the diameter of the pupil.

What about the little flash units that are built into many of the midrange SLR cameras? They do not have enormous power (guide numbers of 40–55 are common), but they are pretty good. They are mainly intended for taking photographs of people at a distance of 10 to 12 ft. They are useful for patient photography, photography of small crime scenes, and recording of the interiors of vehicles. They will certainly get you off to a good start. They are often capable of filling shadows outdoors in bright light, but you will eventually need a larger, more powerful, add-on flash for larger, remote, or difficult subjects.

To obtain the best results with flash photography, you must move the flash away from the camera lens and position it above the lens axis, on a bracket attached to the base of the camera or on a separate stand nearby. The pocket-size "point-and-shoot" cameras, with a flash built in next to the lens, will be perfectly satisfactory for amateur and pleasure purposes and for getting started in biomedical or crime scene photography, but as you advance they cannot give you optimal lighting for scientific work. As you progress you will want to add a separate flash unit and buy a cord to go between it and the camera to give you the option of moving the light farther away and/or choosing its position with respect to the lens so as to pick up texture.

Another basic concept of lighting is the size of the light source in relation to the subject. If we place a small bright light in a suitable place and try to photograph a patient, we will get shadows with very well-defined or sharp edges. Photographers call this "hard" lighting. From this we should learn that on-camera flash is only a convenience—it does not necessarily provide the best lighting.

Therefore, as your skill increases, you will need a special cord to go between your camera and the flash unit to enable you to put the light source where you want it while retaining all the helpful features, such as automatic exposure. In the authors' opinion, an off-camera cord, such as the Nikon SC-17 (Fig. 17.11) or the Canon Off-Camera Shoe Cord 2, is one of the few "must have" accessories.

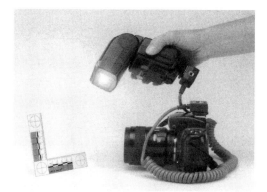
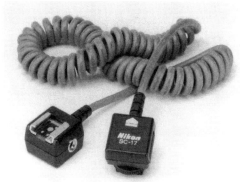

FIG. 17.11   A flash extension cord permits the emergency department photographer to divert the flash out toward the subject.

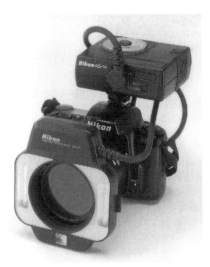

FIG. 17.12   A lens-mounted ring flash (Nikkor SB-21) permits good close-up lighting from 1 to 18 in. The flash tubes on either side of the lens may be fired independently to give the subject more definition. If the flash tubes are fixed simultaneously, they will produce a flatter appearance.

Several manufacturers produce useful and imaginative light sources called *ring lights or ring flashes* (Fig. 17.12). They are small flash tubes formed into a circle to fit around the camera lens so as to produce light on all sides of the subject and thereby give shadow-free illumination. They are ideal for close-up (within 18 in.) detail shots, such as gunshot wounds in the mouth, bite marks, teeth, and vaginal injuries and for the rapid recording of small items, such as bullets and trace evidence (Fig. 17.13), but they are not a cure-all for biological subjects. The problem is not with the lights but rather with the subject being photographed. Much medical and biologic subject material is wet or shiny. Ring flashes result in glare under these conditions, often in the middle of the most important thing in the photograph. Ring

flashes should be regarded as a tool and are therefore helpful in some, but not all, situations.

Some of the best ring lights have two separate flash tubes, one on either side of the lens, which can be operated together or independently for better results. You can achieve much the same by covering parts of a ring light with opaque adhesive tape or a card, provided you allow for the loss of light.

Background

What background is desirable for photography of an injured person? Will the background detract from the subject of the photo (e.g., a crowded resuscitation room with ten medical providers surrounding the patient)? What color of paper or paint or curtains will you place behind the injured warm-skinned persons you are photographing?

The ED photographer must take steps to limit the amount of extraneous material or information contained in the photograph. The presence of bloody clothes, dressings, or medical instruments will distract the viewer and may be deemed inflammatory by a judge rendering an opinion as to a photo's admissibility to evidence. The placement of surgical drapes or towels behind the subject or over the dressings is the easiest way to mask the distractions if it is not possible to physically remove the objects (Fig. 17.14).

EQUIPMENT FOR FORENSIC PHOTOGRAPHY IN THE EMERGENCY DEPARTMENT

Any photograph is better than no photograph, so the ED photographer may be tempted to purchase a "point-and-shoot" camera; however, the 35-mm SLR and, increasingly, the digital SLR are considered the standard for forensic ED photography. The SLR has multiple advantages over the point-and-shoot models:

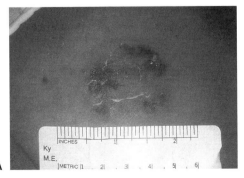
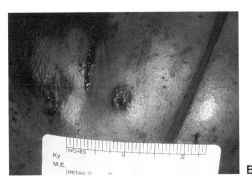

FIG. 17.13   Good use of ring-flash lighting on injuries. **A:** Healing bite mark on breast. **B:** Gunshot entrance wound with the associated abrasion collar (see color plate).

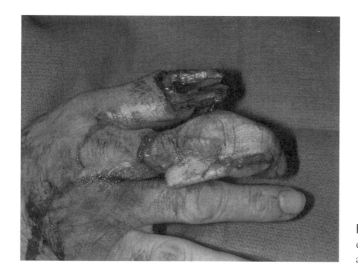

FIG. 17.14 The placement of surgical drapes clarifies the subject of the photograph and covers extraneous details.

- Through-the-lens (TTL) viewing permits the photographer to see exactly what the film sees.
- Interchangeable lens, 55 to 105 mm, macro.
- Ability to control shutter speed and aperture settings.
- Ability to have off-camera flash.
- Ability to select the "film" ASA rating with a digital camera.

Camera Body

The camera body, using a film or digital format, is the "brains" of the photographer. A number of camera manufacturers produce adequate photographic equipment for work in the ED (Table 17-1). In particular, Nikon and Canon have excellent selections of equipment dedicated to medical photography. Expect to spend at least $300 for the body of an SLR film camera and $700 to $1,000 for a digital camera body with a minimum of 6.0 megapixels.

Lens

The photographer must have a lens capable of rendering clean images with fine details at close range, as well as sharp images of larger subjects at varying distances. The macro lens, also called micro lens, provides these features because it can produce a wide range of reproduction ratios (1:1 to infinity.)

Very little about the human body is flat. When imaging wounds on a rounded surface, the photographer will need a lens with very small aperture capabilities (f/22–f/45) to increase the depth of field. When using smaller aperture settings (larger f-number), depth of field is increased, giving an expanded breadth of focus. This is essential for images on curved surfaces such as bite marks on the hand or wrist (Fig. 17.13A). The most popular

lenses for medical and forensic photography are manufactured by Nikon and include the Micro-Nikkor 55 mm, f/2.8; the Micro-Nikkor 60 mm, f/2.8; the Micro-Nikkor 105 mm, f/2.8 (Fig. 17.10); and the Medical-Nikkor 120 mm, f/4. Other camera manufacturers produce macro lenses with similar features. The 105-mm and 120-mm lenses have an

TABLE 17-1

SUGGESTED EQUIPMENT LIST FOR THE EMERGENCY DEPARTMENT

Nikon SLR film camera body: F100, N55, N65, N70, N75, N80, N100

Nikon SLR digital camera body: D50, D70s, D100

Canon SLR film camera body: EOS Rebel K2, EOS Rebel T2, EOS ELAN 7N/7NE

Canon SLR digital camera body: EOS-1D, EOS-350D, EOS-20D, EOS-300D

Nikkor-Micro 55 mm f/2.8, AF-Micro 60 mm f/2.8D

Canon EF-S 60 mm f/2.8 Macro

Nikkor-Micro 105 mm f/2.8, AF-Micro 105 mm f/2.8D

Canon EF 100 mm f/2.8 Macro

Nikon Ring Flash: SB-29s Macro Speedlight

Canon Macro Ring Lite MR-14EX, Canon Macro Twin Lite MT-24EX

Nikon Flash: SB-600 AF, SB-800 AF, SB-27 AF, SB-50 DXAF

Canon Flash: 580 EX, 430 EX, 220 EX

Nikon Databack (varies with camera model)

Nikon flash extension cord SC-17

Nonglare, rigid scale (without advertisement)

Background towel or drape

Adhesive scale for wound/subject size determination and on which the patient's name and record number can be clearly written increased focal length compared with the 55-mm lens and enable the photographer to double the film-to-subject distance and obtain the same image. This increased focal length may be advantageous when attempting to take photographs over the back of the treating medical staff during a resuscitation or in the operating room.

Camera Bag

In a busy ED, a camera bag is essential to protect your equipment. The bag should be large enough to leave some space for other items, such as lens shades, flash, batteries, an off-camera cord, a note pad, and spare film.

In general, the older looking and less attractive your bag, the less likely your equipment is to be stolen. Some photographers carry expensive equipment in diaper bags! A lockable drawer or cabinet in the ED is ideal.

Electronic Flash

An electronic flash is a must for any medical or forensic photographer. The photographer will be able to capture essential details if the flash has enough power to illuminate subjects when using f-stops in the 22 to 32 range. Preferably, the flash should be a dedicated electronic flash with TTL metering. TTL metering permits the camera to communicate with the flash to modify flash intensity, given a selected shutter speed or aperture.

The well-designed camera and flash combination positions the flash several inches above the lens. This causes shadows to fall below and behind the average subject and eliminates hard shadows on the right and left.

Ideally, the flash should be attached to the camera by a bracket that allows the light to come from 8 to 10 in. above the lens and slightly off to the side. Unfortunately, this makes the camera somewhat bulky and not well suited for hospital situations. The built-in and top-mounted flash units are suited to effectively illuminate subjects 24 in. to 15 ft from the photographer. These flash options are inadequate, as most forensic photography is performed at a distance of less than 24 in.

The forensic photographer must have the ability to photograph at distances ranging from several inches to infinity. The light generated by a built-in or a top-mounted flash will not adequately illuminate a subject at distances less than 24 in., because of the angle of the flash (Fig. 17.15). A lens-mounted ring-flash unit (Fig. 17.12) or a flash with a cord extension (Fig. 17.11) directs the flash on the subject and corrects for this close-up deficiency of top-mounted flashes.

A ring flash and the combination ring/point flash units mount directly on the end of the lens. These flash units properly illuminate a subject within inches of the lens. Most lens-mounted flash units work well in the range of 1 to 18 in. from the subject. A ring flash creates its own set of challenges. It generates a round reflection on shiny surfaces and produces a flat image without shadows on areas with depth.

A point light source attached to the camera by a synchronization cord allows the flash to be handheld at an angle to the subject (Fig. 17.11B). This casts shadows, giving the image depth. The point source has a smaller reflection than a ring flash and imposes less distraction from the image.

Databack

A databack (Fig. 17.16) is an electronic device that replaces the standard camera back and enables the photographer to imprint the date, time, or frame number onto the slide or negative. This imprint assists the photographer and the court to determine the date, time, and order in which the photographs were taken. Newer databacks perform advanced functions, such as exposure bracketing, timed photography, and automatic shutter release when a subject enters a predetermined focal position. The databack should be standard equipment for the forensic photographer. With digital cameras, the camera settings and the date and time are automatically embedded in the digital image code.

Film

The ED photographer must decide whether to use print, slide, or digital film. Each offers advantages and poses disadvantages.

In the amateur market, print (negative) film is by far the most popular, reportedly accounting for 90% of films sold. Forensic pathologists, physicians, and functional photographers historically used more slide (transparency) film but are quickly moving to digital images. Which should the ED photographer choose? To oversimplify, if you usually want prints, use negative film. You can always scan a print and import it into a digital presentation. If you usually want slides, use slide film, but fewer and fewer physicians are using this medium. A slide can also be scanned and converted into a digital image. Table 17-2 provides some pointers to help decide between the two types of film. Until recently, most police departments and investigative agencies used negative (print) film but, like many pathologists, they are quickly abandoning film for digital media. If you plan to create PowerPoint presentations, then a digital image is the answer.

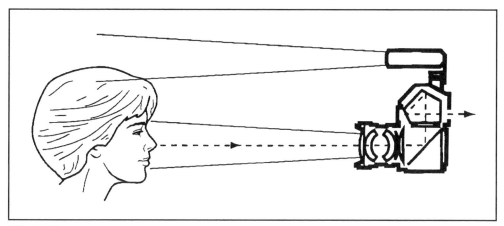

FIG. 17.15   Top-mounted electronic flashes may not illuminate subjects adequately within 6 in. of the lens. The light passes over the subject, leaving an underexposed photograph. (Reprinted from Smock WS. Forensic photography. In: Stack L, Storrow A, Patton D, eds. *Physician's handbook of clinical photography*. Philadelphia, PA: Hanley & Belfus, 2000, with permission.)

Film is rated by speed, or an ASA or ISO (International Standards Organization) number, which describes its sensitivity to light. For forensic purposes, the film must deliver sharp resolution and proper color. A "slow" film, with a lower ISO number, responds slowly and needs a lot of light to produce a satisfactory image. A "fast" film, with a higher ISO number, is more sensitive to light and therefore needs less light to do its job. One advantage of digital "film" is the ability to change the ASA number (50–3200) with each shot.

If you occasionally need large prints (poster size), you are probably better off using properly exposed slow-speed (ISO 25–100) negative film and having the prints made from negatives rather than from slides, but it can be done either way.

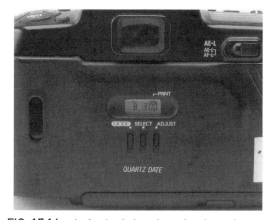

FIG. 17.16   A databack imprints the date, time, or sequence number on the film. This option assists the emergency department photographer in dating the photograph.

ASA (ISO) ratings between 50 and 200 support the function of ED photography to document wounds and injuries. These speeds will give the photographer the sharpest images and saturated color.

You may see the letters "DX" on a film box and notice that the metal film cassette has some small light silvery squares on it. This is the digital index (DX) coding, which in many cameras sets the camera mechanism to the film speed automatically, as soon as the film is inserted. This is helpful because it makes it harder to change film speed and then forget to reset the camera meter; however, good-quality equipment incorporates a means of adjusting the exposure up and down to allow for deviations, manufacturing tolerances, personal preferences, and so on. If you insert a film cassette that has no DX code into a camera that looks for it, the camera will usually default to a film speed of ISO 100, but some point-and-shoot cameras default to ISO 25. The DX code also tells the camera something about the exposure latitude of the film and has a bar code adjacent to it, which can be scanned by the photofinisher to identify the type of film and number of exposures.

Kodak and Fuji produce both commercial and professional grade slide film. The commercial grade films are more than adequate to meet the needs of the forensic photographer in the hospital. Professional grade films also produce excellent results but require constant refrigeration and are less forgiving when exposure mistakes are made. Each type of film has a slightly different color balance and may be affected by ambient light in the hospital. The photographer should select the type and speed of the film that most accurately depict the wounds and injuries as they were seen at the time the images were obtained.

TABLE 17-2

SLIDE VERSUS NEGATIVE FILM

Slide (Color Reversal, Transparency) Films	Negative (Print) Films
Projecting slides onto a screen gives the best color and range of brightness.	Prints have less brightness range and less inherent sharpness.
An original slide can be used to check the quality and color of any copy made from it.	You cannot compare a negative to the original by eye.
Slides are easy to see with a magnifier and easy to evaluate for exposure, color, and sharpness.	Negatives are harder for most people to evaluate because of the distracting yellow-orange backing.
Slides are easy to sort, store, file, and shuffle to make up or alter a presentation.	Negatives are not as easy to number and file.
Slides have a paper or plastic mount on which information and case numbers can be written or added by means of an adhesive label.	Negatives have to be marked on their edges or filed in an envelope or sleeve, from which they may become separated.
There is a wide choice of slide films, each with its own capabilities and way of depicting color.	There is a choice of negative films, some of which are good at certain things (e.g., skin color in portraiture), but it is not as extensive as for slides.
Slides cost less per image for film processing and mounting.	Prints generally cost more per image for film processing plus printing, and much more when large prints are made.
Slides are less tolerant of errors in exposure and therefore help evaluate the performance of automatic exposure systems.	Negative films are more tolerant of errors in exposure and therefore help ensure image acquisition. There is even a color negative film that has an extra wide exposure latitude by design.
Prints can be made from slides, but the process has some technical limitations. For instance, if a slide has contrast or is in some other way less than ideal, it may be necessary to make a special internegative from which to derive prints.	It is easy to print negatives on an automatic machine. Many amateurs make prints at home with good results. It is generally less expensive to make custom prints from color negatives than from slides.

For slides/transparencies, in daylight or with electronic flash, start with

- Fujichrome Astia 100 (accurate skin and fabric tones)
- Fujichrome Provia 100F (very fine grain)
- Fujichrome Sensia II 100 (excellent color)
- Kodak Ektachrome E100G (very fine grain)
- Kodak Ektachrome E100GX (warm color and fine grain)
- Kodak Ektachrome E100VS (vivid color and high sharpness)

For slides under tungsten lighting indoors, use Type B film, 3,200 K.

For color negatives and prints, start with

- Kodak Gold 100, 200
- Kodak Ultra Color 100
- Fuji 100 Superia Reala

Kodak is replacing the most professional negative films at speeds between 100 and 400 with Portra 160NC and 400NC (natural color), 160 black-and-white VC, 400VC (vivid color) for slightly enhanced color, and Ultracolor 100 and 400.

Ideally, to stop the slide film from degrading, it should be stored in a refrigerator. This is particularly important for the professional film. This type of film is generally not designed for ED use.

On the other hand, films marked "professional" are generally manufactured to closer tolerances and aged until they have reached an optimum color balance. They are then refrigerated and delivered to critical professional users. They must be kept cold until just before use, allowed to warm up, and exposed and developed almost immediately. In this way, the critical user is more likely to obtain optimal color balance. Storage at 50°F to 55°F or less is suggested.

Likewise, color-printing papers maintain their color balance better if stored in the cold. All films store better away from heat and humidity.

Regardless of the type, you must let the film warm up before you unwrap it or open the plastic container.

As a guide, allow 1 hour for 35-mm cassettes to warm up after refrigeration and $1\frac{1}{2}$ hours after freezing. Keep a 35-mm cassette in its plastic container until it has warmed up, to prevent condensation. To prevent cardboard boxes from getting soggy, store them in plastic bags with a desiccant inside. You can take the film in and out of a refrigerator or freezer repeatedly without harming it, provided the container remains sealed to exclude moisture.

In general, it is usually safe to use a film that has been well stored approximately 6 months past the printed expiration date, a film that has been refrigerated 12 months past the expiration date, and a film that has been frozen at or near $0°F$ approximately 24 months past the expiration date. This is only a guide for ordinary outdoor and indoor applications, not for recording subtle changes of color on the human body or in the laboratory. The point is that there is no reason to discard a roll of film because it is a few days outdated.

Two of the greatest threats to undeveloped film are heat and humidity. Therefore, do not leave unprocessed film or your camera in the glove box or trunk of your car on a hot sunny day, where the temperature can easily reach $140°F$ and lead to visible color shifts. Inside a car parked in the sun, surface temperatures are even higher, often approaching $200°F$. Once again the advantages of digital storage media shine through: they are not nearly as sensitive to heat and humidity as is the film.

Processing

Photographs, slides, or digital images from the ED or clinical forensic facility should be developed according to a standard protocol for your department. You will have films from important cases, many of which are sensitive and depict unpleasant scenes, or scenes and subjects beyond the daily experience of the average person. With sensitive subject matter such as sexual assault photographs, an in-hospital, medical school, or professional laboratory is preferred. You do not want to be in the position of needing to explain to your local police or drug store why you have photographs of a sexual assault victim or gunshot wounds. These issues are avoided with the use of digital imaging when downloaded to a secure departmental computer.

You should anticipate the possibility of questions about chain of custody during processing and whether standard processing methods or procedures were used. If you selected negative film and the last half of a dozen frames were left unexposed at the end, will you discard them, and risk being asked questions about lost or concealed photographs? It is for such reasons that some EDs prefer to record a case card or serial number at the beginning and end of each sequence. It does not matter greatly what procedure you decide to follow, so long as you do the same thing all the time and can easily show and testify that it is your routine. Simply stated, be prepared for questions from the opposing attorney, who will be looking for every opportunity to throw doubt on your procedures, opinions, and credibility.

Scales of Size and Frames of Reference

If a photograph is to be used for forensic purposes to demonstrate the exact size of a wound, it is necessary to include a scale (Figs. 17.17 and 17.18). If you take a very close-up photograph of a bullet wound on a chest, it will be difficult to know if the wound was $\frac{3}{8}$ or $\frac{3}{4}$ in. in greatest dimension, unless a familiar object or scale is included in the image (Fig. 17.19). Pictures of wounds and injuries need a scale of size to demonstrate, months or years later, the size of their various features.

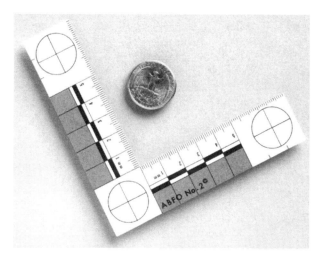

FIG. 17.17 An ABFO No. 2 is an excellent scale and provides measurements in two dimensions. The quartered circles permit the photographer to check for perspective distortion.

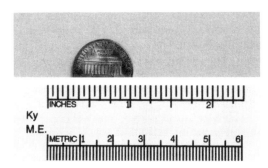

FIG. **17.18** Adhesive scales permit the photographer to write identifying information, such as medical record number, date, or name. On a curved surface, the scale may be bent out of the plane of focus. The scale should be devoid of advertisements.

To properly document an injury, the photographs should show where it was located on the body surface, how big it was, and what it looked like. This is usually achieved by photographing in three views:

1. A view to show its location and orientation, sometimes called an overall, staging, or orientation photograph (Fig. 17.20A).
2. A second but closer view to show the location and identify the wound (Fig. 17.20B).
3. A third close-up photograph, including a scale of size to show the details (Fig. 17.20C). If a traditional ruler or scale is not available, then a familiar object with a standard size, such as a coin (Fig. 17.21), may be placed in the photograph.

If a scale is not included in a photograph, an attorney might complain that the size of the images of interest is not apparent. However, if a scale is incorporated into a photograph, the attorney could suggest that it covers something important.

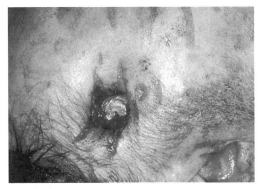

FIG. **17.19** Failure to place a scale in this photograph of a contact gunshot wound to the right temple will prevent the photographer or the court from determining the exact size of the wound or injury.

Therefore, a wound should be photographed with and without a scale. For example, the overall positioning shot could have a scale at the bottom but not next to the wound being documented. Then the close-up view could show a scale next to the wound. This approach reduces or eliminates the ability of an attorney to claim that the scale is covering a feature of the injury.

General guidelines for using scales of size are listed in the subsequent text:

1. The scale should be sized in proportion to the subject: an inch or two in length (3–5 cm) for cartridges and small wounds, 6 in. for people, 2 ft for tires, and 6 ft for car doors.
2. The numbers indicating inches or centimeters must be large enough to read in the end product. Many scales use very small numbers, which are not easy to read in a print.
3. The scale must be in the plane of interest, not behind it (further away from the camera) or in front of the plane (nearer to the camera). In either event, errors will arise when measurements are derived on the basis of a comparison with the scale.
4. The units must be familiar. "Familiar" means inches for most jurors in the United States and centimeters in most other parts of the world. It must be absolutely clear whether inches or centimeters was used. If in doubt, use both, provided they do not take up too much space with a small subject.
5. None of the numbers or letters should be upside down with respect to the subject matter or other numbers. In other words, do not use the kind of ruler that has one set of numbers down one edge, and then along the other edge in reverse, upside down. When you hold the scale in your hand, everything should be in a single orientation, the right way up for reading.
6. The scale should be placed in a natural orientation, so that it is in a normal reading position as you look at the subject just before you take the picture.
7. The scale should not cover part of the subject. If it does, for any reason, another photograph without the scale should be taken.
8. Ideally, there should be no advertising material on the ruler or scale (Fig. 17.18). There should be room on the scale for essential identifying data, such as the case number and/or date and/or initials of the photographer. These numbers must be written carefully, to give a professional appearance, because they may be magnified in the final print.
9. The scale of size should not compete with the subject matter for attention and should be

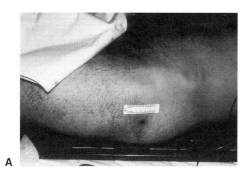
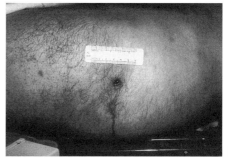
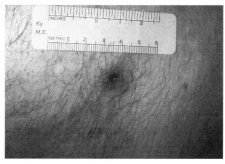

FIG. 17.20   The orientation or overall shot demonstrates the anatomic location of the wound.
A: A gunshot wound to the left hip. **B:** A closer view, which identifies the wound. **C:** A close-up that depicts the entrance gunshot wound, with an abrasion collar.

aesthetically pleasing (Fig. 17.22). For instance, a bright red scale should not be used in most clinical situations.

10. The scale should be generally helpful. For instance,
    - It should not be unduly shiny or reflective.
    - It should not be curved or bent unless you wish it to be.
    - It should be easy to clean and dispose of.
    - It should be easy to position.
    - It should be darker if the subject is dark, and lighter if the subject is light, to avoid exposure problems.

Scales and adhesive labels for use in forensic photography are available from a number of distributors, including

- The Lightning Powder Company, Inc., 13386 International Parkway, Jacksonville, FL 32218, (800) 852-0300, (904) 485-1836, http://www.redwop.com.
- Lynn Peavey Company, P.O. Box 14100, Lenexa, KS 66285-4100. (800) 255-6499, http://www.lynnpeavey.com.

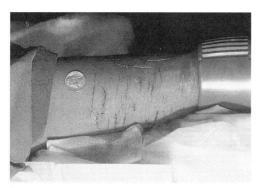

FIG. 17.21   Placement of a coin can serve as a reference if a scale is not available.

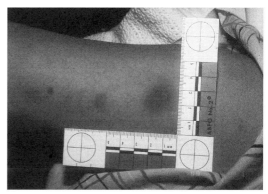

FIG. 17.22   A photograph with a scale and without perspective distortion permits accurate measurement of a wound. These fingertip contusions on the upper left arm are from a domestic assault (see color plate).

Filters

Regarding filters, there are two schools of thought: (i) anything placed over the lens is another potential source of reflection, dirt, or image degradation and therefore should be avoided; (ii) lenses are expensive and it is a good idea to protect the front lens element with something that can be replaced at low cost. Use of a filter is a very good idea in a dirty or gritty environment, like the ED. If you do decide to protect your lens with a filter, and intend to leave it on, make sure its optical quality is as good as the camera lens, or you will inevitably lose sharpness. There is no sense in using an uncoated $5 filter on the front of a $500 lens.

Filters are used to increase apparent sharpness, intensify colors (e.g., enhance foliage), and reduce glare. The apparently clear haze and ultraviolet (UV) filters used with film and digital cameras remove UV light, which we cannot see. The slightly pink skylight filter removes UV as well as a little blue light. In general terms, a skylight filter removes the least UV, then a Haze No. 1, then a UV filter, and finally a Haze No. 2. Manufacturers vary in their use of names, so purchasers should check if the difference will matter. If the fabric brightener in white bed sheets causes them to look blue, the cure is to put a UV filter over your flash so the flash will not affect the fabric brightener.

Filters, whether for digital images or color film, fall into several categories:

- Conversion filters are placed over the lens to let you switch from one kind of light to another, for example, the use of tungsten (indoor) film in daylight.
- Balancing filters make small changes for lighting color, such as between noon and the redder light of sunrise or sunset.
- Neutral-density filters cut down on the amount of light but, in theory, do not alter the color at all. They look gray.
- Color-compensating filters correct the exposure in only one color layer (yellow, magenta, or cyan).
- Polarizing filters are used to reduce reflections from nonmetallic objects, to increase color saturation, and to reduce haze when photographing distant objects. Other common applications include copying, reducing glare from road surfaces when recording skid marks, and taking photographs through glass windows. Good-quality polarizing filters do not appreciably alter color, but inexpensive ones may do so to a limited extent.

The light metering systems of some cameras are adversely affected by polarizing filters. Many see the reduced light intensity and adjust correctly, but others, which use beam splitters to send light to the photocells, are unable to react properly when a linear polarizer is used. This may result in very large exposure errors. Check the instruction manual for the make and model of your camera to see which type is the best. When in doubt, put a polarizing filter on your camera and focus on a sheet of plain white paper or suitable directionally lit subject. Then rotate the filter. A slight change in the exposure reading is normal as reflections are controlled, but if there is a sudden large change in the exposure indication, you will probably need a circular polarizer (a linear polarizer combined with a $\frac{1}{4}$-wave plate).

DIGITAL PHOTOGRAPHY

Digital cameras with storage cards are quickly replacing film photography as the forensic photographic medium of choice. With near photo-quality digital SLR cameras (6–8 megapixels) (Fig. 17.23) now selling for less than $1,000, law-enforcement agencies, SANEs, and emergency physicians have moved into the digital age. The digital camera offers significant advantages over traditional slide and print films, especially for forensic and educational purposes (Table 17-3). Digital images are easily stored, copied, viewed on a computer, e-mailed, and exported into multimedia presentations. The

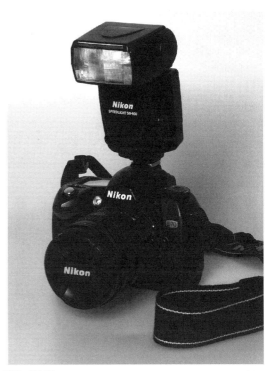

FIG. 17.23 The Nikon D70 produces a near-film-quality photograph with a 6.0 million pixel image.

TABLE 17-3
ADVANTAGES OF DIGITAL IMAGES

No development costs
Chain of custody is simplified
Images are easily copied to a CD or DVD and given to
law enforcement
Immediate review of image for quality, clarity, and focus
Image is easily enhanced to improve the visibility of
details
Easily duplicated and electronically transferred anywhere
in the world
Easily presented in court with computer screen or data
projector
Environmental impact is less than that of films
Ease of advanced scientific applications
Storage media can hold hundreds to thousands of images

TABLE 17-4
APPROXIMATE NUMBER OF RAW IMAGES PER STORAGE CARD CAPACITY

Resolution	512 MB	1 GB	2 GB	4 GB	8 GB
4 megapixel	256	512	1024	2048	4096
6 megapixel	160	320	640	1280	2560
11 megapixel	43	86	168	336	672
14 megapixel	27	55	106	213	426

Estimated number of pictures in RAW mode. The actual
number of images per card will vary and depends on the camera
model and complexity of the scene being photographed.
MB, megabytes; GB, gigabytes.
From Lexar High Speed Professional Compact Flash, Lexar
Media, lexarmedia.com, 2004.

photographer knows within seconds if the image is in focus, adequately illuminated, and well composed and displays what was intended. The digital image can also be easily converted to a color print. The potential disadvantage for legal purposes is that the image can be easily manipulated or altered.

The Digital Camera

Digital cameras, like traditional film cameras, have a camera body and lens with varying shutter speeds, focal lengths, and apertures. Instead of on a film, the image is captured on an electronic sensor—a CCD or a CMOS. The image is then transferred from the sensor and recorded on a removable disk or storage card. Storage cards have multiple names, depending on the camera: "FlashCard," "CompactFlash," "Memory Stick," and "SmartMedia" (Fig. 17.24).

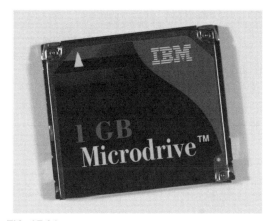

FIG. 17.24 The "FlashCard" can hold hundreds to thousands of digital images.

Storage cards can hold hundreds to thousands of digital images, depending on their resolution (Table 17-4). The image on the sensor, actually a long numeric code, is called a *primary image*. The camera's sensor, either a CCD or a CMOS, has a number of light-sensitive picture elements (pixels) that determine the maximum resolution of an image. Each pixel converts light and color into a discrete numeric code. The greater the number of pixels, horizontally and vertically on the sensor, the greater the resolution and detail of a printed photograph. A 35-mm, ASA 200, color-print negative has the equivalent of 8,640,000 pixels per frame versus 6,104,320 pixels for a 6-megapixel digital camera. For educational, nonforensic, ED photography (for example, lesions, rashes, wounds, interesting cases, and radiographs), a camera with a minimum of 3 megapixels is strongly recommended. The 3-megapixel minimum exceeds the highest resolution possible on a computer screen or data projectors but, more importantly, permits a high-quality 8×10 photographic print for educational posters. For forensic purposes, a 6-megapixel CCD or CMOS is the minimum resolution required to obtain near-photo-quality prints and enlargements.

When the storage card with the primary images is removed from the camera and downloaded to a computer or other storage device, the images are called *original images*. An image intended for forensic or legal purposes must be stored in its own file and must not be altered or modified in any way. A separate file for all original images must be created on a hard drive, a CD-R, or DVD-R if the photograph is to withstand any legal challenge concerning chain-of-custody or image enhancement. Duplicates of the original images should be placed in a separate file and become a "working image." It is from the file of duplicates that traditional enhancements, brightness adjustment, color balancing, contrast adjustment, and dodging and burning can be done. The courts permit traditional enhancements of photographs, whether to negatives in a traditional photo lab darkroom or of working images on a computer screen. The final image should be referred to as an "enhanced image" (Table 17-5).

Image Compression

Digital images stored on the camera's storage device can be preserved in different file formats. The three most common are TIFF (Tagged Image File Format [.tif]), JPEG (Joint Photographic Experts Group [.jpg]), and RAW. To be able to answer questions regarding the admissibility of a digital image, the forensic photographer should understand the basic differences between each of the three formats and how each process stores an image.

Just as a roll of film is limited to a certain number of images based on the length of the film, the digital camera is limited by the amount of digital memory within the storage device. To increase the number of digital images on a memory device, "compression" programs were written to squeeze more images on the storage space. The advantage of compressing digital images is that you are able to put hundreds of images on the device. The disadvantage, from a forensic perspective, is that with large amounts of image compression, changes in the digital code may cause some photographic detail to be lost. This loss of detail may result in legal challenges on admissibility (7).

Two of the three file formats—TIFF and RAW—can store images with minimal compression in a format that does not result in the loss of photographic detail from changes in the image's digital code. TIFF is termed *lossless* because images can be compressed, stored, and reconstructed without any change in the images' digital code. With RAW (unprocessed) digital images, there has been no in-camera processing that adjusts white balance or color and, most importantly, image quality has not been altered by compression. TIFF and RAW images require considerably more space on the storage device but eliminate any legal challenges on the grounds of changes in the image's original digital code. The third format, JPEG, is termed *lossy*. When compressed, stored, and reconstructed, lossy images may "lose" some of the digital code, which can slightly alter the image. The loss of some digital code may insert some minor artifact or reduce some slight degree of fine detail or color variation, which may or may not be visible to the human eye (6). These insignificant changes may provide the basis for pointed questions directed at the photographer and form the legal challenge for the inadmissibility of an image.

The possible loss of some small portion of digital code through the compression of an original JPEG image taken in the ED and its reconstruction or printing at a later date is **not** clinically significant. The photographer must understand that the reconstructed JPEG image is a "copy" of the image, not a true "duplicate" (Table 17-5) (6). If an attorney asks, "Is the picture you are showing the jury an exact duplicate of the image you took in the ED?," the photographer must acknowledge that the JPEG image is a copy, not an exact duplicate, but should also clearly state that the photo does fairly and accurately represent what was seen. If asked, "Has the digital code of the JPEG image been altered in the compression and reconstruction process?," the photographer should answer that "Yes, the digital

TABLE 17-5

DIGITAL IMAGE DEFINITIONS

Primary Image	Digital code of image captured on the camera's sensor (CCD or CMOS) and transferred to the camera's storage card
Original Image	Digital code of image downloaded from the camera's storage card to computer hard drive or other physical medium, i.e., CD or DVD
Working Image	Digital code of image that is processed with enhancements, i.e., color balancing, brightness adjustment, contrast adjustment
Final Image or Enhanced Image	Digital code of image that is used to produce visible image, usually after enhancements, for forensic purposes
Copy	Reconstruction of image after the digital code has been compressed and slightly altered, e.g., a JPEG file. Usually not clinically significant, as the human eye may not be able to perceive any alteration in the image
Duplicate	Exact duplication of the image's digital code, i.e., a TIFF file. JPEG files are **not** duplicates because parts of the code are lost during file compression

Adapted from Blitzer HL, Jacobia J. *Forensic digital imaging and photography.* San Diego, CA: Academic Press, 2002.

code may have been slightly altered by the compression but it did not change what the photograph fairly and accurately depicts." Although the amount of storage space required for the TIFF images is larger than for JPEGs, the TIFF is an exact duplicate of the digital code and would preclude this type of questioning. For this reason some forensic photographers recommend the storage of forensic digital images as TIFFs and RAW and not as JPEGs (6,7).

Admissibility of Digital Images

In June 2002, the Scientific Working Group on Imaging Technologies (SWGIT), sponsored by the US Department of Justice and the Federal Bureau of Investigation, published a document titled *Recommendations and Guidelines for the Use of Digital Image Processing in the Criminal Justice System* (9). This report gave guidelines for the successful introduction of forensic imagery as evidence in a court of law. The document stated, "the successful introduction of forensic imagery as evidence in a court of law is dependent upon the following four legal tests: (i) reliability, (ii) reproducibility, (iii) security, and (iv) discovery." It also stated, "when using digital imaging processing techniques, use caution to avoid the introduction of unexplainable artifacts that add misleading information to the image and the loss of image detail that could lead to an erroneous interpretation. Any processing techniques should be applied only to the working image" (9).

Because the digital image is easily manipulated or altered, the forensic photographer may be asked to provide to the court a duplicate of the original images and of the working images being introduced as exhibits. The purpose for this request is to compare the original with the working image to determine if the image has been altered or enhanced. Some alterations or enhancements in film, slides, or digital images are acceptable to the court, because they do not involve a change of content and are similar to accepted darkroom techniques. These include the following:

1. Making improvements in contrast by slightly darkening or lightening areas with a view to improving the printing or reproduction characteristics, or making selected details a little easier to see.
2. Dodging or burning in areas to lighten a face or bring something out, such as a license plate.
3. Correcting technical defects, such as dust spots or a skipped scan line in a TV picture.
4. Making slight changes in color to reduce adverse effects of artificial lighting or errors in processing.

Unacceptable alterations, unless everyone has agreed to and is fully aware of them, are listed in the subsequent text:

1. Removing objects from a photograph.
2. Making radical changes in color, for instance, the color of a car or human skin.
3. Adding new or repeated images by cloning pixels.

Photoshop 7.0 and, now version 8.0, from Adobe is the most powerful image processing and editing software available to the public. Because of Photoshop's ability to track all changes, enhancements, additions, and deletions made to an imported digital image, the courts have accepted the software's image applications in the forensic arena. The "Action" palette automatically tracks any editing to the image and, if requested by the court, a list of changes and enhancements can be provided by the photographer. Some forensic photographers recommend maintaining a detailed log of image manipulation beyond the accepted enhancement tools of adjustment of brightness, contrast, and color (6,7). It is doubtful that any attorney will ever challenge a forensic photograph taken in the ED, but the photographer must be ready to address any possible challenge, including the chain of custody. Passwords protecting the computer files containing the original and working images address accessibility and chain-of-custody issues. The bottom line will be the integrity and honesty of the photographer when he or she states in court that the image has not been significantly manipulated and it does "fairly and accurately represent the injury."

Storage of Digital Images

To archive and store digital files, standard operating procedures must be developed so the primary image on the camera's storage device can be downloaded as soon as possible to create the original image. Once the original image is recorded on a hard drive, it is recommended that another long-lasting, "write-once medium" (a CD-R or DVD-R) be kept separate and secure, with the original images as the backup file. Whatever method you select, always follow standard procedures and protocols to remove all doubt that the image has been altered.

Erased Forensic Images

Digital cameras with liquid crystal displays (LCDs) permit the photographer to review and, if necessary, delete an image within seconds of capturing the subject. With film negatives, the loss, deletion, or failure to print an image from the negatives could catch the attention of a sharp attorney and require the photographer to, under oath, explain its loss. The same can be said for digital images. Digital cameras (Nikon, Canon) can embed a unique or sequential number within the image's digital code, that is, 0000 to 9999. The photographer should be ready to openly explain why the image was deleted. Possible explanations include "the image was out of focus," "lighting was inadequate," "technical problems with the camera settings," or "my fingers got in the way." An open and honest response should quiet any ill-mannered attorney.

NUMBERING AND IDENTIFYING PHOTOGRAPHS

Always write identifying information, such as the case number, hospital number, patient number, and/or the name and initials, on the slide mounts or negative envelopes immediately after your films are developed or you download digital images. Creating separate file folders for each group of original and working images will facilitate retrieval of negatives, slides, or working digital images at a later date.

COURTROOM PRESENTATION

Emergency physicians and nurses should never purport to be or agree to be qualified as an expert in forensic photography when in a court of law or be permitted to act as one. Even people who do or teach photography for a living are reluctant to allow this identification. Instead, be qualified as a health care provider who is experienced with photography and uses it a great deal. Acknowledge that you have taken some instruction or have knowledge over and above that of the general public. Be qualified as a practitioner, if that is appropriate, as opposed to an expert, and stay well within your field of expertise, just as you would in a specialty of medicine. The intricacies of digital photography make the issue even more complex and certainly one to be avoided. When presenting digital images, the photographer is well advised to have a basic understanding of image definitions: "primary" versus "original" versus "working" and the difference between a reconstructed "copy" of an image and an exact "duplicate" image (Table 17-5). The photographer must also be ready to address chain-of-custody and image storage and reproduction questions. Most importantly, the photographer must be able to answer "yes" to the question, "Does the photograph fairly and accurately represent what you saw?"

Print versus Computer Screen versus Data Projector

Until the turn of the 21st century, color prints and projection of color slides were the standards for courtroom presentation. With the rapid acceptance and expansion of digital media, software, and video output devices, today's judges and juries are comfortable with PowerPoint presentations and computer

TABLE 17-6
DIGITAL IMAGE OUTPUT DEVICE

Device	Screen Resolution	Pixels
17″ LCD computer screen	1280 × 1024	1,310,720
55″ plasma screen	1366 × 768	1,049,088
High-definition TV	1280 × 720	921,600
Data projector	1024 × 768	786,432
Standard digital TV	640 × 480	307,200

LCD, liquid crystal display.

screens. An 8 × 10 color print from a negative, slide, or digital image (minimum 6 million pixels) provides the highest level of resolution and visual detail. When using other media, the photographer must be aware of the limitations associated with the output device (Table 17-6). No output device, plasma display, data projector, or computer screen can provide the detail of the printed photo. Data projectors and computer screens are adequate for showing general images, but do not rely on them to provide the same visual detail as with a photograph. A combined approach of both color prints and a computer presentation can provide the visual detail required and adequately inform the court.

SUMMARY

Your success as a functional ED photographer depends in large part on your ability to look critically at your own photographs, learn from your mistakes, improve with experience, do better the next time, and thereby slowly improve your technique. Good technique, common sense, and an understanding of the technical aspects of photography will enhance your ability to capture meaningful medical information that will benefit patients and their attorneys.

REFERENCES

1. Gove PB, ed. *Webster's third new international dictionary of the English language*, unabridged. Springfield, IL: Merriam-Webster, 1986.
2. Smock WS. Clinical forensic medicine. In: Rosen P, ed. *Emergency medicine: concepts and clinical practice*. St. Louis: Mosby, 2002:828–841.
3. University of Louisville Hospital. *Operative consent form*. Louisville, Kentucky, 1999.
4. Osborne TL. Demonstrative evidence. In: Osborne TL, ed. *Trial handbook for Kentucky lawyers*, 2nd ed. Rochester, NY: Lawyers Cooperative Publishing, 1992.
5. West Group. *Kentucky rules of evidence, Kentucky rules of court*. St. Paul: West Group, 1999.

6. Blitzer HL, Jacobia J. *Forensic digital imaging and photography*. San Diego, CA: Academic Press, 2002.
7. Russ JC. *Forensic uses of digital imaging*. Boca Raton, FL: CRC Press, 2001.
8. The Committee on the Judiciary House of Representatives. Federal rules of evidence. *108th Congress 2nd Session*, Washington, DC: No. 8, December 31, 2004.
9. Scientific Working Group on Imaging Technologies (SWGIT). Recommendations and guidelines for the use of digital image processing in the criminal justice system. Version 1.2, June 2002. *Forensic Sci Commun* 2003;5(1): January 2003. Available at http://www.fbi.gov/hq/lab/fsc/backissu/jan2003/swgitdigital.htm. Accessed on September 26, 2005.

ADDITIONAL RESOURCES

Evidence Photographers International Council (EPIC). Jennings RF. Executive Director, 600 Main Street, Honesdale, PA: 18431-0351; phone: (717) 253-5450, (800) 356-3742; fax: (717) 253-5011; http://www.epic-photo.org, 2006.

The Fujifilm Sensitized Products Technical Hotline: (800) 788-3854, ext. 73; The Fuji ProNet™Hotline: (800) 332-FUJI, and Fuji ProNet™; Fuji Web site access: www.fujifilm.com; Fuji consumer information: (800) 800-FUJI, 2006.

Kerr N. *Lighting techniques for photographers*. Amherst: Amherst Media, Inc., 1998.

The Kodak Information Center (800) 242-2424. (8 a.m. to 8 p.m. EST). Web site: http://www.kodak.com (online information) and http://www.kodak.com/go/professional. Information by mail: Eastman Kodak Company, 343 State Street, Rochester, NY 14650-0519, 2006.

The Nikon School of Photography, 300 Walt Whitman Road, Melville, NY: 11747-3064; phone: (516) 547-8666 (8:00 a.m.–4:30 p.m. Monday through Friday EST); fax: (516) 547-0309; http://www.nikonusa.com, 2006.

Pasqualone GA. Documentation in the ED: forensic RNs as photographers. *J Psychosocial Nurs* 1996;34 (10):47–51.

Pasqualone GA. Forensic photography. In Lynch VA, ed. *Forensic nursing*. St. Louis: Elsevier, Mosby, 2005:170–186.

Polaroid Corporation Technical Support Line: (800) 225-1618; customer care: (800) 343-5000.

Redsicker DR. *The practical methodology of forensic photography*. Boca Raton, FL: CRC Press, 2001.

Vetter JP. *Biomedical photography*. Stoneham, MA: Butterworth-Heinemann, 1992.

Warren B. *Photography*. West Publishers, 1992.

Williams RA, Williams GF. Part 1: Introduction and reflected ultraviolet techniques. *J Biol Photogr Assoc* (now *J Biocommun*) October 1993;61 (4):115–132.

Williams RA, Williams GF. Part 2: fluorescence photography. *J Biol Photogr Assoc* (now *J Biocommun*) January 1994a;62 (1):3–19.

Williams RA, Williams GF. Part 3: reflected infrared photography. *J Biol Photogr Assoc* (now *J Biocommun*) April 1994b;62 (2):51–68.

Note: Page numbers followed by *f* indicate figures; those followed by *t* indicate tables.